African
Doctors of World War I

African American Doctors of World War I

The Lives of 104 Volunteers

W. Douglas Fisher *and*
Joann H. Buckley

McFarland & Company, Inc., Publishers
Jefferson, North Carolina

LIBRARY OF CONGRESS CATALOGUING-IN-PUBLICATION DATA [new form]

Names: Fisher, W. Douglas, 1938– author. | Buckley, Joann H., author.
Title: African American doctors of World War I : the lives of
104 volunteers / W. Douglas Fisher and Joann H. Buckley.
Description: Jefferson, North Carolina : McFarland & Company, Inc.,
Publishers, [2016] | Includes bibliographical references and index.
Identifiers: LCCN 2015038580 | ISBN 9781476663159
(softcover : acid free paper) | ISBN 9781476623177 (ebook)
Subjects: LCSH: World War, 1914–1918—Medical care—United States. |
African American physicians—Biography. | African American physicians—
History—20th century. | United States. Army—African American
troops—Biography. | United States. Army. Division, 92nd—Biography. |
United States. Army. Division, 93rd—Biography. | World War,
1914–1918—Medical care—France. | World War, 1914–1918—
Participation, African American.
Classification: LCC D629.U6 F57 2016 | DDC 940.4/7573092396073—dc23
LC record available at http://lccn.loc.gov/2015038580

BRITISH LIBRARY CATALOGUING DATA ARE AVAILABLE

On the cover: *counterclockwise from top left* Capt. James L. Leach (courtesy Meharry Medical College Archives); Capt. John Q. Taylor (courtesy University of Texas at San Antonio Libraries Special Collections); Lieut. Jonathan N. Rucker (courtesy Rucker family); Lieut. William H. Dyer (courtesy Schomburg Center for Research in Black Culture, The New York Public Library, Astor, Lenox and Tilden Foundations); Lieut. Urbane F. Bass in France (courtesy U.S. National Library of Medicine); Capt. T.E. Jones (*Who's Who in Colored America*, Yenser, Sixth Edition, 1940–1944); Lieut. George I. Lythcott (courtesy Michael J. Lythcott); Maj. Joseph H. Ward (*Scott's Official History of the American Negro in the World War*, Emmett J. Scott, 1919)

Printed in the United States of America

McFarland & Company, Inc., Publishers
Box 611, Jefferson, North Carolina 28640
www.mcfarlandpub.com

Table of Contents

Acknowledgments

The help and encouragement the authors received over the years from total strangers is remarkable. Librarians, archivists, historians, genealogists, curators, family members, and physicians at research centers, archives, museums, historical societies, universities and other special collections provided invaluable help and guidance.

The Ruckers welcomed us to their family and spent many hours talking about their father. Michael Lythcott wrote the account of his Lythcott grandfather and got us started on the research about his Wilson grandfather. We met with Ballard's son and grandson to learn more about him. All gave generously of their time.

Many members of the World War I Historical Association have provided encouragement. The Fort Des Moines Museum and Education Center had us there twice to share our research.

Wilma Moore at the Indiana Historical Society gave us our first opportunity to publish our biographies in Indiana's *Traces* magazine. Her support emboldened us to approach Henry Louis Gates, Jr., who then invited us to contribute 15 biographies to the African American National Biography. That led us to decide we could and should profile all 104 men.

And, special thanks to Kayle Tucker Simon for patiently proofing, editing and polishing our work.

Researching the book has been an exhilarating journey of discovery. We have met amazing people and learned many remarkable things. We are pleased to share them with our readers and look forward to our readers sharing more about these extraordinary men with us.

Preface

During the First World War, author Doug Fisher's grandfather, Captain John North Douglas, commanded the 317th Motor Supply Train of the 92nd Division, a black combat unit. In his diary and reports he wrote about Dr. Jonathan N. Rucker, an African American physician who cared for his 500 troops. For years Fisher's focus was on getting to know Dr. Rucker. What the man was able to accomplish in the Jim Crow South was extraordinary.

In 2010, co-author Joann Buckley became involved. Her initial contribution was to begin the search for other African American physicians who must have served with the 92nd and 93rd divisions. No one, including the curator of the Fort Des Moines Museum where the physicians received their basic military training, knew their names or even how many there were.

After months of combing through files in the National Archives, Buckley discovered *the list*. It was in an ancient folder of the U.S. Army Surgeon General records. It was so old that its identification tab had disintegrated. It was typed by some clerk a hundred years ago on many sheets of paper and then, because there were so many columns of information on the backgrounds of these 104 physicians, their hometowns, medical schools, graduation years, and ages, the sheets were glued together to make a kind of a display piece. The resulting document was four feet long and 18 inches wide. It was virtually hidden because it had been folded inward on itself several times to

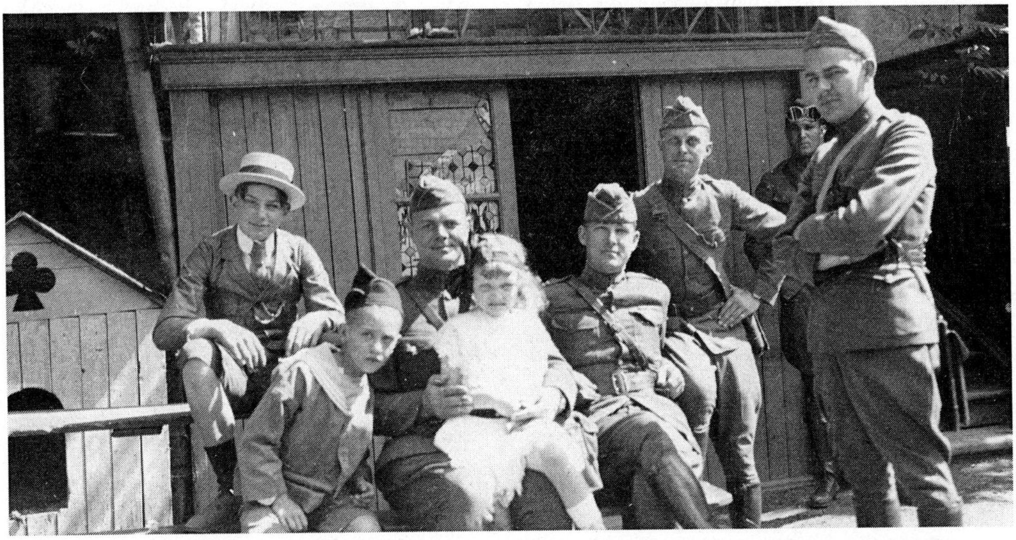

This carte postale shows two unidentified boys at left in August 1918 with Major Fred Carruthers, "Little Suzanne" (the little girl in his lap), Captain John N. Douglas, Lieutenant Fred Wilmont, Lieutenant J.N. Rucker and Lieutenant Parker of the 317th Supply Train, 92nd Division (W. Douglas Fisher collection).

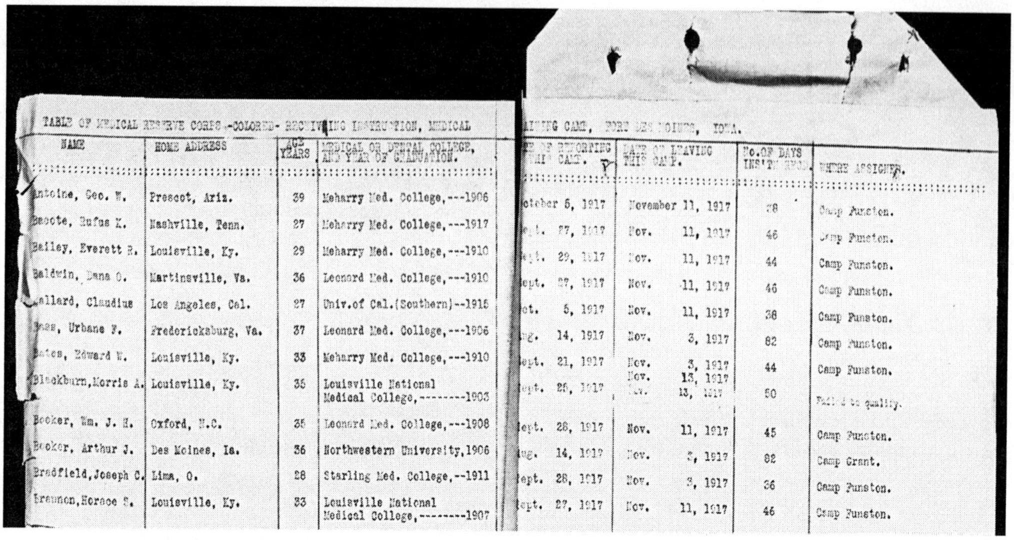

TABLE OF MEDICAL RESERVE CORPS -COLORED- RECEIVING INSTRUCTION, MEDICAL [illegible]ING CAMP, FORT DES MOINES, IOWA.

NAME	HOME ADDRESS	AGE YEARS	MEDICAL OR DENTAL COLLEGE, AND YEAR OF GRADUATION.	[illegible] OF REPORTING THIS CAMP.	DATE OF LEAVING THIS CAMP.	No. OF DAYS INS'T'N [illegible]	WHERE ASSIGNED.
[illegible]ntoine, Geo. W.	Prescot, Ariz.	39	Meharry Med. College,---1906	October 5, 1917	November 11, 1917	38	Camp Funston.
[illegible]scote, Rufus K.	Nashville, Tenn.	27	Meharry Med. College,---1917	[illegible]. 27, 1917	Nov. 11, 1917	46	Camp Funston.
Bailey, Everett R.	Louisville, Ky.	29	Meharry Med. College,---1910	[illegible]. 29, 1917	Nov. 11, 1917	44	Camp Funston.
Baldwin, Dana O.	Martinsville, Va.	36	Leonard Med. College,---1910	[illegible]ept. 27, 1917	Nov. 11, 1917	46	Camp Funston.
[illegible]allard, Claudius	Los Angeles, Cal.	27	Univ. of Cal. (Southern)--1915	[illegible]ct. 5, 1917	Nov. 11, 1917	38	Camp Funston.
[illegible]ss, Urbane F.	Fredericksburg, Va.	37	Leonard Med. College,---1906	[illegible]g. 14, 1917	Nov. 3, 1917	82	Camp Funston.
[illegible]tes, Edward W.	Louisville, Ky.	33	Meharry Med. College,---1910	[illegible]ept. 21, 1917	Nov. 3, 1917 Nov. 13, 1917	44	Camp Funston.
Blackburn, Morris A.	Louisville, Ky.	35	Louisville National Medical College,--------1903	[illegible]ept. 25, 1917	[illegible] 13, 1917	50	Failed to qualify.
Booker, Wm. J. H.	Oxford, N.C.	35	Leonard Med. College,---1908	[illegible]ept. 28, 1917	Nov. 11, 1917	45	Camp Funston.
Booker, Arthur J.	Des Moines, Ia.	36	Northwestern University, 1906	[illegible]ug. 14, 1917	Nov. 3, 1917	82	Camp Grant.
Bradfield, Joseph C.	Lima, O.	28	Starling Med. College,--1911	[illegible]ept. 28, 1917	Nov. 3, 1917	36	Camp Funston.
Brannon, Horace S.	Louisville, Ky.	33	Louisville National Medical College,--------1907	[illegible]ept. 27, 1917	Nov. 11, 1917	46	Camp Funston.

A small portion of "the list," 1917 Medical Officers Training Camp roster (National Archives).

make it fit into the otherwise unidentified folder. Once opened, it was so fragile that it nearly blew totally apart at the seams on the first attempt by the Archives staff to copy it.

So now the quest began for information about each of these men. The two authors spent the next five years in the files at the National Archives, at numerous state and city historical associations, libraries and archives, and utilized a variety of online sources of newspaper articles. The authors also interviewed a number of the children and grandchildren of these extraordinary men.

Initially the authors shared their information in articles in historical journals and magazines like Indiana's *Traces*. Then, after a chance meeting with Professor Henry Louis Gates, Jr., in the elevator of the Hay Adams Hotel in Washington, D.C., and a brief chat about the project, several biographies were included in his African American National Biography. Through the course of development, the authors have shared some of these biographies with historians and the African American community. Following their PowerPoint presentations, they would hear comments like the one by retired African American three-star general Lieutenant General Earl Brown, USAF, "This is my history and I knew nothing about it."

The book begins with the doctors gathered together at the only Medical Officers Training Camp (Colored) in U.S. history. It then presents a chronicle of this period in African American history through their individual biographies. The authors' approach was to gather individual biographies to help illuminate significant events, challenges and the times at the end of the 19th century and the first half of the 20th. The goal is to provide more depth than a biographical dictionary and more color than an historical narrative, by using illustrative examples. By reading through this series of biographies, the authors believe the reader can gain a firsthand appreciation of a critical piece of American history through the lives of these African American doctors who fought for the nation and their communities.

All of these men succeeded in gaining advanced education and training at a time when that was problematic for African Americans. All volunteered to serve their nation in war. Some rose to greatness, and many were recognized for their achievements and contributions. Others, as one might expect in a group exposed to the ravages of war, died young, or later succumbed to the economic and social challenges of the times. Most of their lives ended before the modern Civil Rights Movement of the 1950s and 1960s, but the success of later generations is built upon important groundwork laid by these men who brought so much to their communities.

Introduction

One hundred years ago, in the era of racial segregation, discrimination, lynching and Jim Crow laws, 104 of the nation's estimated 3,000 African American doctors[1] answered their country's call and left their practices to provide medical care to the fighting men of the 92nd and 93rd divisions of General Pershing's American Expeditionary Force (AEF).

In 1917, as the United States formally entered the First World War, mobilizing the army and establishing the draft, the army was coaxed into organizing two divisions for African American combat troops, the 92nd and 93rd. The 92nd Division came to be known as the "Buffalo" Division and was commanded by white officers. It was made up primarily of draftees. The 93rd Division (Provisional) was made up of existing African American National Guard units and draftees. The National Guard units even contained a few African American officers in command positions.

Despite the fact that black soldiers have served in every major American war since the 1700s, officers of African American descent were almost non-existent in the regular army until the First World War. Until the late 1940s, African American officers were not permitted to command white officers and in almost all cases they reported to white commanders.

The scale of everything in the First World War was historic and dramatic. The experience of being part of one American combat division, and there were many divisions, dwarfs the prior experience of all of the individuals involved.

Of the four million Americans who served in the army during the First World War, 400,000 were African Americans and 200,000 of them served in the AEF in France. Roughly 40,000 African Americans in France served in combat with the 92nd or 93rd Division. The remaining 160,000 served in critical support roles such as stevedores, laborers, and medics.

Interestingly, the four infantry regiments of the 93rd Division (369th, 370th, 371st, and 372nd) were split up and served under French command. The 93rd with its 10,000 men spread across the four regiments was never formed into a full division. The 92nd Division did constitute a complete division with 27,000 troops. It served under American command as members of the AEF First Army, and later the AEF Second Army.

The 27,000 men in each army division represented more than the entire populations of the towns and cities from where most of these men came. The logistics of simply feeding and caring for that many men each day was

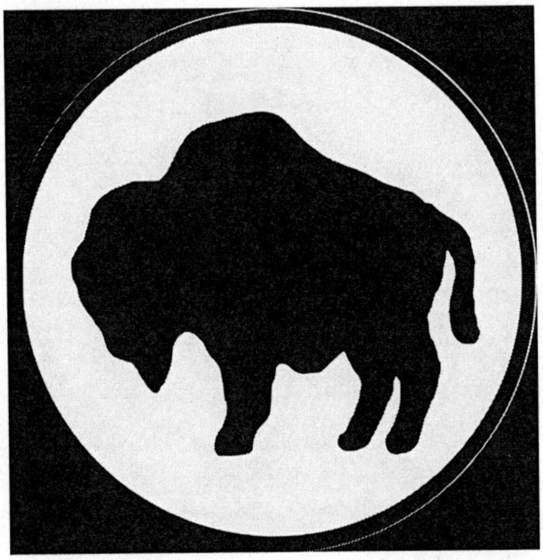

The 92nd "Buffalo" Division shoulder patch.

extraordinary. The area where each division was deployed covered miles of front and miles of depth behind the front. Thus, the communication and transportation challenges were enormous as well. When the 92nd Division was assembled in the 11th Training Area in France, it took the entire city (Bourbonne-les-Bains) and numerous surrounding towns just to house the men. In fact, whole tent cities had to be built because there were not even enough facilities within the city and all the surrounding villages. It was an eye opener and education for all the men involved, and it had never been done before.

Once approval was given for the creation of the two combat divisions, there was a great deal of political hell-raising and banging on doors of the War Department to recruit and train African American doctors for the divisions' medical arm. The effort was led by a Howard University group and sparked by Prof. Montgomery Gregory, a teacher of drama, with the support of the NAACP. Finally, it was Secretary of War Newton Baker who directed army surgeon general William C. Gorgas to create a separate colored medical training camp.

Because of segregation, it was considered not desirable to send African American medical and dental officers to the existing three medical officer training camps (MOTCs) for white officers then in operation. Fort Des Moines in Iowa had been selected as the main site for training black line officers, and so it was decided the medical officers would be sent there too. In this way no extra facilities would be required to implement the segregated training policy and the existing post medical officers, in addition to their other duties, could take over the training.

As America mobilized for war, almost 1,400 volunteers arrived at Fort Des Moines, Iowa, to be trained at the U.S. Army's first training camps for African American officers. Two groups trained there. The first, and best known camp, was for line officers for the infantry, with a few designated for artillery. It was called the 17th Provisional Officer Training Camp (OTC) and opened in June 1917. The second, and virtually unknown camp, trained medical and dental officers. The Medical Officers Training Camp (MOTC)–Colored opened in late July 1917. In total, 639 combat officers, 104 medical officers and 12 dental

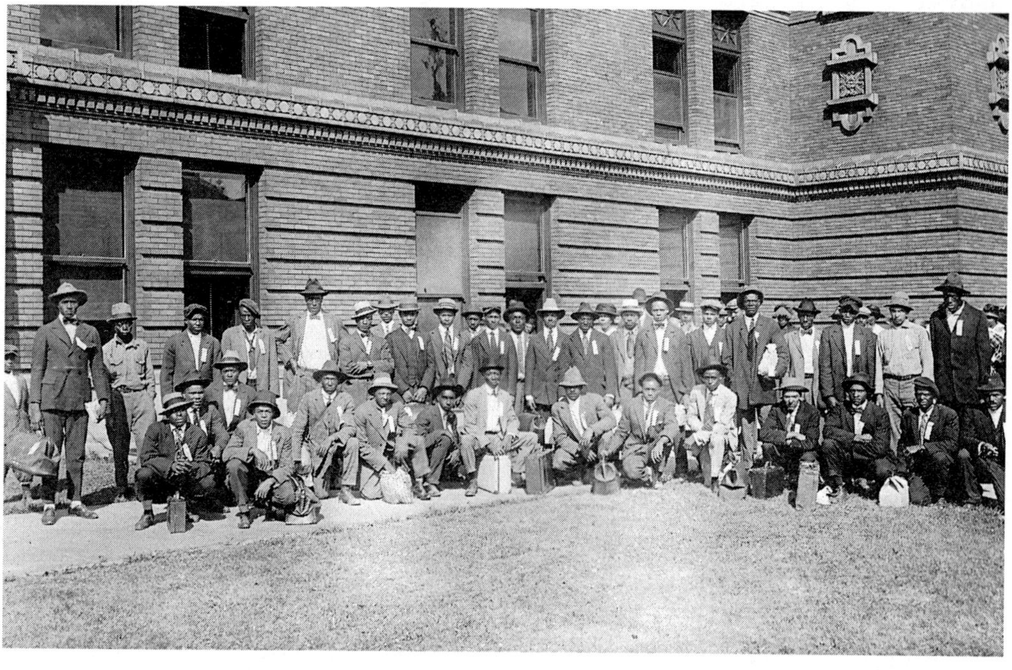

African American draftees ready for service (National Archives).

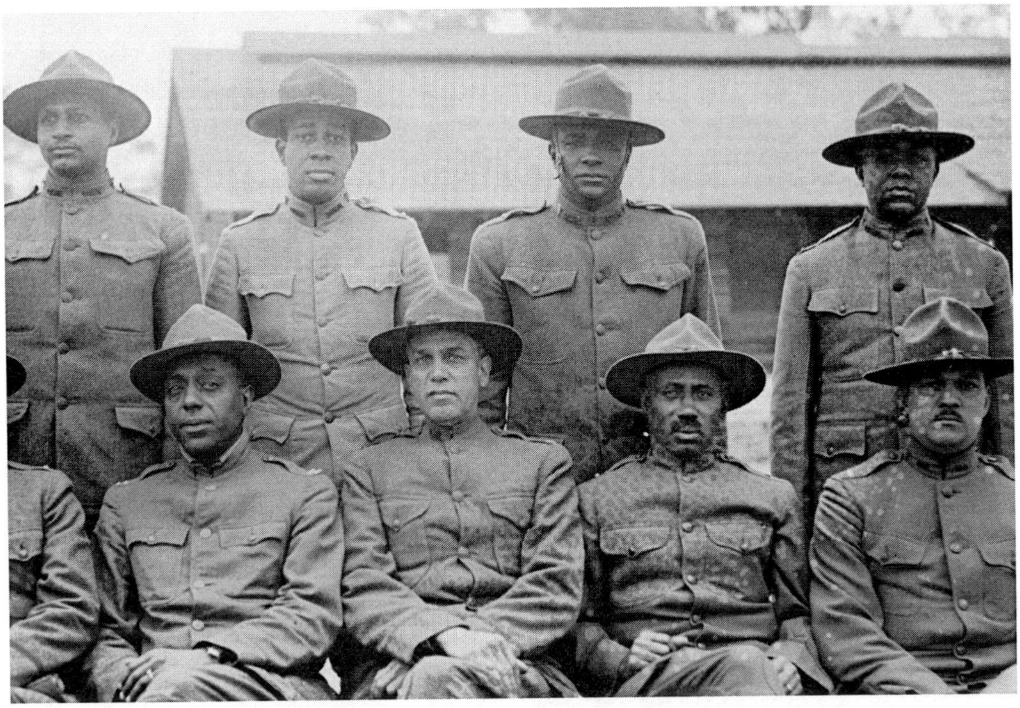

The 370th Infantry Regiment, Camp Logan, Houston, Texas. Top row, left to right: Lieutenants Rufus Bacote, Claudius Ballard, George W. Antoine and Dan M. Moore (all four doctors qualified at Ft. Des Moines). Bottom row, left to right: Captain Leonard Lewis, Major James R. White, Lieutenant Spencer Dickinson, Lieutenant James Lawson (Chicago *Daily News*, courtesy Chicago History Museum).

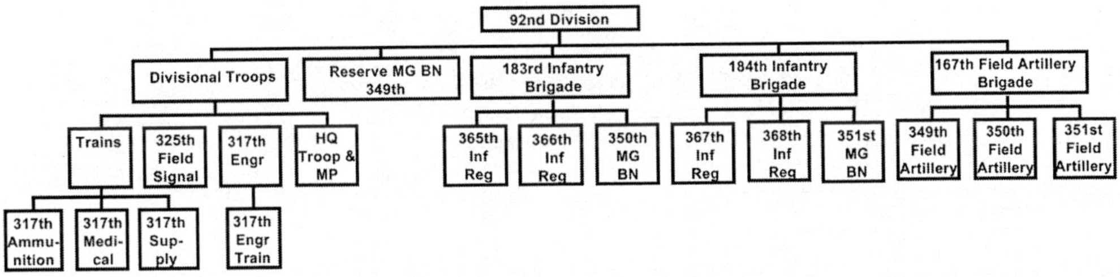

The 92nd Division World War I organization chart.

officers qualified and graduated from both camps in October and November.

Who Were These Doctors?

They came largely from east of the Mississippi River (89 out of 104). Most had roots in the South. Many had moved to the North because their opportunities in the South were limited. They graduated from medical school between 1898 and 1916. They ranged in age from 23 to 47 with an average age of 32. Some were experienced practitioners while others had barely completed their internships. Their average years in practice were six. Tennessee contributed the greatest number (16).

There were very few medical schools for African Americans in the late 19th and early 20th centuries, and very few white medical schools would accept them. Sixty percent of the MOTC doctors came from just three African American medical schools. The largest contingents were from Meharry Medical College in Nashville, Tennessee (34), Howard University Medical School in Washington, D.C. (16), and Leonard Medical School (13) at Shaw

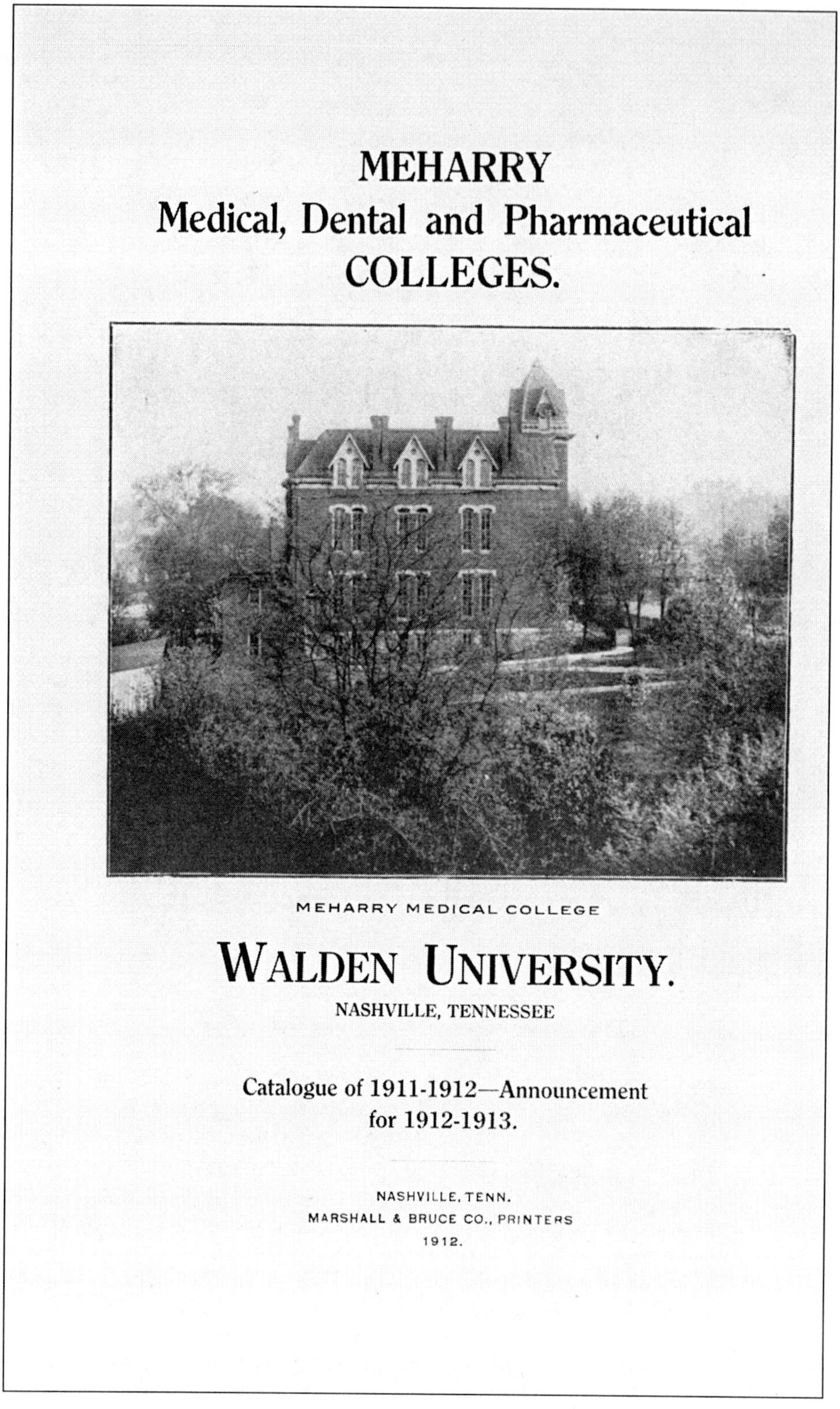

MEHARRY
Medical, Dental and Pharmaceutical
COLLEGES.

MEHARRY MEDICAL COLLEGE

WALDEN UNIVERSITY.
NASHVILLE, TENNESSEE

Catalogue of 1911-1912—Announcement
for 1912-1913.

NASHVILLE, TENN.
MARSHALL & BRUCE CO., PRINTERS
1912.

Meharry Medical College, Nashville, 1912 catalog (courtesy Meharry Medical College Archives).

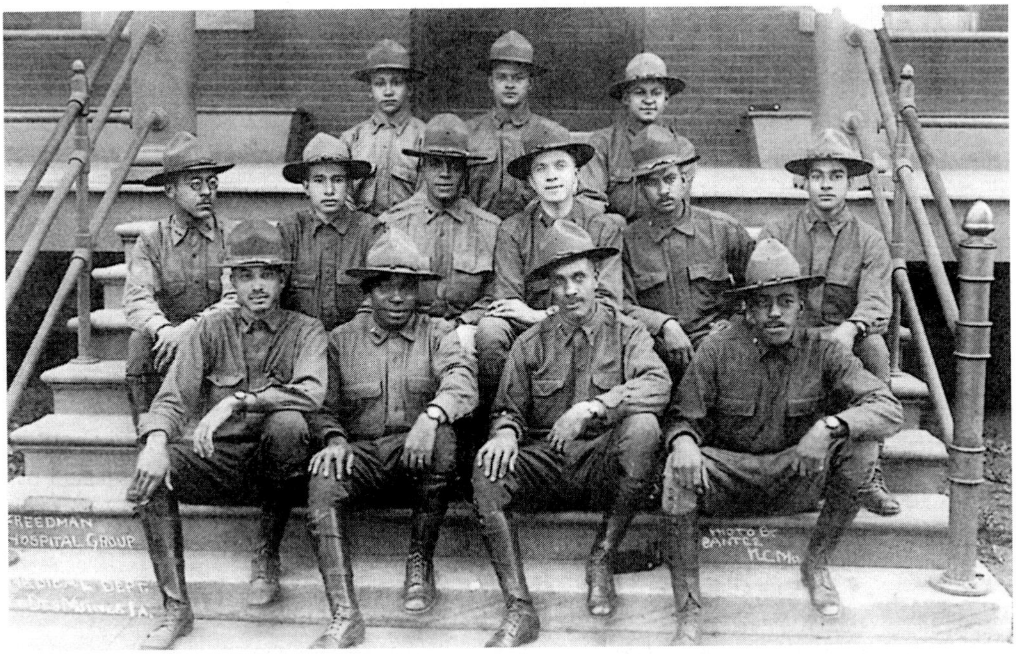

Freedmen's Hospital alumni physicians at Ft. Des Moines. Front row, right, Dr. T. E. Jones. Second row, left, Dr. Arthur L. Curtis; second row, fourth from left, Dr. William J. Howard; second row, right, Dr. Hudson J. Oliver. Third row, left to right, Dr. Louis T. Wright, Dr. Jack Lee, and Dr. Charles H. Garvin (in Robert C. Hayden, *Mr. Harlem Hospital*, courtesy Barbara Wright Pierce).

University in Raleigh, North Carolina. Those schools actively recruited army volunteers from among their alumni. Others had attended smaller African American medical schools that no longer exist, largely due to the 1910 Abraham Flexner Report on medical education in the U.S. and the medical education reforms that it generated.

African American graduates of traditionally white medical schools were represented in very small numbers: the University of Illinois (3), Harvard University (2), the University of Michigan (2), Northwestern University (2), and the University of Southern California (2). One each had graduated from medical schools at Columbia University, the University of Vermont, and the University of Pennsylvania. They represented barely 12 percent of the total.

It can be said that all the doctors were educated, intelligent men who voluntarily joined the Army Medical Reserve Corps. Of the 104 physicians who successfully completed the MOTC and served, 89 of them saw duty in France, where one died on the battlefield.

They performed well and many were promoted to higher rank. Two even became majors before the war's end. Their leadership experience was invaluable and served the nation well in many ways following the war.

Training at Fort Des Moines

Fort Des Moines was a permanent cavalry post that was built in 1901. It covered 400 acres just south of today's downtown Des Moines. It replaced cavalry forts built during America's early westward expansion in the 1800s. The main buildings surrounded an enormous rectangular grass-covered field used for cavalry exercises and training. Many were quite large and permanent, two stories of red brick. They included buildings for administration, mess halls, a chapel, officer quarters, barracks, stables, and warehouses.

In his book *African American Army Officers of World War I,* Adam P. Wilson reports that in 1903, the black infantrymen of the 25th Infantry were trained here, and no race relations' crises were reported.[2] John L. Thompson,

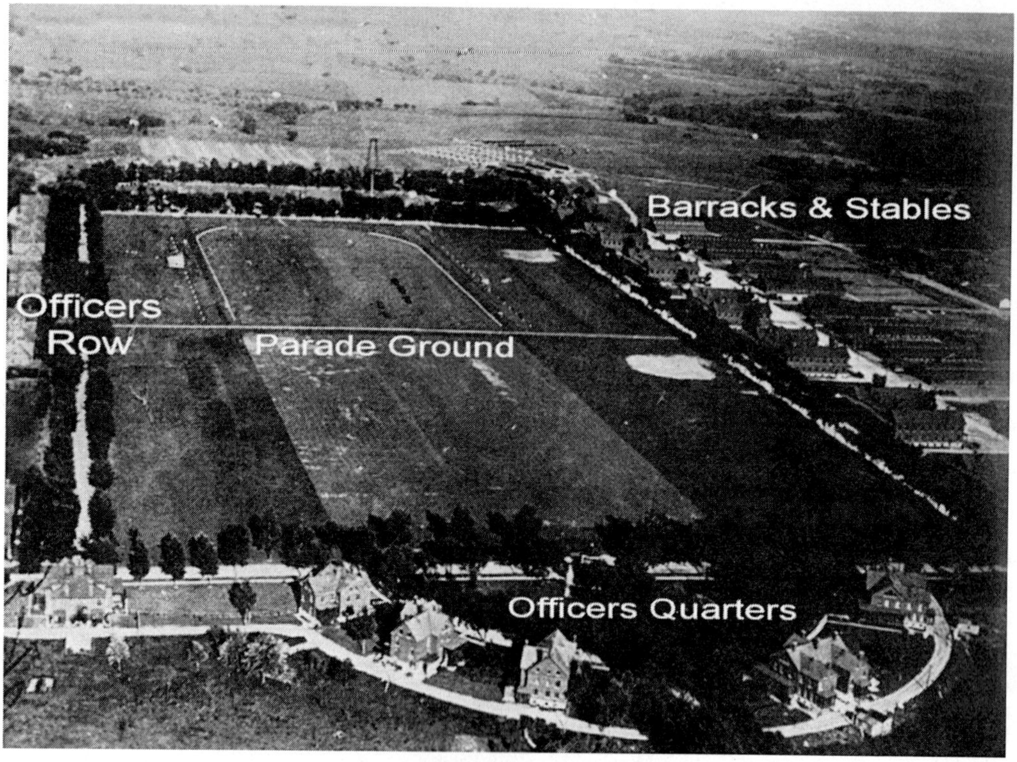

Aerial photographgraph of Fort Des Moines, ca. 1921 (National Archives).

editor of the local *Iowa Bystander*, and one of the leaders of the city's more than 5,000 African American citizens, lobbied in 1917 for use of the fort for the training of the line officers.[3] The medical officers training camp was an afterthought.

The list, uncovered at the National Archives, shows physicians arrived continuously at the camp during August, September and October. The training program was not finalized, and the camp's commander did not arrive until late in August. Training, which was to cover 10 weeks (60 days), ranged from as few as 30 to as many as 96 days. One very late arrival, Lieutenant Royal W. Grubbs, was in camp only 19 days.

In November 1917, the 92nd Division, comprised of 27,000 African American troops when fully staffed, was formally established. Fear, mostly among white Southerners, of creating so large an armed division of African American line officers caused the army to fragment the 92nd Division across several states.

Basic training at Fort Des Moines MOTC ended in early November. More than two-thirds of the physician trainees were sent directly to the 92nd Division headquarters at Camp Funston, Fort Riley, Kansas, for further field training and service with the 317th Sanitary (Medical) Train. The remaining third of the doctors were parceled out to various infantry, artillery and machine gun medical detachments of the 92nd Division located in six different camps spread from Iowa eastward to the Atlantic Ocean. While virtually all of the MOTC doctors remained with the 92nd Division, eight were assigned to the 93rd Division.

MOTC camp commandant Lieutenant Colonel E. G. Bingham, Medical Corps, prepared a lengthy and detailed 11-page "after action" report entitled "Report of Activities, Medical Officers' Training Camp, Fort Des Moines, Iowa, July 26th, 1917–November 13th, 1917." Bingham arrived as commandant on August 20 and remained until the camp closed in November. The authors found his original typed report with handwritten edits in the files of the 92nd Division at the National Archives.

In his report, the colonel noted he found on his arrival there were only three white medical instructors on duty. He recognized that this was inadequate. He requested and received three additional white Medical Reserve Corps officers. He also added four assistant instructors from his African American doctors: Julian Dawson, Raymond Jackson, George Lythcott and Louis Wright. These four men were among the 12 that the colonel recommended for promotion to the grade of captaincy because of their exceptional ability and qualifications.

His report tells us: "Due to the lack of quarters, instructors, mess and sanitary facilities and the daily arrival of officers, the camp's intensive instruction was limited to 10 weeks."

Bingham reported, "Instructions from the Surgeon General's Office were to train regimental sanitary (medical and hygiene) detachments only." The medical detachments usually ranged in size from 10 to 20 men. "We found it necessary because of the lack of adequate study halls to expand the hours of instruction in paperwork and the Manual of the Medical Department. Three night periods of two hours each were added in practical paperwork each week. Each officer was required to prepare the more commonly used forms and medical blanks, and these were carefully graded and criticized."

The following observations contained in the good colonel's working draft of his report (also at the National Archives) were omitted in his final report.

> Discipline was expected to be a problem from raw recruits. There was talk that it would be especially bad among colored troops.... The discipline of the men and officers was uniformly very good. No difficulty presented itself in the camp. Passes to the city of Des Moines were freely granted and did not result in any abuse of the privilege or disorder in the city. Fewer of our men were arrested by the local police authorities than is normal among regular troops.
>
> There were only 30 convictions of enlisted men in this camp. This is a very good record for old and seasoned troops—but when it is considered that practically all of the men at this camp were raw, undisciplined, green lads from civilian life, the record becomes unusually good. Among

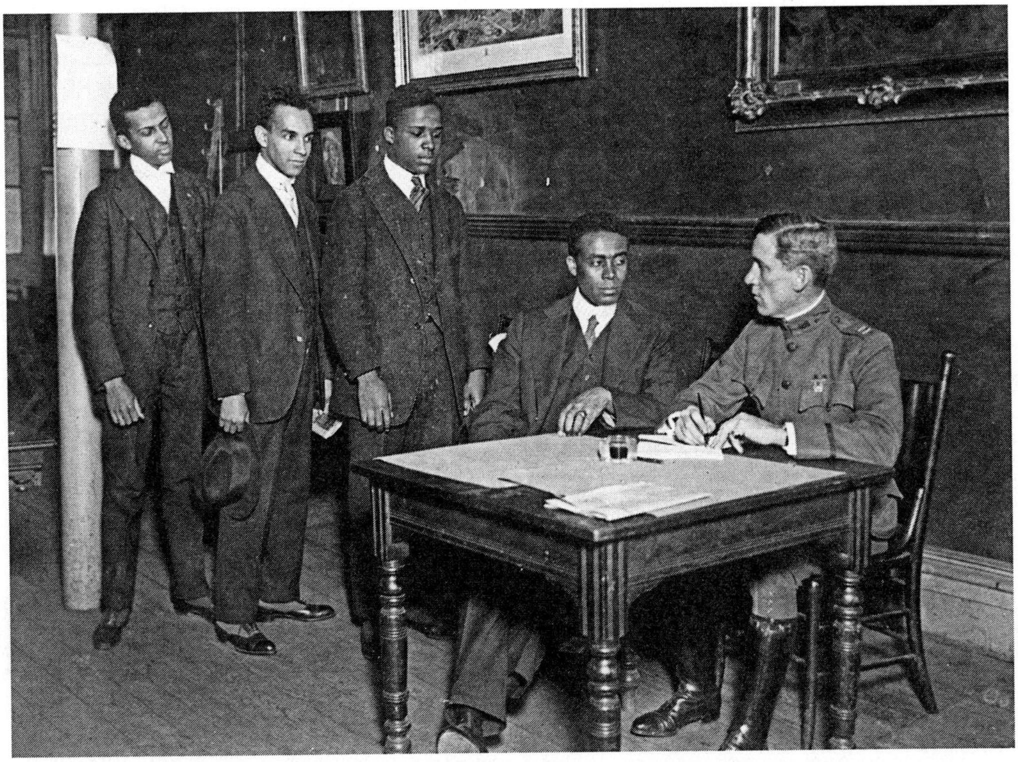

New officers enroll at World War I training camp (National Archives).

officers, none were arrested or reported to us by the Des Moines police.

Everything was done in a hurry in World War I. Many of the training camps had to be built by the very soldiers who were arriving for training. The MOTC was setting up in a camp that was already occupied by the African American line officers training camp (OTC). The medical corps was getting leftovers, whatever facilities remained.

> Messing and Cooking were seriously defective. Due to the fact that all barracks were occupied by the line officers training camp, no provisions could be made to take care of the thousand odd men of this medical camp. To remedy this defect, an estimate was submitted to the Army for the erection of four fly-proof kitchens and mess halls. At the close of camp no appropriation had been made.
>
> As a makeshift we secured from an abandoned National Guard Camp enough material to erect four screened kitchens which served the purpose as well as could be expected. No provision for a screened mess hall could be secured. The men were required to eat as if under field conditions. This was regrettable (as well as unnecessary) for two months was too long a time to wait for the small sum of $7500 needed to correct a very glaring defect.

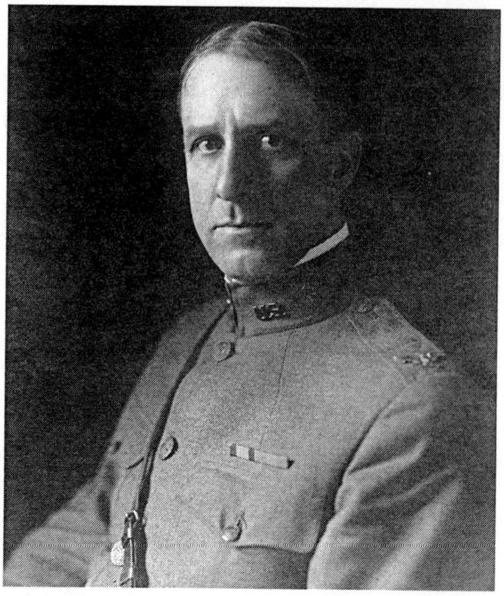

Colonel Ernest Grey Bingham, U.S. Army Medical Corps, commander of Medical Officers Training Camp (Colored) at Fort Des Moines, Iowa (Alabama Department of Archives and History, Montgomery, Alabama).

> The same remarks as to cooking apply in a measure to bathing.—**four** showerheads were all that were provided for 1,000 men, which is not consistent with proper bathing facilities. By a

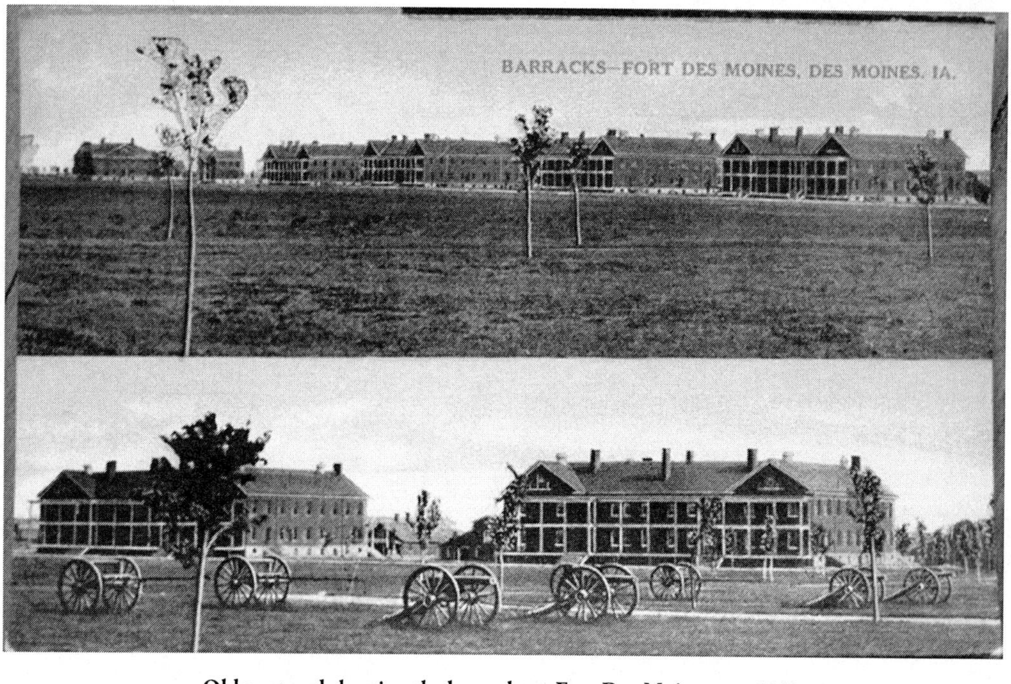

Old postcard showing the barracks at Fort Des Moines, ca. 1910.

mutual agreement between some of the company commanders of the line officers training camp and the Commandant of this camp, certain days were allotted to the bathing facilities of our companies. This tided over an emergency that could have become a grave sanitary defect of the camp.

The report included, "The total expenditures for this camp was but $1,830 which was principally to cover the cost of flooring the stalls of the four stables used as sleeping quarters for the enlisted men."

The colonel reported, "A feature of the training camp much enjoyed by officers and men was a practice march and three day field encampment. The entire command was taken on a ten-mile march to the State Fair grounds and lived under canvas (shelter tents) for three days, October 3 to October 6, 1917. Practical instruction was given in camp making, sanitation, regimental detachment administration, camp infirmary work, packing, bearer work and field work in general." At the Meharry Medical College Archives in Nashville there is a photograph of the actual event and one can see the Iowa State Fair roller coaster in the background.

> The health of the command remained uniformly good during the entire period of camp. No epidemic or any disease of any kind appeared during camp. No case of measles developed in any man who had been in camp more than two weeks. In all, 34 cases developed among 1021 men and 130 officers. I believe a large contributing factor in the relative freedom from measles was the use of open cavalry stables as barracks, for a variety of ventilation was obtained by necessity superior to that possible in a cantonment or under canvas.

Much of their basic U.S. Army training focused on fieldwork and administration. The physicians were being prepared to "conduct the service of the Medical Department without either the supervision of experienced medical officers or the aid of well-qualified noncommissioned officers."[4]

They were expected to become leaders and organize mobile medical hospitals and infirmaries, supervise medics, submit regular re-

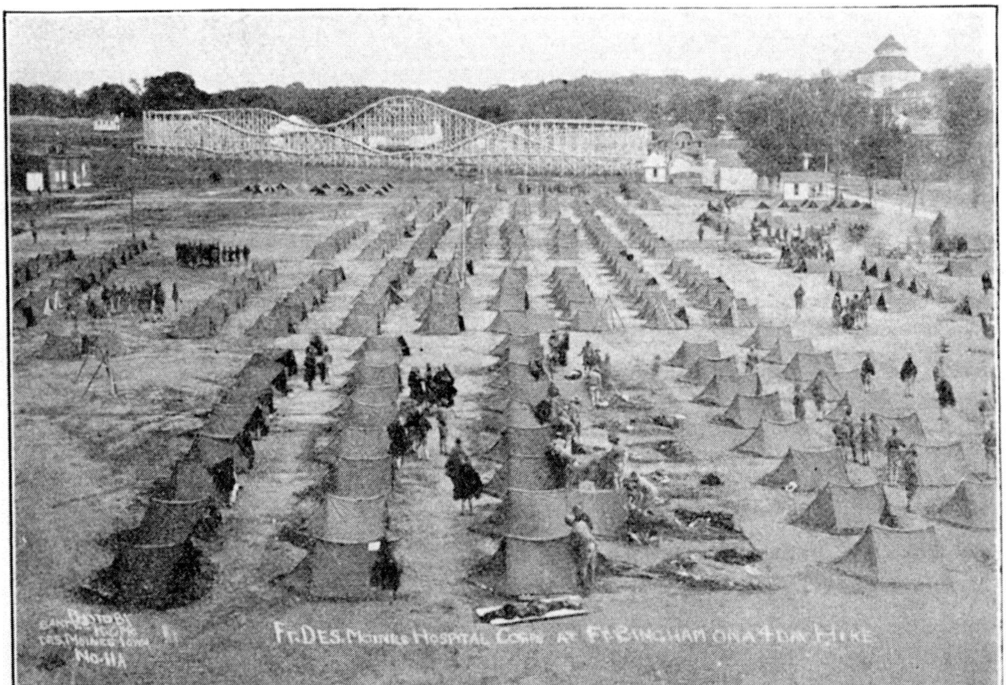
No-11A
Ft. DES. Moines Hospital Corps at Ft. Bingham on a 4 day Hike

Camp Bingham at state fairgrounds (courtesy Meharry Medical College Archives).

ports, track and order supplies, and maintain combat readiness by caring for the health of the troops.

In the end, all those who graduated from the camp departed by November 11, 1917 (which was, coincidentally, exactly one year to the day before the Armistice ended combat in France).

The vast majority of the 104 doctors (69) served at Camp Funston, Kansas, where the 92nd Division headquarters and the division's 317th Sanitary (Medical) Train were formed. The 35 physicians not sent to Kansas were assigned to camps in Illinois, Iowa, Ohio, New York, New Jersey, and Maryland. None were sent to southern states, with the exception of the eight doctors assigned to the 93rd Division. They were sent to either Camp Logan near Houston, Texas, or Camp Stuart at Newport News, Virginia.

The MOTC was an experiment. It was the first time a separate medical training camp was set up for African American doctors, dentists and medics. It was certainly a success judging by the large number of men who went on to serve with the 92nd and 93rd divisions in France. Of the 104 MOTC graduates, 89 actually served in France. With the battlefield death of Lieutenant Urbane F. Bass, 88 of the doctors returned to the U.S. to resume their lives and professions.

The physicians who received their military training at Fort Des Moines and served abroad returned with new skill sets that they were able to use to serve themselves, their communities and their country for decades afterward. They were intelligent, self-selected, volunteer physicians and leaders. Their year and a half of army training and war experiences certainly equipped them well beyond anything they had learned in medical school. They had been given command of medical detachments, which taught them leadership, discipline and responsibility. They experienced military organization, planning and training, and participated in grand and small-scale field operations.

Each AEF combat division included a Sanitary (Medical) Train composed of roughly 930 officers and men, physicians and medics. They were organized to provide care for troops in camp and on the battlefield.

In battle, each division provided three basic echelons of care from the front line to the rear. The closest to the fighting was the regimental aid station, staffed by doctors and medics of the fighting regimental medical detachments. Next were dressing stations manned by division doctors and medics of the ambulance companies who treated and evacuated casualties. Finally there were the four division field hospitals. The doctors trained at Fort Des Moines were distributed at every level of the 92nd Division. Excellent descriptions and images of the organization and processes American doctors experienced can be found at the University of Kansas Medical Center website.[5]

These physicians also experienced painful and unpleasant racism in the army. Despite their efforts to aid America, many white Americans failed to give them the credit they deserved. Their horizons were broadened in many ways, but because of serious racial discrimination in the army, their experiences were not always positive.

At War in France

93rd Division

The first African American combat units to arrive in France, with roughly 10,000 men, were the four infantry regiments of the 93rd Division. They arrived several months before the 92nd Division with its 27,000 men. The 93rd lacked both division support units and artillery, and thus was declared a "Provisional" division. Its regiments were all turned over to the French army by the AEF to fight separately under the French. Their American equipment was surrendered and replaced with French fighting equipment, including French Adrian helmets. The 93rd Division soldiers, with far fewer men than the 92nd Division, suffered more than twice as many killed and wounded and served longer in combat.

The regiments of the 93rd were made up largely of a core of experienced African American National Guard units with draftees filling out the ranks. That allowed them to mobilize quickly. The soldiers of one of these regiments, the "Harlem Hell Fighters" from the 93rd Division's 369th Infantry, earned high praise from the French and were prominent in the U.S. press. The regiment was formerly known as the 15th New York National Guard, and its troops were the first African American combat soldiers to arrive in France. Not only did the 369th arrive first, it served in battle longer than any other American regiment. It suffered many killed and wounded and its activities were widely reported in the United States.[6] While none of the 104 Fort Des Moines doctors were assigned to the 369th, eight of them were assigned to two other regiments, the 370th and the 372nd.

Four of the Fort Des Moines doctors were assigned to the 370th Infantry Regiment of the 93rd, formerly known as the 8th Illinois National Guard. They were Lieutenants George W. Antoine, Rufus Bacote, Claudius Ballard, and Dan M. Moore. According to Lieutenant Claudius Ballard, the 370th Infantry Regiment won more medals than any other American regiment in France, black or white.

Four other Fort Des Moines doctors were assigned to the 372nd Infantry Regiment. The 372nd was composed of various National Guard units from the District of Columbia, Maryland, Tennessee, Ohio, Massachusetts, and Connecticut. The doctors were Lieutenants Urbane F. Bass, Clarence S. Janifer, Sylvanus H. Warfield and Charles H. Laws. Warfield did not accompany the unit overseas. The only battlefield death among all the African American doctors from the Fort Des Moines MOTC occurred in October 1918, when First Lieutenant Urbane F. Bass of the 372nd Infantry died from a mortar blast that severed his legs while he was caring for wounded troops in the field.

92nd Division

The 92nd "Buffalo" Division was not permitted to assemble as a single fighting force until it reached France in mid–1918. The division, less its artillery units, then went to a training area at Bourbonne-les-Bains, where it assembled for the first time and began to receive equipment. From there it departed to engage in combat operations in three different sectors. First, in August, it entered French trenches in the St. Dié sector of the Vosges Mountains of eastern France. There the soldiers were involved in skirmishes, trench raids, and a German counterattack at Frapelle, which they repulsed successfully. It was their baptism by fire, and while casualties were light, artillery and aerial bombardments were very real and conditions were difficult. Troop movements were done at night, without lights. It was there that

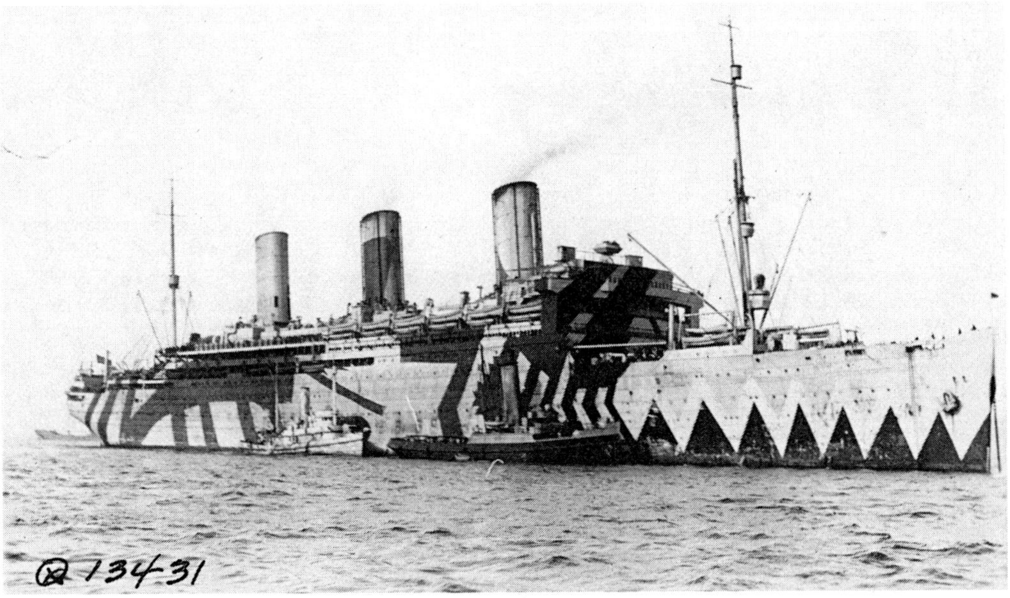

Troopships were camouflaged to elude German U-boats. The SS *Leviathan* arrives safely in Brest, France, May 2, 1918 (National Archives).

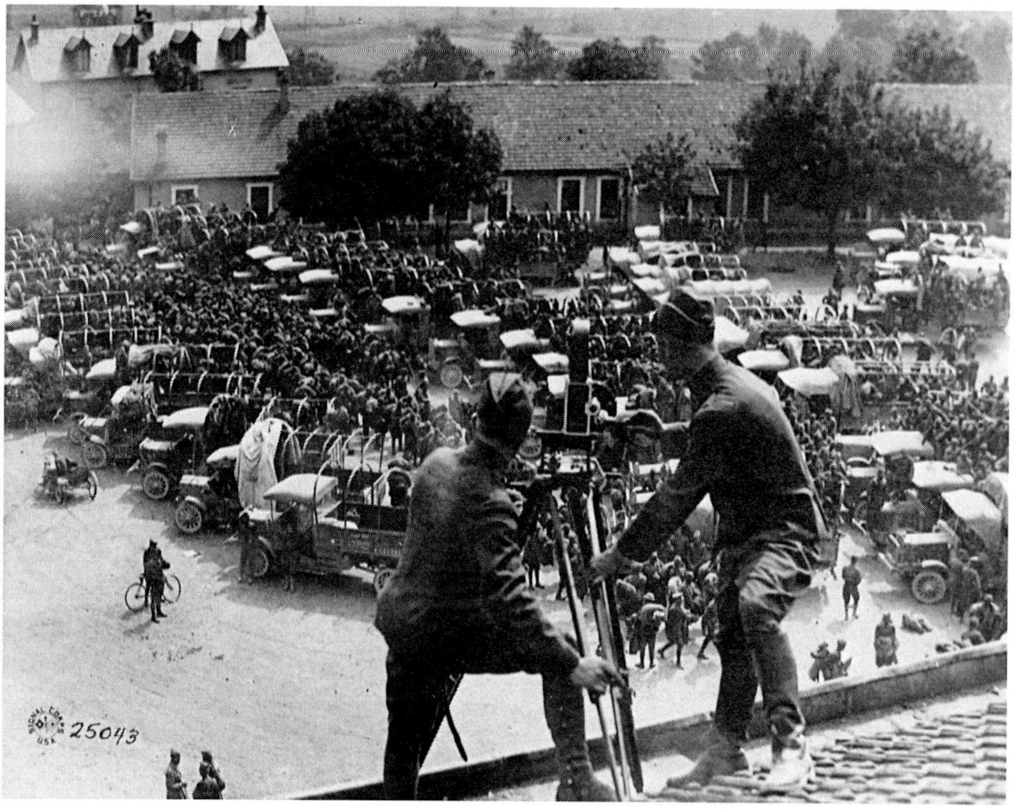

The 92nd Division trucks unloading at Bruyères in the Vosges (National Archives).

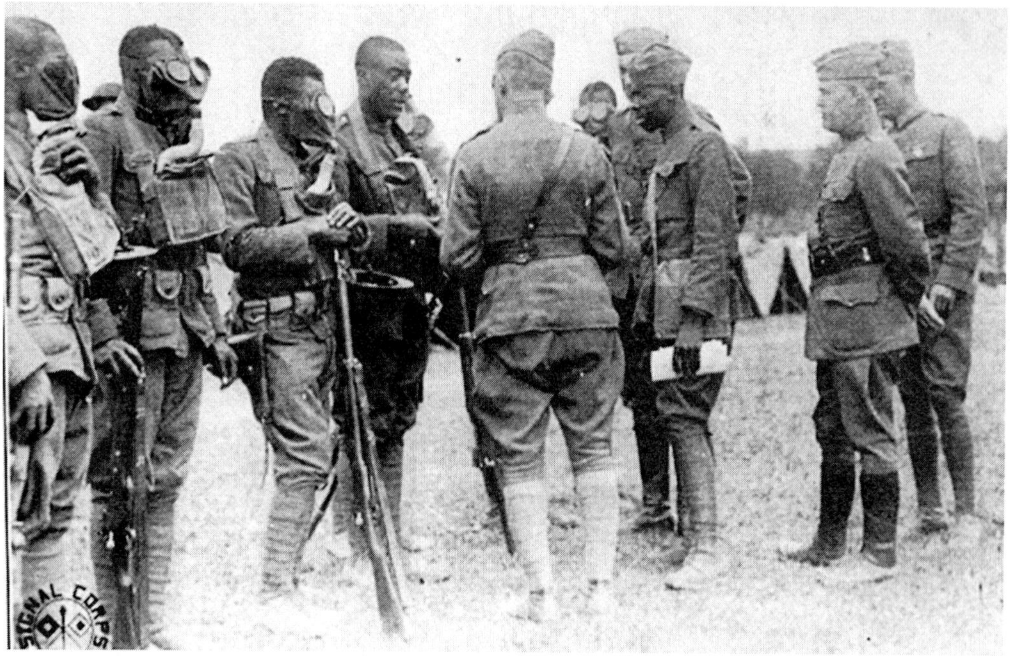

The 92nd Division in the Meuse Argonne, September 1918 (National Archives).

they encountered their first battle deaths and casualties.

At the end of September, on extremely short notice, they were rushed to the Meuse-Argonne for what became the biggest American battle of the war. The AEF First Army attacked German defensive positions that had been hardened over four years. One of the 92nd Division's infantry regiments, the 368th, was assigned to a French brigade to plug a gap on the left flank of the AEF forces. The rest of the division was held in reserve. The 368th saw fierce combat from September 26 to October 3 when it was withdrawn from the fight. The doctors had plenty of work to do with 323 casualties, 260 wounded and 63 dead.

After the division was withdrawn from the Meuse-Argonne in early October, it was sent to join the newly formed AEF Second Army near Pont-à-Mousson on the Moselle River, in what was called the Marbache Sector. The Second Army was preparing to attack near the great fortress city of Metz, which had been a German stronghold and critical railhead since the beginning of the war in 1914. By now the 92nd Division, totally complete for the first time and joined by its artillery units, undertook its greatest offensive action and suffered its greatest losses on November 10–11, as the war was drawing to a close. By the end of the war, the 92nd Division had suffered 250 killed or died of wounds, and nearly 1,200 more wounded and gassed.[7]

Because American army doctors had little battlefield experience, the British and French who had been at war since 1914 shared their hard earned knowledge and techniques with them. For example, the British Orthopaedic Department at the War Office under the leadership of Sir Robert Jones made major contributions to surgical procedures. Without antibiotics, amputation had been the most often used treatment for broken bones of the lower limbs. Jones brought to the physicians at the front the aseptic surgery techniques of Scottish surgeon Henry Gray as well as Gray's use of

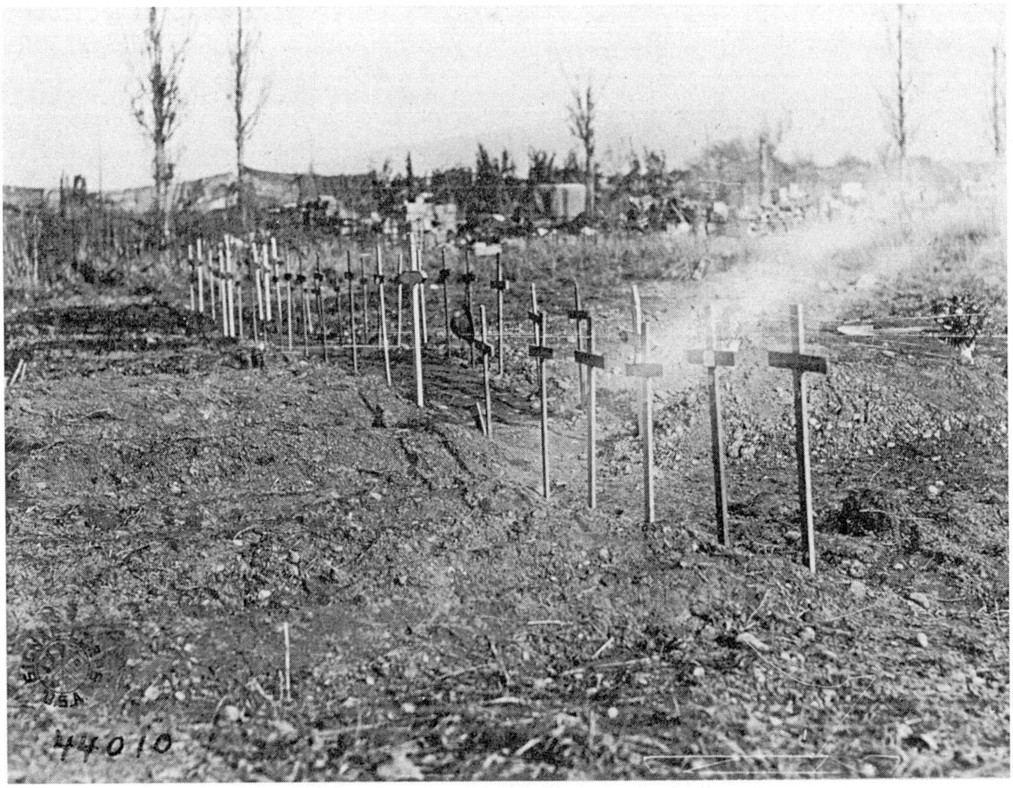

The 92nd Division grave markers (National Archives).

local and general anesthesia. In 1917 surgeons were even sent from the United States to learn these orthopedic surgical techniques.[8]

Sir Jones also brought the bone setting procedures of his uncle Dr. Hugh Owen Thomas into general practice during the war. The most important for the wounded in the First World War were the Thomas Splints, which are still in use today for setting broken hip, femur, knee and ankle joints.[9] These surgical techniques that the army doctors saw early on spread through American orthopedic surgery after the war.

Throughout the AEF's time in Europe, illness caused more deaths than combat. The Spanish Influenza pandemic took a terrible toll on the AEF. The 92nd Division was fortunate to have avoided the very worst of that, perhaps, ironically, because of the army's policy of segregation of black troops. Nevertheless, phosgene and mustard gas disabled many officers and men. Some were back in action within hours or days, while others suffered injury that affected them for the rest of their lives.[10]

The lives and experiences of these African American doctors that follow are a chronicle of largely forgotten leaders at the turn of the 20th century.

NOTES

1. *The Meharry Annual Military Review 1919*, The Record, 16, Harold D. West Collection, Meharry Medical College Archives, Nashville, TN.
2. Adam P. Wilson, *African American Army Officers of World War I* (Jefferson, NC: McFarland, 2015), 50.
3. Ibid.
4. Ibid.
5. *Medicine in the First World War, Military Medical Operations*, www.kumc.edu (accessed May 25, 2015).
6. Frank E. Roberts, *The American Foreign Legion* (Annapolis, MD: Naval Institute Press, 2004), 3–19, 53–62, 98–121, 193–202 and Appendices A, B and C.
7. The 92nd Division, Summary of Operations in the World War, Prepared by the American Battle Monuments Commission, United States Government Printing Office, Washington, DC, 1944, www.history.army.mil/topics/afam/92div.htm (accessed June 8, 2014).
8. Thomas Scotland and Steven Heys, *War Surgery 1914-18* (West Midlands, England: Helion & Company, 2012), 150–151.
9. Ibid.
10. Carol R. Byerly, PhD, *The U.S. Military and the Influenza Pandemic of 1918–1919*, Public Health Report 2010; 125 (Suppl 3): 82–91, http://www.ncbi.nlm.nih.gov/pmc/articles/PMC2862337 (accessed April 12, 2015).

The Biographies

George Washington ANTOINE

26 November 1878–17 August 1939
Meharry Medical College, 1906

Roots and Education

George W. Antoine was born in Texas. Not much is known of his early life until he attended Guadalupe College, an educational institution for African Americans located in Seguin, Texas. He took three sessions of algebra and Latin. Guadalupe was the only black Baptist institution of higher learning in South Texas. It was endorsed by the state of Texas and, by the time Antoine attended, was averaging more than 300 students a semester.

Antoine then made his way to Nashville, Tennessee, and Meharry Medical College. He graduated in 1906, married 19-year-old Lottie Voliver and, according to the 1910 Census, moved with her and her six-year-old nephew William Voliver to Prescott, Arkansas. Prescott is a small city in the southwest corner of Arkansas, about 50 miles from Texarkana, Texas.

Soon thereafter the family moved on to Houston. In the early 20th century, Houston was home to almost 45,000 people, and a railroad hub for the export of cotton. Oil had been discovered nearby in 1901, and the city was developing into a major petroleum center. The population exploded and there were very few physicians to serve the city's African American population. Dr. Henry E. Lee, Dr. Thomas Shadowens and Dr. Antoine, all Meharry graduates, came to Houston and opened practices in the early 20th century. They were generalists and treated patients with broken bones or infectious diseases or delivered their babies. They worked from offices in their homes, at least initially. It was from Houston that Dr. Antoine volunteered for service in the First World War.

Military Service

In 1917 Dr. Antoine volunteered to serve in France during World War I and reported for duty at the Fort Des Moines Medical Officers Training Camp on October 5, 1917. He was only in this training camp for 38 days—one of the shortest times—before his transfer to Camp Funston and then to Camp Logan near his hometown of Houston, Texas. He was assigned to the 370th Infantry Regiment of the 93rd Division, comprised of African American soldiers of the Old 8th Illinois National Guard. First Lieutenant Antoine was assigned to Depot Company K as medical officer.

Camp Logan had been the scene of race riots in early 1917. As a result, the army wanted to move these African American troops out as soon as possible. In March 1918 they were sent promptly to France on the SS *President Grant*. They departed from Hoboken, New Jersey, on April 7, 1918.[1]

AEF headquarters was not ready to deal with arriving troops so General Pershing promptly solved the problem of what to do with them by turning them over to the French, who had been requesting American soldiers.

Once in France, another doctor from Camp Logan wrote home about treating those with flu and conditions there: "We have the men sick in two field hospital tents about 68 in all and full we are sending some to isolation in their companies for isolation there. But hope to be thru with it soon. I didn't lose any time when I had my attack but feel OK now for two days, Capt ... and I had our hands full I tell you that.... I would make 29 or 30 calls and give meds each morning besides inspecting, etc., kept us going."[2]

The 370th was a combat infantry regiment and so while initially treating soldiers with flu might have consumed much of the medics' time, the 93rd fought under the French in a number of campaigns, and battle casualties were significant. "During World War I, the 370th Infantry served with distinction with the French 34th, 36th, and 59th Infantry Divisions, earning streamers for the battles of Lorraine and Oise-Aisne. Sectors occupied and engagements participated in were Saint Mihiel with the French in 1918, Argonne Forest, St. Gobain Forest, Bosi de Mortier, Mont des Signes, Oise-Aisne Canal, Laon, Grandlup, Soissons, and Oise-Aisne and Lorraine offensives. One battalion of the Regiment, under the command of Lieutenant Colonel Otis B. Duncan, was engaged in pursuit of the retreating enemy far in advance, when halted by the Armistice."[3]

Dan Moore, Claudius Ballard and Rufus Bacote were among the doctors who trained with Antoine at Fort Des Moines and were assigned to the 370th's Medical Corps with him. An assessment of the 370th's performance during the fall offensive from September 15 to November 11, 1918, records it fought "hard and well" while sustaining significant casualties of "approximately 560 officers and men wounded and 105 killed in action or dead of wounds."[4]

After the war had ended, Lieutenant Antoine and two other medical officers on December 3, 1918, accompanied 167 wounded warriors of the 92nd and 93rd Division back to Camp Upton in New York. On February 15, 1919, he was further assigned to accompany a detachment on a special train to Camp Travis at San Antonio, Texas, "to insure proper medical care on the journey." When he arrived his discharge and final pay were processed on February 23, 1919.[5]

Career

Dr. Antoine returned to his wife Lottie and their home at 2801 McGowen Avenue in Houston where he practiced for the next 20 years. His office was opened at 409½ Milam (the ½ usually means the office was on the upper floor). The first floor would have been some kind of retail store or restaurant or entertainment for the African American community. He practiced at the Houston Negro Hospital and was active in the Lone Star State Medical, Dental and Pharmaceutical Association, serving as its first vice president in 1928.

In 1925, his daughter Mattie Louise was born. Then on October 5, 1927, his Lottie died. The 1930 U.S. Census tells us that he and Mattie moved into a home close to his cousins, W. C. and Addie Robbins, at 2805 Dennis Street so they could help with her care. He and Mattie lived next door at 2811 Dennis Street. Shortly before his death, he was remarried to a woman named Zella.

In the *Chicago Defender* obituary of Dr. Antoine he was described as "a prominent Houston physician, who died suddenly."[6] He died of heart disease. Funeral services were conducted from his residence in Houston. His widow Zella, daughter Mattie (14), and brother Ed Antoine survived him.

His legacy included a bricks and mortar tribute. One of Houston's American Legion Posts was named in his honor. It hosted many events for veterans and the African American community in Houston. A second tribute included a baby boy born on December 12, 1939 (the same year he died), in Harris, Texas, to Robert Lee Antoine and Minnie Beatrice Williams. They named their child George Washington Antoine.

Dr. Antoine's life was one of giving to his nation and his Houston community. He was indeed a prominent Houston physician. To this day there are several physicians with the first or last name of Antoine on Antoine Drive in Houston. They continue his legacy.

Notes

1. Record Group 120–93rd Division Regiments & Medical Detachments Manifests, National Archives, College Park, MD.
2. http://heroletterswwl.blogspot.com/2009/07/us-army-doctor-wwi-letter-camp-logan.html (accessed June 20, 2014).
3. http://www.globalsecurity.org/military/agency/army/1-178in.htm (accessed June 20, 2014).
4. Frank E. Roberts, *The American Foreign Legion* (Annapolis, MD: Naval Institute Press, 2004), 164–172.

5. Special Orders, Headquarters Camp Travis, Texas, 23 February 1919, National Personnel Records Center, National Archives, St. Louis, Missouri.

6. "Observe Last Rites," *Chicago Defender*, August 26, 1939, 6.

Rufus Herve BACOTE

1 July 1890–13 October 1930
Meharry Medical College, 1917

Roots and Education

Bacote was born in Timmonsville, South Carolina, a very small town located about 10 miles west of the city of Florence in what was a heavily agricultural area. His parents were both born in South Carolina. His father, M. T. Bacote, was a farmer. His mother was Hattie Jackson. Rufus was the second oldest of four brothers. His oldest brother Fred worked as a laborer on the family farm. Fred, who had a sixth grade education, later became an undertaker in a local funeral parlor. A younger brother, Brooks, also farmed and later became a minister. His youngest brother, Minus, was a farmer as well.

Rufus Bacote was educated in South Carolina, perhaps in nearby Florence, and most certainly he worked on the family farm, too. In 1917, at the age of 27, he graduated from Meharry Medical College in Nashville. The path that led Bacote to medicine is not clear, but we know he came from humble beginnings and overcame numerous disadvantages to become a doctor and later serve his nation. When he registered for the draft in May 1917 he was living in Nashville and married to Amanda Bacote. He was a newly graduated physician, and on his draft registration card he still gave his home as Timmonsville.[1]

Military Service

Bacote began his military service as a first lieutenant in the Army Medical Reserve Corps and trained for 46 days at the Medical Officers Training Camp (MOTC) at Fort Des Moines. When he completed his training on November 11, 1917, he was first assigned to Camp Funston, Kansas, and then re-assigned to the 370th Infantry Regiment of the 93rd Division. The 370th was largely made up of soldiers and officers from the Old Illinois 8th National Guard. Many of its members had battle experience. They were veterans of the Spanish-American war. He was assigned to its 2nd Battalion as a medical officer.[2]

Lieutenant Bacote was one of several African American medical officers who accompanied the regiment to Camp Logan in Houston, Texas. From there, the unit transferred to Hoboken and departed for France in April 1918. His unit fought with the French because all four regiments of the 93rd Division were detached from the American Expeditionary Force (AEF) and sent to war under French command. The 370th carried with it a full staff of African American medical officers. Three of them, Dan M. Moore, George W. Antoine and Claudius Ballard, were with Bacote at the MOTC at Fort Des Moines. The medical detachment was composed of 23 men who alternately attended to the wounded. Because of their prompt attention on the battlefield only 105 men in the entire regiment lost their lives and more than 425 recovered from wounds.

The 370th saw extensive combat in France. According to Sweeney, "About fifty percent of the 370th met casualties of some sort during their service in France ... they were singularly free from disease.... Probably 1,000 men were gassed and incapacitated at times, as the regiment had three replacements to make up its losses. The regiment went to France with approximately 2,500 men from Chicago and Illinois, and came back with 1,260. Many of the wounded, sick and severely gassed were invalided home or came back as parts of casual companies formed at hospital bases. The replacement troops that went into the regiment were mostly from the Southern states. A few of the colored officers assigned to the regiment after its arrival in France were men from the officers training camps in this country and France."[3] From this it is obvious that the medical challenges that Dr. Bacote and the other physicians experienced were substantial.

Career

Following the war Dr. Bacote returned to his wife in Nashville where she had been staying at 1220 East Hill Street. From there they moved to Kentucky to practice medicine. In 1920 they lived in a rental at 113 East 4th Street in Maysville, Kentucky, a small, older industrial city on the Ohio River. From there they moved west to Earlington, Kentucky, another small city in the western part of the state about 100 miles north of Nashville, Tennessee. In all likelihood, the need for a physician there probably came to his attention through his medical college, Meharry. They didn't remain long in Earlington before finally moving to Louisville where they resided at 547-B Lampton Street. He practiced there until 1930.[4] Sadly, he suffered from chronic interstitial nephritis (kidney disease) and died shortly after his 40th birthday on October 13, 1930.[5]

He was buried in Nashville. His wife, Amanda, returned to Nashville to live at 1620 Scovel Street. Eventually she moved to Chicago, where she was active with the Pilgrim Baptist Church School. In fact, her picture appeared in the *Chicago Defender* newspaper in 1946 noting she had won an award and was in the May Queen contest at the church school.[6] Pilgrim Baptist Church is an historic church located on the south side of Chicago. It was originally constructed as a synagogue. The church is notable both as an architectural landmark and for the cultural contributions by the congregation of the church. The church is in the heart of Chicago's Bronzeville neighborhood. A Baptist congregation moved into the building in 1922, forming Pilgrim Baptist Church.

The church is credited as the birthplace of gospel music in the 1930s. Thomas A. Dorsey, the "Father of Gospel Music," was the music director at Pilgrim Baptist for decades. Many famous singers such as Albertina Walker (the "Queen of Gospel"), Mahalia Jackson, Aretha Franklin, Sallie Martin, James Cleveland, and the Edwin Hawkins Singers are among those who have sung at the church. It housed a large series of murals painted by the African American William E. Scott between 1936 and 1937.

Pilgrim's charismatic and forward-thinking pastor Junius C. Austin hired both Scott and Dorsey in the 1930s to increase the church's appeal making it one of the largest churches in the country in just a few years. In 1973, the building was listed on the National Register of Historic Places, and the building was designated a Chicago Landmark in 1981.[7]

The Bacotes both served their communities and their country. While we have no evidence that Dr. and Mrs. Bacote had children, clearly they are remembered for caring for many other families.

NOTES

1. World War I Draft Registration Card, Rufus Herve Bacote, ancestry.com.
2. W. Allison Sweeney, *History of the American Negro in the Great War* (New York: Negro University Press, 1969), 153.
3. Sweeney, *History of the American Negro in the Great War*, 161.
4. AMA Deceased Physician Card, National Library of Medicine, Bethesda, MD.
5. Kentucky Death Record, 1930, Rufus Herve Bacote, ancestry.com.
6. "Wins Award," *Chicago Defender*, June 15,1946, 16.
7. "Pilgrim Baptist Church," http://en.wikipedia.org/wiki/Pilgrim_Baptist_Church (accessed March 13, 2015).

Everett Russell BAILEY

30 March 1888–22 October 1932
Meharry Medical College, 1910

Roots and Education

Everett R. Bailey was born in New Castle, Henry County, Indiana, to Reverend John Bailey and Cora (Dempsey) Bailey. New Castle is a city 44 miles east-northeast of Indianapolis, on the Big Blue River. In 1900, when Bailey was 12 years old, only 3,406 people lived in the town, which was surrounded by farms.

By the time Everett went away to medical school in Nashville, his parents had moved to Maysville, Kentucky. It is a very old, small city of the Ohio River. Located on the early pioneer routes westward, it was an early trading center. Small industry developed there as well because of its location on the great river. At the age of 22, Bailey earned his medical degree as a member the 1910 Meharry Medical College class in Nashville. He married Drusilla Bailey. In 1914, the couple was living in Louisville, Kentucky. The city had the largest African American community in the state. That year their infant son died. His parents came from Maysville to spend some time with them.[1]

Military Service

In 1917 Dr. Bailey volunteered for service in the U.S. Army and was commissioned as a first lieutenant in the Medical Reserve Corps.

On November 11, after 44 days of basic training at Fort Des Moines, he was sent to Camp Funston at Fort Riley, Kansas, where he joined 92nd Division's medical unit. On November 15, he was assigned to the 365th Ambulance Company, commanded by Captain Sherman B. Hickman. There were five physician officers and 95 enlisted personnel who spent the next six months at Funston undergoing further training and caring for soldiers as the division continued its mobilization. They worked in an infirmary and in the field. In May 1918 they left for New York and France.

In July 1918, soon after First Lieutenant Bailey arrived in France, he was detailed to the Train's Ambulance Section (consisting of four ambulance companies) as the Battalion Gas Officer. Two non-commissioned officers were detailed to assist him with these duties. Sudden bursts of H.E. (high explosive) gas shells were responsible for a large portion of gas casualties. Constant gas mask drills were essential.[2]

Bailey was sent for specialized training in the prevention and treatment of gas casualties. One of his duties was to provide leadership and training in gas warfare for the medical personnel in the all of the Train's ambulance companies. In August 1918, he was transferred to the 366th Field Hospital.

The field hospital section of the sanitary train consisted of four field hospitals. Each accommodated 216 patients. Divisional specialists were assigned as needed. The equipment at each of these hospitals was initially identical, but later it was specialized as the nature of the wounds and the needs of the patients dictated.[3]

A report Lieutenant Bailey wrote from the 366th Field Hospital on November 1, 1918, indicates the magnitude of the gas problem. During the two weeks from October 14 to October 31, 261 gas cases were treated. The casualties came in from 19 different units. One hundred and thirty-one were diagnosed as Yperite poisoning, with acute conjunctivitis, respiratory problems, vomiting and 45 surface burns. Another 127 cases were diagnosed as Arsene poisoning with eye and respiratory problems, vomiting and sneezing. Of the 261 cases, 135 were evacuated to the Base Hospital, 68 were sent to the Camp for recuperation, 54 were treated and returned to duty with the command, and four cases still remained in the hospital.[4]

Following the end of the war, Lieutenant Bailey returned to the United States in early 1919 and completed his military service. He was honorably discharged on May 28, 1919, and returned home.

Career

In 1920 his home and office were located in Louisville at 716 15th Street.[5] By the early 1920s he moved to Indianapolis, Indiana, where he continued to work as a physician. In 1922 he had an office at 548½ Indiana Avenue and resided at 2628 Boulevard Place.[6] A few years later, the couple moved from Indianapolis to Chicago, where they lived at 299 Prairie Avenue.[7] In 1931, the *Chicago Defender* newspaper carried a photograph of Dr. Bailey with the caption "RETURNS HERE—Dr. Everett R. Bailey, formerly of Chicago but more recently of Indianapolis has returned to the Windy City and opened offices at 456 E. 47th St."[8] He and his wife moved to 6032 Prairie Avenue.

Dr. Bailey practiced medicine in Chicago until his premature death the following year at age 45 from a lung abscess.[9] The effects of gas that he experienced during the war may have contributed to his early death. His body was returned to his birthplace in New Castle, Indiana, where he was buried in the South Mound Cemetery. He lies there under a military headstone provided by the U.S. Army.[10]

Notes

1. The (Maysville, KY) *Public Ledger*, March 16, 1914, 6.
2. Record Group 120, Records of the 92d Division—Box 6, Confidential Memorandum, October 5, 1918, National Archives, College Park, MD.
3. U.S. Army Medical Department, Office of Medical History, Vol. VIII, Field Operations, Chapter IV, Medical Service of the Division in Combat, GPO 1925, Washington, D.C., history.amedd.army.mil (accessed April 23, 2015).
4. Record Group 120, Records of the 92d Division, 317th Sanitary Train, Field Hospital 366 Report, Report of Gas Cases, November 1, 1918, National Archives, College Park, MD.
5. World War I Draft Registration Cards, 1917–1918, and 1920 U.S. Census, E.R. Bailey, ancestry.com.
6. U.S. city directory, 1922, Indianapolis, IN, ancestry.com.

7. 1930 U.S. Census.
8. Photograph—*Chicago Defender*, February 28,1931, A10.
9. Illinois Death Index, 1916–1947, ancestry.com and AMA Death Card, National Library of Medicine, Bethesda, MD.
10. U.S. Headstones Applications for Military Veterans, 1925–1963, for Everett R. Bailey, ancestry.com.

Dana Olden BALDWIN

20 March 1881–9 November 1972
Leonard Medical School, 1910

Roots and Education

Dana O. Baldwin was born March 20, 1881, in Belvoir, Chatham County, North Carolina, to the Reverend Jay Halsey and Mary Crutchfield Baldwin. His father was a Methodist minister. Baldwin began to help support the family at a young age as a farm laborer. Most of his early study was at home until the family moved to town and schooling for more than two months a year was possible. Finally, he was able to attend the Apex Normal and Industrial Institute and graduated in 1897 at age 16. He went on to Shaw University in Raleigh. Throughout college he continued to work as a farm laborer during the summer. He then taught in the public schools during the winter and worked as a private waiter until his mother convinced him to return home and pursue his education. He returned home and entered Shaw's Leonard Medical School. Dr. Baldwin received his medical degree in 1910.[1]

That year he opened Martinsville's first African American medical practice. This small city (still less than 20,000 people) is located in Henry County in rural south central Virginia near the North Carolina border. The city's chief industry was the manufacture of plug chewing tobacco. Furniture construction became more important by the mid–20th century. Throughout its history, Martinsville's racial makeup was about half white and half African American. The early years of his practice were hard, but it grew a little each year.

On December 24, 1911, Dr. Baldwin married Vina A. Flood. They adopted two girls, J. Mae and Rosa B., and raised three boys and a girl as foster children. The family lived at 155 Fayette Street.

Military Service

Dr. Baldwin was 36 when he volunteered and was commissioned first lieutenant in the Medical Reserve Corps. On September 27, 1917, he reported for basic training at Fort Des Moines. After training he was assigned to the 368th Ambulance Company of the 92nd Division, 317th Sanitary (Medical) Train. Either he had problems with his superior, Lieutenant Colonel David B. Downing, or he found military life wasn't what he expected. In any event, he submitted his resignation before ever leaving for France, but the army did not act on this request. He was sent to France where he served until the war ended. Initially, his main responsibility was caring for sick soldiers. His responsibilities included infirmary illnesses and surgical duties, and he was also expected to take on sanitation duties involving waste disposal, water purification and the kitchen inspections.

The cold and damp from the interminable rain meant the soldiers were constantly unwell and ripe for illness. Between September and November 1918, influenza struck. It brought sickness and pneumonia to as many as 40 percent of the U.S. Army personnel.

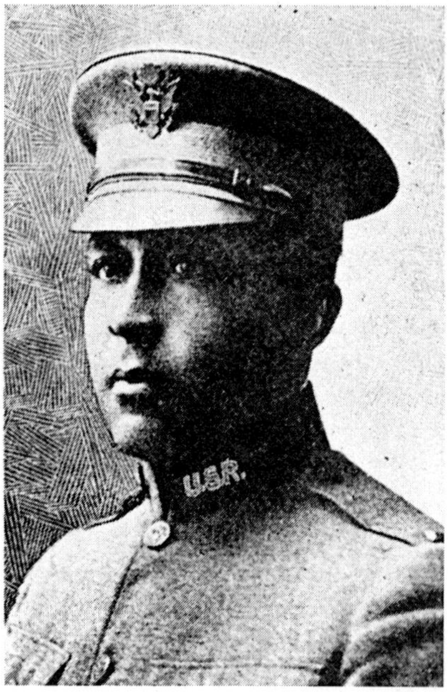

Dana O. Baldwin (national pictorial, members of the National Medical Association, 1925, courtesy Kansas City Public Library).

During the American Expeditionary Forces' Meuse-Argonne campaign, the epidemic diverted urgently needed resources from combat support to transporting and caring for the sick and the dead. Influenza and pneumonia killed more American soldiers and sailors during the war than did enemy weapons.[2] Army physicians learned to deal with extraordinary circumstances, treating hundreds of sick plus the wounded while continuing their mundane but critical sanitation duties (like water treatment or garbage disposal).

On April 2, 1919, he was honorably discharged and resumed his active medical practice in Martinsville.[3]

Career

In the "History of the American Negro," Dr. Baldwin was quoted as saying he believed the best way to promote the interests of African Americans is "by advocating and working for better schools, better churches, better sanitation, by buying and working farms, by seeing to it that the children are instructed in civic duty in the schools and taught the importance and power of the ballot."[4]

Denied privileges at the white hospital, Dr. Baldwin constructed his own 27-bed facility in 1929. He named it St. Mary's after his mother. His patients were largely poor so he established the Baldwin Business Center to supplement his income. It included Baldwin's Drug Store. His brother, Sam Baldwin, owned the pharmacy. Also located on the Baldwin Block ("The Block" as it was called by locals) were a hotel, a movie theater, a dance hall, bowling alley, pool hall, barbershop, dental office and an ice cream parlor. The medical practice and multiple businesses Dr. Baldwin opened during the 1920s and 1930s formed the heart of Martinsville's African American business district along Fayette Street. A great fire burned down nearly all of the wooden structures that made up the Baldwin Block in 1928, but it was rebuilt.[5]

At a time when Jim Crow laws made most private and many public facilities off-limits to African Americans, Dr. Baldwin helped nurture an independent black economy. He was a Trustee and Steward of his AME Church and member of the Masons, Odd Fellows, Knights of Pythias and St. Luke's Elks as well as the Magic City Medical Society (Roanoke) and the National Medical Association.[6]

In the early 1930s, Dr. Baldwin opened the Sandy Beach Resort, a motel and pool with a stage for concerts just outside the city. He inaugurated an annual June German Ball, a dance party that stretched from the Baldwin Block to Sandy Beach. The likes of Duke Ellington, Cab Calloway, Count Basie, Sam Cooke and James Brown performed at the festival during its 40-year run.

He also built and operated the Baldwin Miniature Golf Course for the African American community. He made it a regulation course, constructed the same as any other.[7]

There was an occasion in 1938 when Dr. Baldwin treated and hospitalized a black man who had his leg broken by police officers. He then took the matter to police court where he submitted a bill for $1 to cover the cost of treatment. This ensured the police actions were reported in the newspaper.

St. Mary's Hospital operated until 1951. The Fayette Area Historical Initiative and the Virginia Foundation for the Humanities' exhibit, entitled "Working and Playing on Fayette Street," have memorialized it.[8]

On June 6, 1953, the *Baltimore Afro-American* reported,

> The Baldwin's Gymntorium was opened with a program honoring Dr. and Mrs. Dana Olden Baldwin, Martinsville's leading citizens.
>
> Dr. Baldwin is responsible for Martinsville's first moving picture theatre, 1911; first ice cream parlor, 1912; first Baldwin's pants factory employing colored men and women; the gymnatorium; first hospital, and first Boosters Political Club.[9]

For 60 years Dr. Baldwin worked hard to improve the lives of Martinsville's African America community. He saw patients until his death from a stroke in 1972.

NOTES

1. Joseph J. Boris, editor, *Who's Who in Colored America*, New York, NY, 1928–1929, Second Edition (New York: Who's Who in Colored America Corp., 1929) 422.
2. Carol R. Byerly, Public Health Rep. 2010; 125 (Suppl 3):82–90, ncbi.nim.nih.gov (accessed February 21, 2015).
3. Thomas Yenser, ed. and pub., *Who's Who in Colored America, 1938–1939–1940*, 5th ed. (New York, 1940) 38.

4. Arhur Bunyan Caldwell, Editor, "Dana Olden Baldwin," *History of the American Negro and His Institutions* (Atlanta, 1921), 289.
5. "Fire Loss Greater than First Estimated," *The Bee*, December 27, 1928, 7.
6. Joseph Boris, *Who's Who in Colored America* (New York: Who's Who in Colored America Corp., 1929), 422.
7. *The Bee*, June 20, 1930, 5.
8. African American Historic Sites, www.aaheritageva.org (accessed June 6, 2012).
9. "Honor Dr. Dana Baldwin as Gymnatorium Is Opened," *The Baltimore African American*, June 6, 1953, 18.

Claudius BALLARD

14 June 1890–1 May 1967
University of Southern California, 1915

Roots and Education

Claudius Ballard was a native Californian from Los Angeles (an Angeleno). His grandfather, John Ballard, was a former slave from Kentucky who it is believed came to California in 1859 as a settler. His father was William L. Ballard, also a native of L.A. His mother was Mary Esther (Tibbs) Ballard. Young Ballard was an only child and was educated in the Los Angeles public schools. His mother was instrumental in ensuring he received a good education. After he graduated from Los Angeles High School he attended the University of Southern California (Los Angeles) and later studied medicine at the University of California at Berkeley, graduating in 1913. He passed the State Board medical examination and began to practice medicine in Los Angeles. At 24 he was said to be the youngest practicing physician in Los Angeles at that time.[1] The local African American newspaper carried a laudatory front-page story about him headlined "Rising Young Physician and Surgeon Who Is Rapidly Taking Front Rank in His Profession in This Section." The article included a large photograph of him standing in front of his new 1915 Model Studebaker 3-Passenger Roadster.[2]

As early as July 1914, he and a friend and close associate, Dr. Leonard Stovall held a meeting at their offices with other physicians and helped establish a permanent state medical society in Southern California.[3] In April 28, 1915, Dr. Claudius Ballard presented a paper, "The Pituitary Body, Its Function and Pathology."[4] In September 1915 a West Coast African American newspaper reported Dr. Ballard had come from L.A. to pay a visit to Oakland, where he had lived as a medical student.[5] In October 1915 Ballard led the discussion of a medical paper on "Official and Unofficial Narcotic Preparations." In December 1915, he presented a paper on "Tonsillitis and Its Sequel."[6] In March 1916, a dentist, Dr. W. H. Browning, joined Drs. Ballard and Stovall in their practice offices.[7]

In 1917, when the government called on doctors to volunteer for the First World War, Ballard, who was still single, volunteered and was commissioned as a first lieutenant in the Medical Reserve Corps.

Military Service

Lieutenant Ballard became a decorated war veteran. He was called to active duty on September 27, 1917, and sent to the Medical Officers Training Camp at Fort Des Moines. He arrived October 5, 1917, and upon completing his training there on November 11, was assigned to the Medical Detachment of the 370th Infantry Regiment (93rd Division). Before his regiment was activated and rechristened the 370th Infantry, it was an experienced African American National Guard unit known as the 8th Illinois. Lieutenant Ballard reported to Camp Logan in Houston, Texas, and was assigned to lead the medical team for its 3rd Battalion. He, George W. Antoine, Rufus Bacote, and Dan Moore were among the army's first African American physicians to arrive in France. Once there, his regiment served under French command and in a number of tough battles. It distinguished itself in combat, and Ballard was awarded the French Croix de Guerre medal for his courageous actions at a forward aid station. Though wounded during the fighting, Ballard continued to administer to the wounded and refused to be evacuated. One report said he rescued ten wounded men on the battlefield, even though he was himself wounded.

His regiment was one of the first fighting regiments to return from France and it received a glorious welcome in New York at the harbor, and later in Chicago, as it paraded through the streets to great crowds.

Military records show he was officially

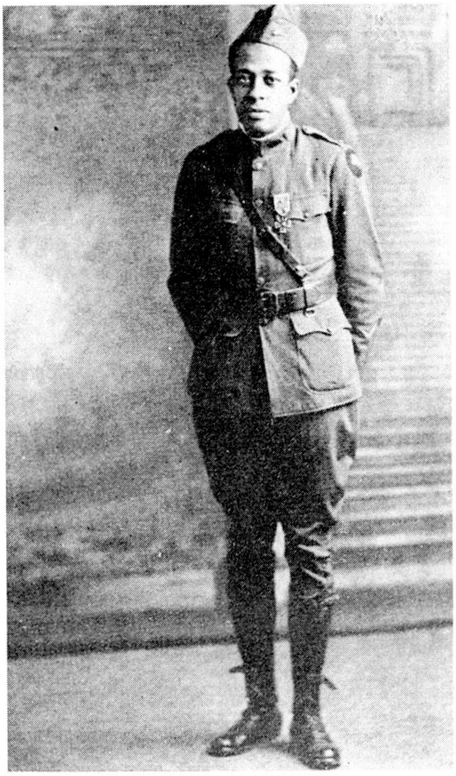

Claudius Ballard with French Croix de Guerre medal (courtesy Ballard family).

honorably discharged February 21, 1919, at Camp Lee, Virginia, and his father, William L. Ballard, of 1560 West 36th Street, Los Angeles is shown as his dependent parent.

Career

When Ballard returned to Los Angeles in 1919, he resumed his medical practice and advertised his return in the local newspaper. Dr. Ballard wrote a lengthy column commenting on his military experience. One year after the armistice on November 29, 1919, it appeared in the local *California Eagle* newspaper entitled "After Its Victories":

> Armistice day and the following day we spent in the town of our last battle, Gue d'Hossus, Belgium, the Germans being stationed in the eastern section and the 8th Illinois in the western part of the city. In many instances the Germans would cross over, offering to shake hands and be friendly, but our orders were strictly against fraternizing with them in any manner whatever. As a matter of fact the Germans, although defeated were much more demonstrative in their joy over the Armistice than we were. Most of us were too exhausted from the loss of sleep, forced marching and fighting without food and often water, to indulge in enthusiastic rejoicing such as took place in the back of the lines and at home. True we were happy that it was over, realizing what it actually meant even more than the people at home, but it was fully two days before we could bring ourselves to a real celebration.
>
> The great calm after the sudden cessation of the roaring cannon, bursting shells, and whistling of bullets make it seem as if we had been transferred into a new world altogether and it took a little time before we could adjust ourselves to our new condition.
>
> The French and Belgians were indeed grateful to us, wining and dining us at every chance. Women and children turned out to greet us.
>
> On the afternoon of the 12th, we turned our first steps homeward. Retiring from Belgium, we began our march through the devastated areas of France, over the ground on which we had fought just a few days ago. Tramping over the fields we recalled the point of battle where our heroes and comrades had fallen, small wooden crosses marking the grave of Private Jones here; Corporal Smith here; a French Soldier there and so on throughout the battlefields of France. Heavy shelling had destroyed Town after town we passed through. Nothing remained but piles of stone. In many places shells and gas bombs had plowed the fields up so that they were totally barren. Even grass refused to grow. One often thought, "Oh, if only the German territory could have had a taste of this destructive warfare," but the Armistice came too soon.
>
> Marching by easy stages, we arrived in the vicinity of Laon on November 16th. We remained here until December 12th and engaged in repairing roads and villages in the immediate vicinity. Leaves of absence were given freely to points of interest in France. Every officer and many enlisted men were allowed a stay in Paris.
>
> Leaving Laon, we marched to Soissons and remained there until December 23rd when we entrained for the American Embarkation Center at Le Mans. We arrived there on December 25th. We now passed from under the control of the French and were under American orders. Our French equipment was turned in, and American given in its place. On the 8th of January 1919, the regiment entrained for Brest

where we remained for inspections, etc., until February 2. After being reviewed by General Pershing and thanked for our services, we set sail on the steamer La France and arrived in New York on February 9, 1919.

We were among the first of the fighting troops to return from France, and we were met with great enthusiasm. The mayor and his reception committee met us at the harbor. There were three bands to serenade us. We were stationed at Camp Upton, Long Island, until February 15th when we entrained for Chicago, arriving on the 17th. At 2 p.m. the regiment paraded through the Loop District, a half day's holiday having been declared that all might turn out to welcome the 8th Illinois. After a big reception in their honor, the regiment left for Camp Grant, IL, to be mustered out of service on March 12, 1919.

Fighting in three different sectors, the regiment lost in battle about 100 killed outright and 600 wounded and gassed. The enemy took only one soldier prisoner. We broke through the Hindenburg Line at its strongest point, that is its "key" [Ment des Singes (Monkey Mountain)]. We took part in the final drive against the Germans, driving them back as much as 25 miles in one day, capturing many German cannons and machine guns, ammunition and material.

There were almost one hundred medals awarded to men in the regiment—70 French War Crosses (Croix de Guerre), 21 American Distinguished Service Crosses and two Distinguished Service Medals. All these achievements took place by colored soldiers fighting under colored staff officers who planned and managed their own attacks and maneuvers. Our record is exceptionally high, we won more medals than any other American Regiment in France. This shows that the colored soldier not only fights better under colored officers but that the colored officer is a capable leader and strategist on the battlefield.

Signed, Claudius Ballard, M.D.[8]

He soon married Miss May Lee Paine (or Shaw) of Rome, Georgia. On March 5, 1921, their first son, Albert Lucky, was born and on November 21, 1924, a second son, Reginald, was born.

Unlike many physicians who had their medical offices in their homes in those years, he maintained separate medical offices in downtown L.A. at 12th and Central Avenue and at 28th Street and Griffith with Dr. Leonard Stovall. During the 1920s he served as the Secretary of the Physicians, Dentists, and Druggists Association of Southern California, the group he helped found in 1914. In 1922 he reported the organization had a membership of 28. Different members presented original papers each month and outside specialists lectured from time to time.[9]

African Americans continued to migrate to California during the 1920s. Once there, they found the same strong segregation as in the rest of the country. Real estate covenants prevented them from settling in areas other than those currently occupied by blacks, and although blacks broke into the civil service they were hired for the most minimal positions. By 1928 the state's stature was strengthened by its hosting of the NAACP convention. Notables like Lincoln Steffens, W.E.B. Du Bois and Arthur Spingarn attended the meeting at the new Somerville hotel in a good L.A. neighborhood.[10]

In 1931 Dr. Ballard relocated his office from 1700 Central Avenue to 1104 East 47th Place, at the corner 47th and Central Avenue.

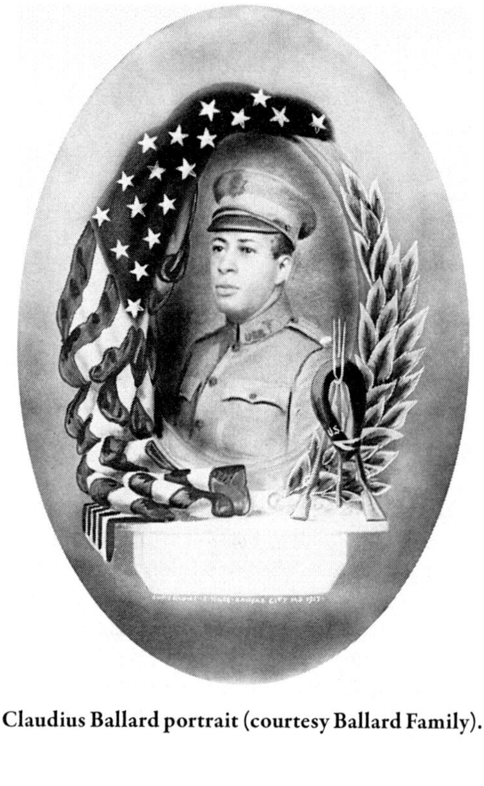

Claudius Ballard portrait (courtesy Ballard Family).

He advertised daily office hours from 11 a.m. to 12 noon, 2 to 4 p.m. and 7 to 8 p.m.[11] In 1932 he was one of the founders of the 28th Street Health Center in south L.A. and maintained his affiliation with it for many years. In 1933 he was one of several speakers providing health lectures during National Health Week in L.A.[12] Ballard was not only active professionally, but also in civic and fraternal circles as well.

In 1933, early in the Great Depression, the Urban League's annual report discussed the heavy toll it was taking on the average American worker, and particularly the Negro worker. The report highlighted a course in hygiene and care of the sick that had been provided by a registered nurse to men in the community, in conjunction with Stovall and Ballard's 28th Street Health Center.

During the Great Depression of the 1930s, the 28th Street Health Center employed girls under the National Youth Administration program, helping them launch careers. During the end of the 1930s, the tuberculosis association chose the Center as the headquarters for survey work because of its x-ray and other facilities.[13]

In November 1938, the local African American newspaper paid homage to Drs. Stovall and Ballard and described their backgrounds and accomplishments. The article carried a large photograph of the two of them at work in their white medical jackets in their medical offices.[14]

On Memorial Day in 1939, on the 21st anniversary of the end of the First World War, a lengthy remembrance was published paying tribute to African Americans who served in the army. In the article, under "Wins French Medal," it notes, "Dr. Claudius Ballard, a physician of Los Angeles, won the Croix de Guerre for bravery in the Belgian Drive."[15]

During the Second World War, West Coast cities such as Los Angeles felt particularly vulnerable to attack by the Japanese and actively prepared. Ballard did his part again, and was active as an instructor in first aid, teaching classes at the Southern California Club and Jefferson High School.[16]

In1944, there was a rising concern with venereal disease and courses were introduced at the University of Southern California to address the subject. Dr. Ballard was one of the dedicated physicians who "night after night for two whole weeks" spent time studying the matter. It was part of an effort to increase professional knowledge of the problem and show what the medical community had to offer.[17]

In 1945, Dr. Ballard's name was listed among the donors to the "Dollars for Victory" campaign fund being run by Charlotte A. Bass of the *California Eagle* newspaper. His community support activities never ceased.

Ballard was a member of the Sigma Pi Phi graduate fraternity and a founder of its local Xi Boulé. Leading professionals, including many in the medical field, were included in the organization's select membership. To be selected an individual must have made some outstanding contribution in his field and also be "a good fellow." In 1946, he traveled across the country to attend a three-day national conclave in Baltimore, Maryland, that drew hundreds of African American leaders.[18]

Dr. Ballard was also active in the National Medical Association, NAACP, YWCA, and the Catholic Church.[19] He was also a registered Republican.

In 1952, he and his friend Dr. Stovall were honored at a small formal dinner as the 28th Street Health Center they helped found in 1932 marked its 20th anniversary. It had grown, relocated to 806 East Jefferson Avenue, and was named the Stovall Clinic.

When Dr. Ballard died in May 1967, his obituary reported his two sons, Albert and Reginald, and his wife, May Lee Ballard, from whom he was separated, survived him.[20] His son Albert became an engineer for a chemical company and died in 2011. His youngest son, Reginald, had six children and later retired in 1978 from the Los Angeles City Fire Department as a captain and opened a real estate business.

According to his grandson, Ryan Ballard, an educator, Dr. Ballard is buried in the Calvary Cemetery at 4201 Whittier Boulevard in East Los Angeles. It is a Roman Catholic cemetery and he rests there among other notable figures including actors, actresses, producers, politicians and industrialists.

NOTES

1. "Angelenos Last Rites Completed," *Los Angeles Sentinel*, May 11, 1967, B11.
2. "Rising Young Physician and Surgeon Who Is Rapidly Taking Front Rank in His Profession in This Section," *California Eagle*, January 16, 1915, 1.
3. "Dentists and Pharmacists Unite with Physicians to Form State Society," *Journal of the National Medical Association (JNMA)*, July–September 1914, Vol. 6, No. 3, 212.
4. "Program of the Doctor, Dentist and Druggist Association of California," *Journal of the National Medical Association (JNMA)*, July–September 1915, Vol. 7, No. 3, 238.
5. "Oakland Jottings, Local," *The Western Outlook*, September 4, 1915, 3.
6. "Society and Personal," *Journal of the National Medical Association (JNMA)*, April–June 1916, Vol. 8, No. 2, 124.
7. *Ibid.*
8. "After Its Victories," Letter to the Editor, *California Eagle*, November 29, 1919.
9. "NMA Communications, California," *Journal of the National Medical Association (JNMA)*, January–March 1922, Vol. 14, No. 1, 40–41.
10. Rudolph M. Lapp, "New Black Pride and Pressure Groups," *African-Americans in California*, San Francisco: Boyd & Fraser, 1987, 43.
11. "Removal Announcement, Dr. Claudius Ballard," *California Eagle*, May 22, 1931, 11.
12. "California News, Los Angeles," *Chicago Defender*, April 22, 1933, 18.
13. "Clinic Marks 20th Anniversary," *Los Angeles Sentinel*, December 25, 1952, A2.
14. "Today, by Charles Edwards," *California Eagle*, November 10, 1938.
15. "War Made Them Heroes," *New York Amsterdam News*, May 27, 1939, 13.
16. Negro Who's Who in California, 1948, 41.
17. "Medical Men Here Attend Graduate Courses at USC," *California Eagle*, January 20, 1944, 3.
18. "18th"Boule" Get-Together Draw's Nation's Leaders," *The Afro-American*, August 31, 1946, 13.
19. Negro Who's Who in California, 1948 Edition, 41.
20. "Angelenos Last Rites Completed," *Los Angeles Sentinel*, May 11, 1967, B11.

Urbane Francis BASS

14 April 1880–6 October 1918
Leonard Medical School, 1906

Roots and Education

Urbane F. Bass was born in Richmond, Virginia, to Rosa and Richard J. Bass. His father was a salesman—shoes and clothing in the 1880s, insurance in the 1900s. His mother stayed home with their six children. The family lived on East Duval St. in Richmond. Urbane worked as a clerk while in school. He graduated from Virginia Union University in Richmond in 1902[1] and Leonard Medical School of Shaw University in Raleigh, North Carolina, in 1906.[2]

Leonard was the first African American medical school in the United States to offer a four-year curriculum. It was named after Judson Wade Leonard, the brother-in-law of Shaw University's founder Henry Martin Tupper. Shaw University is the oldest historically black college in the South and often called the "mother of African American colleges in North Carolina" because its alumni founded other colleges. The first six men to receive degrees from Leonard did so on March 31, 1886.[3] The medical school existed for only 36 years. During that time it graduated nearly 400 physicians. Like most African American medical schools of the time, Leonard faced financial difficulties, and these ultimately lead to its closure in 1918. The building still stands on the Shaw campus. In 1994, it was designated a North Carolina Historic Landmark.[4]

After graduation from Leonard, Dr. Bass began his practice in Richmond, Virginia, but by 1909 he moved north to Fredericksburg. He became that city's first African American physi-

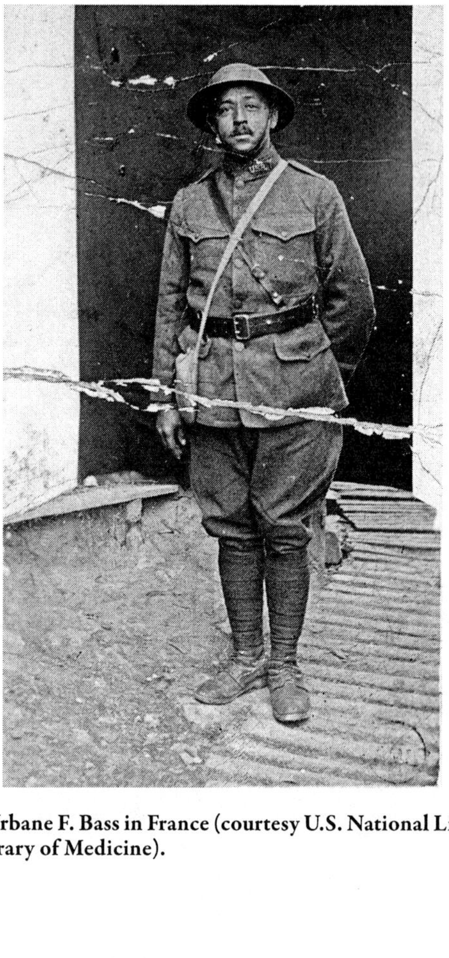

Urbane F. Bass in France (courtesy U.S. National Library of Medicine).

cian since Reconstruction and established a medical practice and pharmacy. The practice on Amelia Street was well received by the African American community in spite of the local hospital's denial of privileges. Ruth Fitzgerald described his practice in *A Different Story*, writing, "Bass often treated Fredericksburg-area patients in their own homes, doing surgery on kitchen tables if necessary."[5]

By 1916, his practice was growing, as was his family, but this father of four wrote to Secretary of War Newton Baker offering his services. One of Bass' friends, J. B. Morris, told his family, "Dr. Bass was dedicated to serving his country in a time of critical need. He knew our men were going to die in France and told me he would give his life to save them, if he had to. I could see the sincerity in his eyes. He was committed to the end."[6]

He received a commission as a first lieutenant in the Medical Reserve Corps and was 37 years old when he reported for duty at Fort Des Moines on August 14, 1917.

Military Service

After basic medical officer training at Fort Des Moines, Iowa, he was sent to Camp Funston, Kansas, on November 3, 1917. His brother-in law Dr. Rufus S. Vass also trained at the same Medical Officers Training Camp (MOTC). Bass went to France with the 372nd Infantry Regiment of the 93rd Division aboard the SS *Susquehanna*. It departed Newport News, Virginia, on March 30, 1918.

From his friend J. B. Morris we learn:

> Dr. Bass had been transferred to the all-black 93rd [Division] under French command as a First Lieutenant. On October 17, 1918, he was frantically working on wounded soldiers at a forward aid station under heavy German fire. He was hit with shrapnel when a shell exploded near him, and both legs were severed. He died before he could be taken from the field on October 17, 1918.[7]

Bass was awarded the Distinguished Service Cross posthumously, "for extraordinary heroism in action near Monthois, France, October 1–5, 1918. Lieutenant Bass administered first aid in the open and under prolonged and intense shell fire, until he was severely wounded and carried from the field."[8]

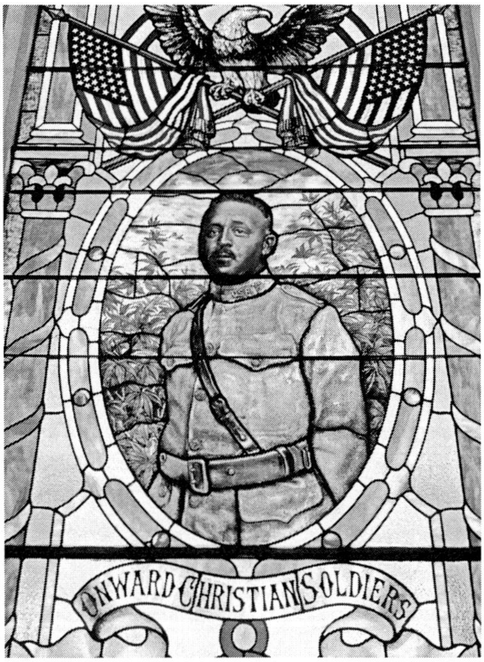

Urbane F. Bass stained glass window memorial (courtesy Shiloh Baptist Church New Site, Fredericksburg, Virginia).

His body was returned home for reburial on July 23, 1921. He became the first African American commissioned officer to be buried in the Fredericksburg National Cemetery. He lies on "Officer's Row" near the entrance to the cemetery. The Social Service Building in Fredericksburg is named Bass-Ellison, honoring him and Richard C. Ellison, Sr., another African American doctor who served the community for many years. The Shiloh Baptist Church installed a large stained glass window of Bass' image in recognition of his heroism.[9]

After the War

Dr. Bass had found a love worthy of envy when he married Maude Vass. The couple had four children, three daughters (Anne, Frances Mae, and Ruth) and one son (Urbane F. Jr.). After his death, Maude was a widow at 32. She had quite a difficult time accepting his death. In 1922 she was staying with family in Washington, D.C., when she was "taken to the Washington asylum because of her violent nervous state." A few weeks before this episode, she had attempted suicide by jumping from a two-story window. It was her father, the Reverend Samuel N. Vass, who had her committed.[10]

Early in 1923 she and the four children moved to her hometown, Raleigh, North Carolina, to be close to her family. There she raised her family and taught music to the blind for 30 years at the North Carolina State School for the Blind.

Maude and her Vass family saw that all four children were well educated and set for productive lives.

Daughter Frances Mae Bass had been born on August 24, 1908, in Fredericksburg. Mae married Charles Clinton Spaulding of Durham (general counsel of North Carolina Mutual Life Insurance Company), on September 1, 1936.[11] Charles graduated from Clark University where he was a member of the Omega Psi Phi fraternity . Mae graduated from Shaw University where she was a member of the Alpha Kappa Alpha sorority and completed some graduate work at Columbia University. Mae worked in the Durham city school system for almost 30 years. She was also a member of the Links, the Quettes, Little Slam Bridge Club, and Model Mothers Club. Mae died in Durham, North Carolina, on February 1, 1959.[12]

Ruth graduated from Shaw University and obtained a master's degree from the University of Michigan.[13] She, like her sisters, was a member of the Alpha Kappa Alpha sorority. She joined the faculty of Mary Allen Teachers' College in Crockett, Texas. Ruth married the Reverend Moses Newsome on June 11, 1942. Reverend Newsome also graduated from Shaw University, receiving the A.B. and a B.D. degree. He also held a master's degree from Oberlin College and was a member of the Alpha Phi Alpha fraternity. The couple moved to Charleston, West Virginia, where he was pastor of the First Baptist Church.

Anne married Mr. Sterling and moved to Washington, D.C.

Urbane Bass, Jr., had been born on February 20, 1910.[14] He followed in his father's footsteps and became a physician. He set up practice in Cairo, Illinois, at the southernmost tip of the state where the Ohio and Mississippi Rivers meet. In 1952, racial tension flared over efforts to end racial segregation in the local public schools. Four African American children were to attend Cairo schools for the first time. Dr. Bass Jr.'s home was bombed on January 29, 1952.[15] His family (including his four children) was able to escape injury when dynamite was thrown through a window. The rear of his home was demolished. Several African Americans and one white person were arrested on charges of conspiring to endanger the lives of children by forcing African American children to attend the all-white Cairo schools. Additionally, four men were arrested in the bombing of Dr. Bass' home.[16] Racism grew in Cairo, and city facilities were completely segregated. Several years later in 1958 Dr. Bass moved his family to Los Angeles, California.[17]

Maude never remarried in the almost 70 years between their deaths. She died at 100 and is buried next to her husband in Officer's Row in Fredericksburg.

NOTES

1. Dr Urbane Bass Is Killed—February 1919, Flickr.com (accessed 21 April 2015).
2. Robert V. Morris, *Tradition and Valor: A Family Journey* (Manhattan, KS: Sunflower University Press, 1999), 33–36.
3. Leonard Hall (Shaw University)—Wikipedia (accessed February 22, 2015).
4. *Ibid.*
5. Ruth Coder Fitzgerald, *A Different Story: A Black History of Fredericksburg and Spotsylvania, Virginia* (Unicorn Press, 1979), 169–170.
6. Morris, *Tradition and Valor*, 33–36, 53.
7. "The Negro Doctor and the Door," *Journal of NMA*, 1919, 11(4), 195–196.
8. "The Push Beyond Bellevue Signal Ridge," *The American Foreign Legion: Black Soldiers of the 93rd in World War I*, muse.jhu.edu (accessed February 23, 2015).
9. Fitzgerald, *A Different Story*, 169–170.
10. *Ibid.*
11. "Spaulding-Bass Wedding Unites Noted Families," *New Journal and Guide*, September 12, 1936, 4.
12. *Ibid.*, "Mrs. Spaulding, Wife of Durham Insurance Official," February 14, 1959, 3.
13. "Daughter of World War Hero Married in Raleigh," *Pittsburgh Courier*, June 13, 1942, 10.
14. Social Security Death Index—ancestry.com.
15. "Correct Error of Indictment in Cairo Blast," *Chicago Daily Tribune*, May 16, 1952, A6.
16. "Jury Clears All Concerned in Cairo Row," *Chicago Defender*, March 1, 1952, A5.
17. "Protest Violence in U.S.—CRC Head," *Baltimore Afro-American*, February 9, 1952, 3.

Edward Willard BATES

5 November 1884–7 August 1930
Meharry Medical College, 1910

Roots and Education

Edward W. Bates was born to John W. and Tyria Norwood Bates on November 5, 1884, in Dallas, Texas. His parents were both from Texas. His mother came from Tyler, in East Texas. He was raised in Texas and was educated at Bishop College in Marshall, Texas, 150 miles east of Dallas near the Louisiana border. The school was founded in 1881 by the Baptist Home Mission Society. It was part of a movement to build colleges for African American Baptists. Nathan Bishop, who had been the superintendent of several major school systems in New England, led the effort. Bates later graduated from Meharry Medical School in Nashville in 1910, where he was a classmate of Dr. Everett R. Bailey, with whom he served in the army.

Dr. Bates started his medical practice in Louisville, Kentucky, in 1912. There he joined the Quinn Chapel AME church. He became upset with the pastor, the Reverend J. R. Harvey, for reserving seats for "white people" at the expense of prominent African American members of the church. Harvey also selected all white judges for a choir contest. Dr. Bates led the criticism of his pastor.[1]

Military Service

In 1917, when he was 33 years old and living and working in Louisville, he volunteered for service in the U.S. Army. He reported to Fort Des Moines on September 21 and upon completing training there, he was sent to Camp Funston, Kansas. He was assigned to the 368th Ambulance Company of the 317th Sanitary (Medical) Train of the 92nd Division. One report in the YMCA news of Camp Funston said that first lieutenants Bates and Pearl joined their commander, Captain H. H. Walker, and the men of the 368th in giving a "swell" party. It was also reported that Lieutenant Bates joined other medical officers with an interest in religious work while in camp.[2] He remained in Kansas until June 1918 when his unit departed for France.

Shortly after arriving in France, Lieutenant Colonel David B. Downing questioned Bates' surgical ability "based on report of written examination held in July 1918. Papers were examined and marked by a board of three officers." His grade on military and medical subjects was 58½ out of 100.[3] By command of Major General Ballou, Bates and another lieutenant, John D. Carr, were provided with counsel (Major McClure of the 317th Supply Train) and put before an efficiency board of their peers for a follow-up proficiency examination. Apparently successful, the following day, August 10, 1918, Bates was ordered back to his unit by General Ballou.[4] On September 7, 1918, he received orders and attended a Gas Defense School. He again returned to duty with his unit on September 18. In early October, the entire division was sent to the Marbache sector near Pont-à-Mousson on the Moselle River, where they remained and fought until the November 11 armistice.

On November 10–11, 1918, during the closing days of the war, Lieutenant Bates proved his mettle, and showed that General Ballou was absolutely correct in keeping him in France. He was commended for meritorious conduct in action near Heminville, France. His Division had taken part in a major assault near Metz and had taken many casualties. In 1919 the Meharry annual reported that it was Bates and his ambulance unit "who carried Captain Kennedy's gassed and wounded [body] under shell fire, from the Aid Station to the Ambulance Station." Captain Kennedy recommended Bates for the Distinguished Service Cross (DSC). He was cited in orders for bravery under fire. The men in Bates' medical unit were also cited for bravery.[5]

On January 3, 1919, a special board of the 317th Sanitary Train convened at Mayenne, France, "for the purpose of adjudging the responsibility and justness of claims for damages by residents of Jezainville, France for loss of wood during the period that the Sanitary Train was billeted there." Captain Ulysses G. B. Martin, who trained with Bates at Fort Des Moines, was commanding officer of the 367th Ambulance Company, one of the units billeted there. He supported Bates' testimony that the company did not have sufficient wood for heating purposes from the Quartermaster so they gathered barbwire entanglement stakes and dead wood on the forest floor. Special orders had

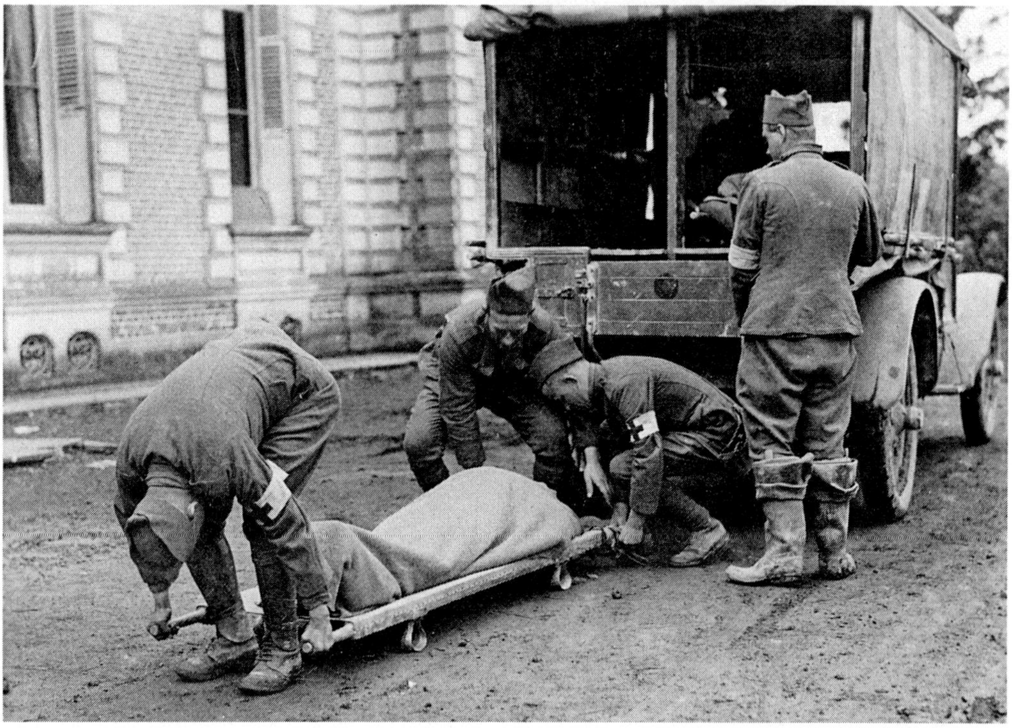

Transporting the wounded, France, 1918 (courtesy U.S. National Library of Medicine).

been issued not to take any personal property of the inhabitants. Bates asserted he had no knowledge of disobedience to orders not to disturb "hop poles, fence poles, live trees or any personal property of the inhabitants ... I am Supply Officer and had frequent inspections of the men's billets. For the most part of the time, there was sufficient fuel issued to the men to be comfortable, so no rustling would be necessary."[6]

Career

Following his discharge from the army in 1919, Dr. Bates returned to Louisville where he tried to resume his medical practice. It appears he may have experienced problems there. His obituary would later refer to "shell shock" he had suffered during the war.[7] He and his wife, Sadie B. Bates, 31, from Alabama, lived on the ground floor of 518 Breckenridge Street. They had a man who worked as a driver living with them as a lodger to help defray their living expenses. Another couple lived above them on the second floor of the house. Not long afterward, Edward and Sadie moved to Chicago.

Dr. and Mrs. Bates rented a place at 5741 Calumet Avenue in Chicago. By the end of the 1920s, Sadie has left him. His mother Tyria Ward and his stepfather Shelby Ward moved into the house. In 1928, Dr. Bates and his "mother Ward" were reported showing the widow Daisy E. Harvey around Chicago. Interestingly, she was the widow of the pastor in Louisville he had criticized in 1917. By 1930, Bates was living with his mother and stepfather at 5622 Prairie Avenue. His stepfather was employed as a cook by the railroad. His cousin George Caldwell, a railroad laborer, also lived there.[8] His medical office was at 3541 Michigan Avenue, in the Bronzeville section of the city.

Bronzeville was located at the crowded corners of 35th and State Street and 47th Street and South Parkway Boulevard. It was a perfect location for a physician. People came to this center of Chicago's African American community to see and be seen, shop, conduct business, dine and dance. The crowds reflected the diverse mix of people living in the black belt: young and old, poor and prosperous, professionals and laborers.[9]

Dr. Bates was an active member of the Olivet Baptist Church at 31st and South Parkway. The church's roots were in community activism. It was at one time the largest Protestant church in the world, with 20,000 members. Before the Civil War, it was an active station on the Underground Railroad. During the Chicago Riots of 1919, African American leaders met here to plan how to best restore peace to the city. Social reform and assistance for new migrants was such a big aspect of the church's work during the 1920s Great Migration that it served as a community center and maintained 40 different organizations for social, cultural, and economic purposes.[10]

Suddenly on August 7, 1930, this "popular physician" experienced a heart attack and died at his breakfast table.[11] He was only 45 years old. One news report said his death was attributed to shell shock from his service in France. The official medical cause of his death that was given was mitral stenosis and nephritis (heart disease and renal failure).[12] His mother, an aunt and two cousins survived him.[13] He and Sadie never divorced. His Cook County death certificate listed her as his wife.[14]

Notes

1. "Accuse Pastor Quinn Chapel of Drawing the Color Line," *Chicago Defender*, September 15, 1917, 1.
2. Russell S. Brown, *Y.M.C.A. No.11 (Colored Service)*, March 9, 1918, Jesse Moorland Papers, Box 126–72. Howard University Manuscript Archives, Washington, D.C.
3. RG 120 Records of the American Expeditionary Forces (World War I) Headquarters, 317th Sanitary Train, 92nd Division, Box 210, Memorandum, 31 July 1918, National Archives, College Park, MD.
4. *Ibid.*, RG 120 Records of the American Expeditionary Forces, Memorandum, France, August 9, 1918, Subject: Counsel and Witnesses.
5. Meharry Medical College Annual Report, 1919, 42.
6. RG 120 Records of the American Expeditionary Forces, 92nd Division, Box 1, NM-91 1241, Declassified Holdings, "Doc. Board Appointed for Investigation of Responsibility of Property in Jezainville," January 3, 1919, National Archives, College Park, MD.
7. "Dr. Bates Dies at Breakfast Table," *Chicago Defender*, August 16, 1930, 7.
8. 1930 U.S. Census.
9. wttw.com (accessed April 26, 2015).
10. http://www.blackpast.org/aah/olivet-baptist-church-obc-chicago-illinois-1850 (accessed April 26, 2015).
11. *Chicago Defender*, August 16, 1930, 7.
12. AMA Deceased Physician Card, Bates, Edward Willard, National Library of Medicine, Bethesda, MD.
13. *Chicago Defender*, August 16, 1930, 7.
14. Illinois, Deaths and Stillbirths Index, 1916–1947, Edward Willard Bates, ancestry.com.

Arthur John BOOKER

31 October 1881–25 August 1952
Northwestern University, 1906

Roots and Education

Arthur Booker was born in San Antonio, Texas, to Anderson and Carrie Raglan Booker. Early in his life, his father Anderson was a farmer on Hilton Head Island, South Carolina. His father left there and enlisted in the Union army during the Civil War. He served in the 34th, 46th and 108th U.S. Colored Infantries and later was a Buffalo Soldier in Company H of the 9th U.S. Cavalry. He was posted in the western states during the Civil War and stayed there. He had made his home in San Antonio by 1877.

The Civil War Pension Index has Anderson declared an invalid on August 20, 1887. He was then employed as a city engineer in San Antonio, which has long been a military town. He worked at the government depot initially and married Carrie, a woman nearly 20 years his junior. The 1910 Census records show her employed as a laundress in the home at 310 North Marcos Street. Anderson and Carrie had seven children—Arthur, Ola, Ulissia, Allen, Cameron, Leaman, and Melvin. According to the 1910 U.S. Census, Melvin, the youngest, was only four and his father was 69 and still working for the city.[1] Sixteen years later after Anderson's death on November 26, 1926, Carrie was granted military widow benefits.[2] Anderson was buried in the National Cemetery in San Antonio. Carrie died on April 11, 1942, and was buried with her husband.[3]

Arthur, who was their oldest child, attended public school in San Antonio and then went on to graduate from Prairie View College in Texas. He headed north for his medical studies and received his degree from Northwestern University, Evanston, Illinois, in 1906. Dr. Booker then interned at Provident Hospital in Chicago. He took an additional year of medical study in London and Paris before he was licensed to practice medicine in Iowa on January 19, 1909.

Outside In is a wonderful history of African Americans in Iowa. It tells us:

> In the summer of 1910, Dr. Arthur J. Booker shot into Des Moines as if fired from a cannon. He set the local medical establishment on its ear:

Reticent and soft-spoken Dr. Booker was still a man to be reckoned with. Amazingly, he applied for and was appointed to the position of department chair in human anatomy at Drake University's Medical College, where he taught for two years before resigning to tend a growing private practice.

He was an accomplished diagnostician, and was ultimately welcomed by his white colleagues as their acknowledged equal. He was the first African American physician in the state to be accorded such respect.[4]

He married Naomi Coalston in Minneapolis. They lived at 413 Sixth Avenue in Des Moines. The couple would never have children.

In 1915, the journal of the Iowa State Medical Society included an article by Dr. Booker. He published his conclusions (based on 74 cases) on bronco-pneumonia in children. He said, "Fresh air was the most reliable agent in restoring children to health," and, "Many children are nursed to death."[5] He also wrote a weekly column called "Health Hints" for the Des Moines African American newspaper, the *Iowa Bystander*.

In addition to his weekly health columns, Dr. Booker lectured at the local churches on health concerns. In April 1917, he addressed the AME Church on the "Causes and Prevention of Tuberculosis,"[6] a leading cause of death in those years.

Military Service

In 1916, Dr. Booker volunteered for service with the Iowa National Guard. He was refused but not deterred. The Des Moines branch of the NAACP adopted resolutions in support of efforts of its national organization to convince the war department to make provisions for the training of colored men as officers for the colored troops drafted if war were declared. Dr. Booker and his local education committee had been out recruiting. He reported that they had the names of 100 men who were ready to volunteer to serve.[7] He was such an articulate speaker that he was invited to address the citizens of Des Moines at patriotic mass meetings.[8]

Volunteering at patriotic meetings and recruiting others to serve in the military were not enough for Dr. Booker. He wanted in on the action so he volunteered for service in U.S. Army Medical Reserve Corps. First Lieutenant Booker was 36 when he was commissioned.

Just before he reported to training camp, the *Bystander* bid him farewell by highlighting aspects of his life in Des Moines. He was one of the organizers of the YMCA, an active member of the NAACP, the Masonic Lodge, the Knights of Pythias, the white county and state medical associations, and he wrote his weekly newspaper column.[9]

Booker didn't have to travel far for training on August 14, 1917. The Medical Officers Training Camp (MOTC) at Fort Des Moines was just outside the city. In addition to training doctors, a small group of dental surgeons also reported to the camp for training as officers with the U.S. Army Dental Corps. In the end, the army did not meet its goal on the number of dentists. Only 12 volunteered for officer training. This small corps faced the same lack of supplies and housing as the medical officers. Additionally, they were only able to perform the most necessary of dental operations because there was such a shortage of equipment available. They made do, and at the end of camp, all 12 graduated and moved on to the next level of training with the 92nd Division.[10]

After 82 days of training, Lieutenant Booker was assigned to the 365th Infantry Regiment at Camp Grant, Illinois. It was part of the 92nd Division's 183rd Infantry Brigade under Brigadier General Malvern-Hill Barnum.

The atmosphere at each of the training camps reflected to a remarkable degree the feelings and sympathies of those men in control. Regarding Camp Grant, the *Chicago Defender* newspaper reported:

> Many will recall those ringing words of Major Gen. Thomas H. Barry, Commanding General of the 86th Division, in his address to the white officers and men at Camp Grant just before the arrival of the Negro Soldiers. He made it emphatically plain that each soldier is entitled to every courtesy and consideration that his grade demands, and that the "black hearts attempting less would find no easy abiding place in his division."

To take such a stand at the very outset was to discourage the birth and growth of racial prejudice, to encourage the absence of friction of any kind. And the next camp commander,

Gen. Kennon, was none the less insistent that Gen. Barry's policies should be followed.[11]

Camp Grant is remembered as a place where "you feel free to move about in any and every direction without the slightest fear of interference or molestation." The only downside about the camp was that "the mercury does hover around the below zero mark and the icicles of Frigid Zone proportions display themselves in gorgeous splendor."[12]

Booker departed for France with his regiment in May 1918. Fortunately, he left Camp Grant and was already in France when the worst of the Spanish Influenza pandemic affected over 4,000 soldiers there. It took the lives of more than 1,000 soldiers at Camp Grant between the 23rd of September and the 1st of October 1918.

Lieutenant Booker and his fellow physicians did deal with the influenza as he cared for soldiers of the 365th Infantry Regiment throughout the war in France. The 365th Infantry Medical Detachment, which included six doctors from his MOTC, was concerned with training and sanitation, treating various diseases, trench foot, delousing and caring for the sick and wounded. They found themselves particularly busy with battle casualties during the offensive toward Metz. On November 10, during the advance by the 365th and 366th Infantry regiments east of the Moselle River, a large number of men claimed they were gassed. There were numerous reported casualties from mustard gas that came into the battalion aid stations. According to a medical report, "The regimental surgeon of the 365th (himself later gassed) cut at least by 50 per cent the number of gas cases reported and later at the triage hospital a large percentage more were dismissed as only slightly gassed."[13] The job of caring for the troops did not end with the armistice on November 11. It would be three more harsh winter months before they embarked for home. Booker returned to the States with the 92nd Division in February 1919 and was honorably discharged on March 26, 1919.

Career

Dr. Booker returned to Des Moines where he resumed his practice and his community activism. In January 1920, the *Bystander* reported on the Roosevelt Club, a small group of 28 community leaders who met to formulate plans for constructive programs in Des Moines. Dr. Booker was among its members.[14] In 1921 he chaired the Health Bureau of the Negro Business Men's League, and he lectured on healthy living. He was still active from his office at 907 Walnut Street on December 30, 1922, when he applied for his veterans' bonus.

In 1924, when he was 43, Arthur and

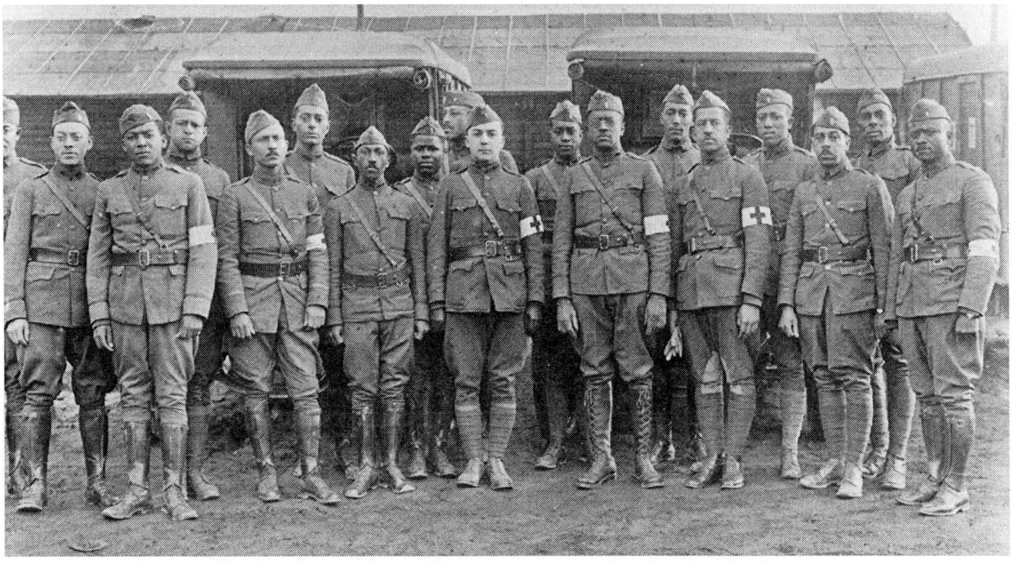

The 92d Division dental officers World War I (National Archives).

Naomi Booker decided to relocate to Los Angeles, California. At this time in U.S. history, Southern California was viewed as an attractive place for African Americans. Jobs were available, the economy was good and home ownership was possible for all.

The *Iowa State Bystander* published an article "Man Among Men" about his 14 years of service to the community and his large surgical practice, and said, "No community can well afford to lose a man of his caliber."[15]

Dr. Booker likely was recruited because he immediately joined the Howard Drew Medical Association. He and his wife Naomi bought a house at 890 East 42nd Street in Los Angeles. Initially his offices were downtown at 1800 South San Pedro, and later at 4122 Central Avenue.

He would become as prominent a citizen and respected surgeon in Los Angeles as he was in Des Moines. He reconnected with fellow veterans of the First World War in the local Southern California Medical, Dental and Pharmaceutical Association. At its November 1927 meeting three veterans who had served together in France presented papers—Drs. A. J. Booker, Whittaker and Smitherman.[16]

He was a lifelong member of the American Legion and the NAACP.[17] On the same day the *California Eagle* reprinted the "Man Among Men" article, it covered his involvement in the local NAACP membership drive. He was the featured speaker at a March 1924 program at the Zion M. E. Church at Pico and Paloma Streets.[18] When the Olympics came to Los Angeles in 1932, Dr. Booker was one of the 50 prominent citizens who organized a grand ball to honor them.[19] By 1934, he was president of the local chapter of the Los Angeles Fellowship League, an organization that fought against racial discrimination and injustice. He brought speakers like Dr. H. Odum from the University of North Carolina who was recognized as one of the greatest sociologists to discuss the economic crisis.[20]

He was a sought after speaker in Los Angeles. In 1934, he gave "one of the most informative talks that was heard for quite a while" at the NAACP annual meeting.[21] Dr. Booker was also active in local politics, endorsing candidates for the Los Angeles Board of Supervisors.[22] When Jesse Owens, the fastest human, came to Los Angeles in 1935, a "committee of big shots" met him. Dr. Booker was among them.

By 1935 membership in the Los Angeles Fellowship League had risen to 700 men. Each year the group presented awards to citizens who contributed most to advance the welfare of African Americans in the city. This was the year they recognized Dr. A. J. Booker in the field of professional advancement.[23] Two years later he was president of the League. One of the programs he organized for the group heard the merits of which union was better for the African American worker—CIO or AF of L.

Booker continued presenting the health talks he started in Des Moines. In 1937, he addressed the members of the Los Angeles' Crusaders Club on "Mental Hygiene."[24]

In 1938, Dr. and Mrs. Booker sailed to Honolulu aboard the SS *Lurline*, a fast and luxurious ocean liner built and launched in 1932. Before departing, the "very prominent Mrs. Naomi Booker" was bid bon voyage by 100 ladies at a Hawaiian themed bridge-luncheon by the Non-Pareil Club at the Clark Hotel. It was judged the smartest affair of the season.[25]

In 1939, the "inimitable Dr. A. J. Booker, with his usual sparkling humor" was still presiding over the Los Angeles Fellowship League.[26] He continued his work with the Fellowship League and other civic organizations for the next several years. He worked especially hard gathering donations for the Fellowship's Kenny Washington Scholarship Fund to aid needy students through college.[27]

He and Naomi continued to live at their home at 1800 San Pedro Street. After three years of intermittent illness and 28 years of practice in Los Angeles, Dr. Booker died at age 70 at Good Samaritan Hospital.[28] His obituary in the *Philadelphia Tribune*, said he was "rated as one of the finest physicians in the West.... With several prominent local leaders serving as pallbearers, the last rites were solemnized by Dr. Howard Kingsley, famous west coast religious figure."[29] The *Los Angeles Times* reported on his internment at Rosedale Cemetery.

For several years after his death, his wife Naomi took out a large "In Memoriam" notice in the *Los Angeles Sentinel* to keep his memory alive.[30]

NOTES

1. U.S. City Directories, San Antonio, Texas 1977–79, ancestry.com.
2. Civil War Pension Index, 1861–1934, ancestry.com.
3. U.S. Veterans Gravesites, ca. 1775–2006, ancestry.com.
4. Silag, Bridgford and Chase, Editors, *Outside In, African-American History in Iowa 1838–2000* (State Historical Society of Iowa, 2001), 249.
5. *Journal of Iowa State Medical Society*, Vol. V, No. 3, 1915.
6. *The Bystander*, April 6, 1917, 8.
7. *Ibid.*
8. *Ibid.*
9. *Ibid.*, "Dr. A. J. Booker," August 3, 1917, 4.
10. John M. Hyson, Jr., *African-American Dental Surgeons and the U.S. Army Dental Corps: A Struggle for Acceptance*, armymedicine.army.mil (accessed May 15, 2015).
11. Dunn, "The Atmosphere at Camp Grant," *Chicago Defender*, March 16, 1918, 4.
12. *Ibid.*
13. RG 120—Records of the American Expeditionary Forces (World War I), 92nd Division, 317th Sanitary Train, S.G.O. 314.7-2, Medical History of the 92nd Division, 16, National Archives, College Park, MD.
14. "Roosevelt Club Elects Officers," *The Bystander*, January 9, 1920, 4.
15. "Man Among Men," *The California Eagle*, March 7, 1924, 1.
16. *The New York Age*, November 12, 1927, 3.
17. *Los Angeles Sentinel*, August 28, 1952, A1.
18. "In the Realm of Society," *California Eagle*, March 7, 1924 6.
19. "Far Western Society," *Pittsburgh Courier*, August 13, 1932, 6A.
20. "Dr. H. Odum Lauds Fisk and A.U.," *Atlanta Daily World*, July 23, 1934, 2.
21. "Santa Monica News," *California Eagle*, February 16, 1934, 6.
22. "Opponents Endorse Mcdonough," *Los Angeles Sentinel*, November 1, 1934, 5.
23. "Los Angeles Citizens Receive Honor Awards," *Pittsburgh Courier*, December 21, 1935, 6.
24. "Dr. Booker Talks to Crusaders Club," *Los Angeles Sentinel*, January 21, 1937, 1.
25. "Los Angeles Society," *Chicago Defender*, May 28, 1938, 14.
26. "Gold Plaque Award Given to Fay Allen," *Los Angeles Sentinel*, December 21, 1939, 1.
27. *Ibid.* "Uppercuts as Blocks," January 18, 1940, 3.
28. "Dr. A. J. Booker Dies in California," *Afro-American*, September 13, 1952, 19.
29. "Deaths of the Week," *Philadelphia Tribune*, September 20, 1952, 13.
30. *Los Angeles Sentinel*, August 26,1954, A6.

William John Henry BOOKER

29 April 1882–24 August 1921
Leonard Medical School, 1908

Roots and Education

William J. H. Booker was born in Concord, New Hampshire. There were two other spellings of his surname before "Booker" became the American family name. His father, William John Henry Booher, was born in German West Africa and immigrated to Canada with Booker's grandfather, Wilhelm Jacomenah Hesslebac Boohah. In Canada, his father met and married Canadian Mary Ann Menafee, but Booker's father died before he was born. As a small boy, Booker attended local public schools in Concord, where practically all his schoolmates were white. Then he and his mother moved south and lived one year in Columbus, Georgia, before moving to Winter Park, Florida.

His own brief autobiography, using the Booher spelling, and appearing in 1921 relates this:

> My father died before I was born. Mother died when I was fourteen years of age.
>
> We lived at the time in Winter Park, Florida. I was left without means, so had to struggle for even a livelihood. I had seen accounts of Tuskegee in different papers, and my mother had expressed a desire for me to go there, so I was determined to go.
>
> I finally consulted a good woman, Miss L. M. Abbott who, after the death of my mother, had been very kind to me and a very valuable help. She encouraged me in many ways, and, knowing I was without money, prepared a list, soliciting aid from friends around the little village. In this way, I secured enough money, with what I earned, to enter Tuskegee. I was compelled to enter night school and work out my board.
>
> The first years were very hard and embarrassing. I had no source whatever from which to get money for clothes and was at times without underwear and other clothing necessary to health. Many times I had to wash a shirt at night in order to be presentable at school the next day. Things went this way for some time, but finally Mrs. Booker T. Washington learned of my condition and sent me to the barrel room to supply myself with clothing. This gave me the push for some years as I began to work at Tuskegee during summers and soon got ahead. I graduated there in 1902.
>
> During the four years at college, I worked in Pullman cars, earning enough during vacations to pay school expenses at the next term. I was graduated in Medicine in 1908 and practiced in Oxford, NC.... While at Tuskegee I won the Joseph Frye prize.[1] [The Frye prize was awarded at commencement each year "to the student,

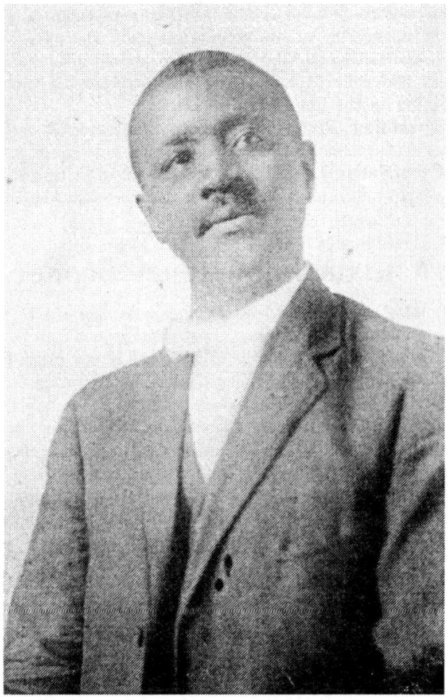

William J. H. Booker (*History of the American Negro: North Carolina Edition*, 1921).

male or female, who makes the most progress at his or her trade and at the same time makes the best record in academic studies."[2]]

I was surprised during the summer of 1902 when Mr. Washington informed me that I had been selected to fill the place of Conference Agent for the school. I accepted the work and remained in it for two years.

While he was at Tuskegee, Booker took a literary course (liberal arts) and learned the tinner trade. A tinsmith makes and repairs things made of light-colored metal, particularly tin ware. He was active in athletics, especially football and tennis. He traveled extensively and toured Europe in 1903.

Later he studied medicine at the Leonard Medical School at Shaw University in Raleigh, North Carolina, and graduated in 1908.[3] He received his medical license from the North Carolina State Board of Medical Examiners in June 1909.[4]

On August 3, 1909, Dr. Booker married Miss Ida May (Mae) Shaw of Montgomery, Alabama. They went to Oxford in Granville County, North Carolina, to set up a medical practice. In 1910, they lived at 77 Penn and then moved later to 85 Hillsboro Street. His wife, originally from Tennessee, became a public school teacher. They soon had two children, Mary Louise and William John Booker.

In 1912, Dr. Booker won an automobile in a contest sponsored by the Hamilton Drug Company. The person receiving the most votes won the "smart little machine." Booker secured enough votes "from friends among his race to land the automobile."[5] Having the car would undoubtedly have helped him serve the medical needs of his community.

Booker was very active in the community and became the school physician at the Mary Potter School in Oxford. He was also the local examiner for the Standard Life Insurance Company. Among his many fraternal memberships were the Masons, Odd Fellows, Gideons, Royal Knights, and Granville Helpers, where he served as president.[6]

Military Service

When America entered the First World War in 1917, Dr. Booker volunteered and was commissioned as a first lieutenant in the Army Medical Reserve Corps. He reported to Fort Des Moines, Iowa, where he trained at the Medical Officers Training Camp (MOTC) from September 28 to November 11, 1917. Lieutenant Booker was then assigned to the 92nd Division's 317th Sanitary (Medical) Train at Camp Funston at Fort Riley, Kansas.[7] On December 17, 1917, he was found to be physically unfit for duty, and he was honorably discharged from the army at Camp Funston. It all likelihood he suffered from a medical condition that was discovered at Camp Funston because he died less than three years later.

Career

Following his army service, he returned home to Oxford. While Booker's role is unclear, we know that in 1919 the African American people in Oxford purchased a lot with wooden buildings for a hospital. Mrs. Spencer, a local African American woman, was put in charge of it. Medical care for the local community was important and news articles from the period refer to concerns about smallpox, influenza, pneumonia and typhoid fever.[8]

According to the 1920 Census, Booker lived in Oxford with his wife and two children.

He was only 39 when he died unexpectedly. He suffered apoplexy (cardiac stroke) on August 24, 1921. A brief obituary described him as a "Highly Esteemed Colored Physician." He was reportedly stricken with paralysis ten days before his death and died at his home on Hillsboro Street.

His wife and two children survived him.[9] His death certificate was signed by one of the other army physicians with whom he had trained and served, Dr. Thomas C. Tinsley of Durham, North Carolina.[10]

After his death, his wife, Ida May (41), and children, Mary (19) and William (17), moved to Atlanta, Georgia, where in 1930 she worked as a public school teacher. They lived in downtown Atlanta at 77 Ashby S.W. in an area near the Booker T. Washington High School and the Atlanta University Center.[11] With Dr. Booker's death, Oxford lost a leading citizen whom they described as "learned and faithful."

NOTES

1. Arthur Bunyan Caldwell, Editor, *History of the American Negro, North Carolina Edition*, Vol. IV (Atlanta, 1921), 451–454.
2. "Annual Prizes," *The Tuskegee Student*, Tuskegee Institute, Alabama, April 26, 1906.
3. W.E.B. Du Bois, Editor, "The Horizon," *The Crisis*, June 1922, Vol. 24, No. 2, 75.
4. *Charlotte Medical Journal* [Serial] Volume 60, 1909, 41.
5. "The Automobile Contest," *Oxford Public Ledger*, May 15, 1912, 1.
6. Caldwell, *History of the American Negro and His Institutions*, 451–454.
7. Table of Medical Reserve Corps—Colored—Receiving Instruction, Medical Training Camp, Fort Des Moines, Iowa, RG-112, Records of the Army Surgeon General, National Archives, College Park, MD.
8. Hays, Frances B., "*Health, Doctors, Hospitals, Nurses*," unpublished manuscript at Granville County Historical Society in Oxford, N.C.
9. Obituary, "Dr. Booher[Sic] Dead," *Oxford Public Ledger*, September 2, 1921.
10. North Carolina Certificate of Death, William J. H. Booker, ancestry.com.
11. 1930 United States Federal Census, s. v. Ida M. Booker.

Frank Erdman BOSTON

10 March 1891–8 February 1960
Medico Chirurgical College, 1915

Roots and Education

Frank Boston was a Philadelphian. He was born, educated, and practiced medicine for more than 40 years in Philadelphia. He came from a poor but industrious family. His father, Charles A. Boston, was variously described in 1910 as a janitor, in 1918 as a clerk, and in 1920 as a plumber at the U.S. Navy Yard. His mother was Julia Sands. The family lived in north central Philadelphia at 821 North 15th Street and later 813 North 16th Street in modest three-story brick row houses. His older brother, Edgar, became a floral decorator. His older sister, Mae, became a hairdresser in the family home.[1] Mae later lived with Boston for many years and assisted in his medical office.

Boston studied at Lincoln University before entering the Medico-Chirurgical College of Pharmacy and Medical School in Philadelphia. He specialized in surgery and graduated in 1915. In 1916, Dr. Boston interned at Roosevelt Hospital.

In May 1916, he was on duty when a child was brought in with a serious brain injury. The child was in shock. Since Roosevelt had no x-ray equipment, he put the child in a car and drove him to Dr. Brady at Medico-Chirurgical Hospital for x-rays. During the 15-minute car ride, the child seemed to recover and then, as they were about to operate, he became unconscious and died. "Dr. Boston resented the coroner's criticism of his action." Boston argued that if Roosevelt had an x-ray machine, the child might not have died.[2] Boston went on join the surgical team at Mercy Hospital. He specialized in diseases of the stomach. He also did anatomy demonstrations at Temple University.[3]

Military Service

Boston responded to the army's call for physicians and became a first lieutenant in the Army Medical Reserve Corps. He was sent to Fort Des Moines, Iowa, in 1917 for military training at the Medical Officers Training Camp (MOTC) for Colored officers. After 84 days of training, First Lieutenant Boston was sent to Camp Sherman, Ohio, where he was assigned as a medical officer with the 317th Engineers Regiment of the 92nd Division.

By the time he left for France in mid–1918, he had been promoted to Captain. Once in France, Captain Boston's medical detachment

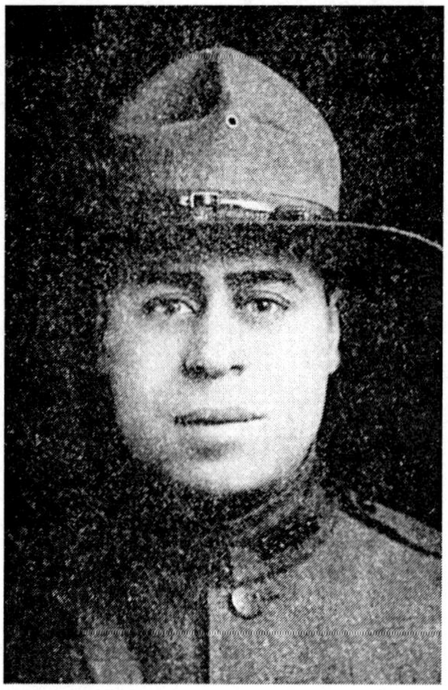

Frank E. Boston (national pictorial, members of the National Medical Association, 1925, courtesy Kansas City Public Library).

was busy caring for sick men and those with injuries that happened as they performed manual labor such as "building a pier at St. Nazaire, constructing barracks and heaving baggage."[4] They saw their first combat at St. Dié when "they were baptized by bombardment and gas attack. The Germans were attacking the town of Frapelle, and the 317th Engineers were at once set to work extending the trench system."[5] The Engineers were engaged in building and maintaining roads, bridges, trenches and fortifications. They continued to face the enemy over the next two and a half months, in the Meuse-Argonne campaign and in the Marbache sector during the Metz offensive in the last days of the war.

Undoubtedly, Dr. Boston learned a great deal about trauma and practicing surgery under less than ideal conditions. When the war ended Captain Boston maintained his commission in the Medical Reserve and rose to the grade of major. He also was a member of the Association of Military Surgeons.

Career

Upon his discharge in 1919, Dr. Boston returned to Mercy Hospital and resumed his practice. He was one of seven surgeons on the surgical staff of Mercy Hospital in 1925. Three other Mercy physicians were fellow army veterans, Drs. Egbert T. Scott, Clarence S. Janifer and James L. Martin.

He was a member of the American Medical Association (AMA), the Philadelphia County Medical Society and the National Medical Association (NMA). When the NMA held its annual national convention in 1926 in Philadelphia, Dr. Boston was chairman of the Committee for Gynecologists and General Surgeons and arranged clinics at Mercy Hospital where surgeons of national fame operated."[6] The following year at the June 1927 meeting of the Pennsylvania State Medical, Dental and Pharmaceutical Association in Harrisburg, Dr. Boston conducted surgical clinics at the Harrisburg General Hospital that were "marvels of scientific skill."[7]

By 1928, Dr. Boston was known to hundreds of veterans because of his work with the Veterans of Foreign Wars (VFW) and the free clinic he ran for them. When one of his hands became infected while performing surgery and "a serious case of blood poisoning developed" he spent some time in Philadelphia's American Stomach Hospital recovering.[8] Major Boston's leadership in the Veterans of Foreign Wars included council membership in the local and state organizations. When Marine general Smedley D. Butler addressed the 1934 annual banquet of Post 1507 in Carbondale, Pennsylvania, Major Boston was also on the program.[9]

In 1934, while still maintaining his staff position at Mercy Hospital, Dr. Boston established a privately owned hospital, Elm Terrace Hospital, in Lansdale, Pennsylvania, located about 25 miles north. It had 23 beds. Five years later, it was established as a non-profit, and renamed North Penn Hospital. He moved his primary residence from downtown Philadelphia north to Hatfield in Bucks County near Lansdale. He also maintained the family home downtown at 813 North 16th Street, where his sister Mae continued to reside.

In addition to working at Lansdale he continued to be on Mercy Hospital's staff. Mercy conducted annual clinical lectures for physicians, dentists, medical students and graduate nurses. They took place over an entire week. In 1936 at the fourth annual series, Dr. Boston was one of ten Mercy staff members presiding at these lectures.[10] When the Lansdale First Aid squad received a call to an auto accident around midnight on June 30, 1938, they took the injured to Mercy Hospital where Dr. Boston treated the three who had survived the accident.[11] On another occasion, he performed an extraordinary feat when a 15-year-old boy was stricken with acute appendicitis while bedridden with scarlet fever on an isolated farm. The family physician could not move the boy to the hospital because of his contagious disease so he summoned Dr. Boston. There was no electricity in the home. Volunteer firemen using a gasoline-powered generator rigged floodlights and a heater so he could operate on site. "Physicians said the operation saved Sylvanus Wambold's life."[12] The story was picked up by Associated Press and ran across the country.

During the 1940s he and his rescue squads responded to many emergencies. Too many of them involved children.

In 1944, Mercy Hospital awarded certificates to 11 physicians on the basis of 25 or more years of service. Boston and the others were honored at a formal banquet at the Pyramid Club. His fellow World War I army surgeon, Egbert T. Scott, was also one of the honorees.[13]

Boston never married and during the intervening years he was an inveterate international traveler, for pleasure and business. Perhaps his appetite had been whetted when he served in France. In 1929, he traveled to France. In 1938, he cruised to Bermuda. In 1941, he took a two-week ocean cruise on a Swedish vessel *Kungsholm* out of New York. In 1950, he flew to London, England. In 1953 he returned from Le Havre, France, aboard the *Mauretania*, and in 1954 he returned from Rotterdam aboard the *Westerdam*.

The rescue squad he founded was all too busy in Lansdale. Bucks County highways were the scenes of many deaths of children hit while riding bicycles. When a five-year-old went into the water after one accident, Dr. Boston went as far as massaging his heart, but the boy could not be revived.[14]

Boston was always very committed to his community. He was a member of the First Baptist Church of Lansdale. In 1957, he was honored along with ten Mercy-Douglas Hospital staff members with a "Gold Feather Award" for 25 years of service to the Community Chest. In 1959, he was named Lansdale's "Man of the Year."

In 1960, he passed away after a long illness. He was 69. At the time he was living on Fairhill Road in Hilltown Township, Bucks County, and had his offices in the Lansdale Medical Center Building, which he founded and owned. His obituary records more good deeds. He "founded the Volunteer Medical Service Corps in Lansdale in 1932.... He was a Boy Scout official and served a chairman of the Health and Safety Committee for the General Nash District, Valley Forge Scout Council."

He was also a member of the Reserve Officers Association of Military Surgeons, the International College of Surgeons and the Montgomery County Medical Society.[15]

When the 40 members of the Bux-Mont ambulance and rescue squads met on February 10, they "observed a moment of silent prayer for their founder."[16] His community members knew they had lost a truly inspirational leader.

NOTES

1. 1910 and 1920 U.S. Census.
2. "'Burn Half of City Hospitals,' Cries Coroner," *Evening Public Ledger*, May 11, 1916, 2.
3. Joseph J. Boris, *Who's Who in Colored America* (New York, 1919), 422.
4. Arthur E. Barbeau and Florette Henri, *The Unknown Soldiers* (Philadelphia: Temple University Press, 1974) 141.
5. Barbeau and Henri, *The Unknown Soldiers,* 145.
6. *Journal of the National Medical Association (JNMA)*, July–September 1926, Vol. 18, No. 3, 156.
7. "Physicians, Dentists and Doctors Holding Record Sessions," *Pittsburgh Courier*, June 25, 1927, 12.
8. "Dr. Boston Ill," *Pittsburgh Courier*, December 8, 1928, 10.
9. "Retired U.S. Marine Leader Accepts Invitation to Attend Affair in Pioneer City," *Scranton Republican,* February 16, 1934, 13.
10. "Mercy Hosp. Staff Plans Clinic Talks," *Chicago Defender*, March 28, 1936, 2.
11. "Pennsburg Man Is Killed; Three Hurt," *Pottstown Mercury*, July 1, 1938, 10.
12. "No Isolation Hospital; Operation Performed at Isolated Farm," *The Gazette and Daily*, March 3, 1942, 1.
13. "Mercy Medics Honored at Pyramid Club," *Philadelphia Tribune*, June 14, 1944, 3.
14. "Physician Tried in Vain to Save Drowned Youth," *Altoona Tribune*, April 17, 1953, 1.
15. "North Penn Hospital's Founder Dies," *The Daily Intelligencer*, February 9, 1960, 1.

16. "Area Rescue Squads Meet," *The Daily Intelligencer*, February 11, 1960.

Joseph Cyrus BRADFIELD

19 February 1889–11 April 1936
Starling Medical College, 1911

Roots and Education

Joseph C. Bradfield was born in Mt. Vernon, Ohio, to Joseph and Elizabeth (Williams) Bradfield. The city is the county seat of Knox County. It was named after George Washington's home, and it was an important railway stop where several railways intersected. By 1900, there were 6,638 people living in Mt. Vernon. Only 1.1 percent of them (less than 100) were African Americans. Joseph spent his childhood there and graduated from Mount Vernon High School.

After graduation from high school, he went on to Starling Medical College in nearby Columbus. Willoughby Medical College had been re-chartered in 1848 under the name Starling in honor of Mr. Lyne Starling. Starling had donated a building site and $35,000 for the building of a medical school and hospital. About two-thirds of the building was assigned to St. Francis Hospital in downtown Columbus. During the 60 years of its career under its original name the medical college graduated 2,600 students. It is now the medical department of Ohio State University. Dr. Bradfield graduated in 1911.[1]

While in Columbus, Bradfield met Edith Payne. After graduation he moved to Lima, Ohio, and opened a practice in 1912. Lima was the county seat of Allen County, and a city of few African Americans. The 1910 census reports Lima's entire population as 38,771. Only 978 were African Americans. It is difficult to say what drew him there, but on December 24, 1912, he married Edith, and the couple found a house at 723 West Spring Street. They had two children, Joseph and Madeline.

Military Service

In 1917 Bradfield volunteered for service in the Army Medical Corps. He reported to Fort Des Moines' Medical Officers Training Camp on September 28, completed his basic training and was reassigned to Camp Funston, Kansas, on November 3. He was assigned to the 365th Ambulance Company, and in July 1918, he was shipped to France with that unit.

Shortly after arrival on August 1, 1918, his assignment was changed to the 365th Field Hospital, which was a triage hospital. Its first combat location was Raon L'Étape. The hospital, which relocated whenever the division did, assessed the injured and ill as they came from the field. When influenza struck, they initially cared for the men and then passed them on to hospitals in the rear. The gassed soldiers also came here. The entire number of casualties of the 92nd division was 1,511. Of that number, 39 officers and 661 soldiers were gassed. The large number has been attributed to the daring exploits of the men of the 92nd coming out of the trenches to make raids on the enemy.[2] The Germans responded to these attack by unleashing poison gas. If the gas didn't kill the soldiers, it affected many of them after the war. A number of them died early of respiratory and lung-related causes.

The living conditions for the medical troops were sometimes difficult, and at other times deplorable. Bradfield's superior, Captain J. A. Barker, MC, described one of the last locations of the 365th Field Hospital in a memo to his superior officer dated December 22, 1918.

> 1. The billets now occupied by the Field Hospital personnel consist of a barn at Rue Rivere.
> 2. It is crowded dark and cold. There are no facilities for heating and not suitable for human habitation for any length of time under existing weather conditions.
> 3. No lights are allowed.[3]

Bradfield was promoted to the rank of captain while in France. Captain Bradfield continued his military involvement as a lifelong member of the American Legion.

Career

Dr. Bradfield returned from the battlefield to Lima, his family, his practice and his civic involvement. "As he worked to establish himself as a doctor, he also began to see to the needs of his fellow blacks, beyond their physical well-being. He believed that political involvement was the answer to many of the ills facing the black community."[4] He was a very active member of the Republican Executive Committee of Allen County. "He was partisan to the core. In a gentlemanly way, urged support of the entire ticket."[5]

He was quoted as saying, "We [Negros] are not strong enough to elect any candidate, but we do hold the power to defeat any candidate. Now is the time for us to exercise that power. We should be proud of our race and should stand together. It is only when a race does cling together that they progress. I'm a Negro, I can't help it and I'm proud of it. I want to work among my people for my people, and I want to see them advance."[6]

The good doctor was involved in a number of civic organizations. He was a member of Alpha Psi Alpha fraternity, the Sigma Pi Phi, and was a 32nd degree Mason. He taught a Sunday school class at the Second Baptist Church every week. The *Cleveland Call* reported, "In a city of relatively few Negroes, Dr. Bradfield extended his activities to all races. He was a member of the Lima Academy of Medicine and a prominent staff member of St. Rita's and Memorial hospitals."[7]

While Allen County's population growth lagged behind the state and nation, the 1920s was a time of industrial expansion in Lima. In 1925, Lima Locomotive Works, Inc., built the "Lima A-1," a 2–8–4 model that became the prototype for the modern steam locomotive. The Locomotive Works also created a new division, the Ohio Power Shovel Company. In 1927, local industrialist John E. Galvin helped found Superior Coach Company. It became the world's largest producer of school buses and funeral coaches within two decades. In 1930, eight railroad companies served Lima.[8]

The darker side of the progressive era revealed itself in the prominence of the Ku Klux Klan in the city. It was a center for the Black Legion, a notoriously violent subset of the Klan. On August 1, 1923, a KKK parade in Lima drew a crowd estimated at 100,000 people.[9] This likely was of great concern to Dr. Bradfield and may have had something to do with his decision to leave Lima. He never discussed his reasons. It was reported that an offer had come to him from a hospital in Springfield to join its staff.[10]

The *Pittsburgh Courier* tells of his aborted attempt to leave Lima by reprinting an editorial first published in *The Lima News*, in 1926. In part it read:

> There will be a mass meeting ... to convince Dr. Bradfield not to leave Lima except under protest from his fellow man. The United States has proclaimed Booker T. Washington the greatest of the Afro-American race. Lima has proclaimed Dr. J. C. Bradfield, the greatest of his race in northwestern Ohio. He is a medical authority, an able surgeon, a keen student of government, a politician insofar as to direct his people toward the safe and sane, a churchman, a publicist upon draft, and the perfect gentleman in the clinic, hospital, or at the bedside of the stricken.
>
> *The Lima News* wishes to add its appeal ... that Dr. Bradfield remain in Lima until his service to his own race, and to all mankind, is finished only when he receives the call and crosses the bar.

The NAACP joined the campaign to keep him in Lima. They rented Memorial Hall (named in honor of those who had fought in the First World War) and invited everyone in town. As the local newspaper reported, 1,000 of Lima's 3,000 blacks turned out, as did many whites, to convince him to stay.[11]

It was more than enough to convince him. He and his family stayed.

Dr. Bradfield and his family remained in Lima until he "crossed the bar" there 10 years later in 1936. He was only 47. He had been ill for two years, but he died on April 14, 1936, after a two-week bout with pneumonia in St. Rita's Hospital.

In his obituary the *Cleveland Call and Post* had written that he "had been an honored and respected citizen of Lima since 1912 when he came there to practice medicine." Tributes included one from Dr. Bushong, president of the Allen County Academy of Medicine: "Dr. Bradfield occupied a high and distinctive place in this community. He was not only a physician to the colored people but also their close friend and advisor. He was one of the most popular men in the local medical societies and well liked for his excellent comradeship as well as professional ability. He will be sorely missed."[12]

A year after his death, the Bradfield Community Center was opened as a place for the city's African Americans to gather for socializing and recreation.

Dr. Bradfield and his wife are buried in Lima's Woodlawn Cemetery.

NOTES

1. http://en.wikipedia.org/wiki/The_Ohio_State_University_College_of_Medicine (accessed September 20, 2013).
2. W. Allison Sweeney, *History of the American Negro in the Great War*, G. G. Sapp, 1919, 202.
3. RG 120—Records of the American Expeditionary Forces (World War I) 92nd Division, 317th Sanitary Train, National Archives, College Park, MD.
4. Kim Kincade, "Bradfield at Center of African-American Life," *The Lima News*, February 16, 2005, Lifestyle C1.
5. *Ibid.*, C2.
6. *Ibid.*, C2.
7. "Noted Medico Dies at Lima; Was War Vet," *Cleveland Call and Post*, Apt 23, 1936, p1.
8. http://en.wikipedia.org/wiki/Lima (accessed September 20, 2013).
9. "Noted Medico Dies at Lima; Was War Vet," *Cleveland Call and Post*, Apt 23, 1936, p1.
10. Kincade, Kim, "Bradfield at Center of African-American Life," *The Lima News*, February 16, 2005, C2.
11. "Dr. Bradfield's Legacy Lives On," *The Lima News*, February 23, 2005, Lifestyle, C1.
12. *Ibid.*

Horace Signor BRANNON

19 January 1884–20 October 1970
Louisville National Medical College, 1907

Roots and Education

Horace S. Brannon was born in 1884 in Louisville in Jefferson County, Kentucky. His father, Charles H. Brannon, was a coachman who died in 1931. His mother's maiden name was Lottie Thurston, and she survived until 1939. The 1900 Census shows he was the oldest of their four children. He had two younger sisters, Susan and Hattie, and a younger brother named Charles. The family lived at 1510 Second Street. Brannon was educated in Louisville schools and graduated from the Louisville National Medical College (LNMC) in 1907.

His college was the first of several independent medical institutions for African Americans when it was founded in 1888. After 20 years the school had a student body that fluctuated between 25 and 35 students annually. By 1908, the school had graduated more than 100 practicing physicians and was well regarded in Kentucky, but between 1908 and 1912 the school faltered and was forced to close. The Flexner Report was published about this time in history. It called for higher national standards for medical education. The school's "inability to raise adequate sums of money for improving facilities and faculty likely caused LNMC's demise."[1]

Military Service

When the United States entered the First World War in 1917, Dr. Brannon volunteered to serve as a physician in the U.S. Army. At age 33, he had been a practicing physician for almost 10 years. He received a commission as a first lieutenant in the Medical Reserve Corps and reported to Fort Des Moines for military training. On September 27, 1917, he joined other African American volunteer physicians at a special Medical Officers Training Camp (MOTC). After 46 days of training he was ordered to the 92nd Division at Camp Funston at Fort Riley, Kansas. Brannon was assigned to the 366th Field Hospital of the division's 317th Sanitary (Medical) Train.

The division was sent to France in June 1918. Soon after arriving in France he was reassigned to the 365th Ambulance Company where he served throughout the war. Ambulance companies were responsible for establishing dressing stations near the front lines and provided first aid to casualties. They also provided transport for the sick and wounded back to field hospitals for further treatment, triage and evacuation and base hospitals as needed.

In August, his company was assigned at Raon L'Étape in the St. Dié sector of the Vosges Mountains of eastern France. There, for the first time, his division entered into the trenches and the troops sustained combat injuries. All personnel, including medical, were exposed to German aerial bombardment and artillery fire. Immediately upon entering the trenches to relieve the U.S. 5th Division, the 92nd Division was embroiled in a battle to hold the village of Frapelle against a German counterattack. "Two men were killed and six severely wounded before the relief was completed. In this sector the 'doughboys' of the 366th [Infantry Regiment] were first introduced to a flame-projector at-

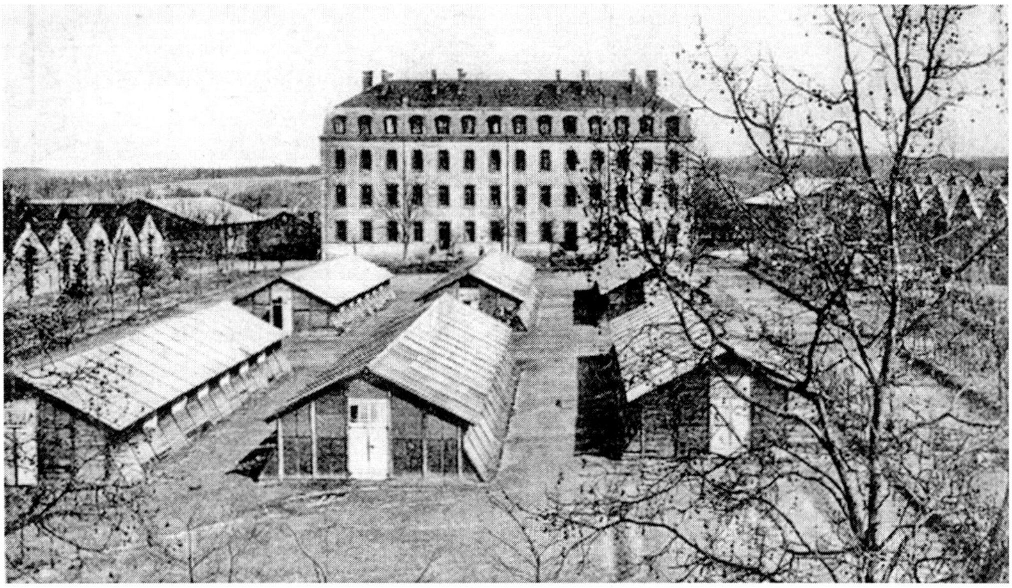

French postcard showing Sainte Menehould, Valmy barracks, Argonne.

tack. The Germans also had air-superiority there. When the weather was clear the front line trenches were bombed from above. In addition to being subjected to systematic daily programs of artillery fire by the Germans, they experienced one, and at times two, heavy barrages over their front-line positions. Airplanes flying above often directed the fire for more than thirty minutes at a time before being driven away by French anti-aircraft guns. The roads traveled by the supply trains were bombed, shelled with shrapnel, high explosive and gas shells every night."[2]

After its baptism of fire in the St. Dié Sector, the division moved hurriedly to Ste. Menehould in the Argonne Forest in late September. There it became a reserve corps for the Meuse-Argonne campaign, which became the greatest American battle of the war. One infantry regiment of the division, the 368th, was committed to the battle near Binarville, under the command of the French, and it sustained many casualties over a period of several days before it was withdrawn.

In early October, the division moved once again, to the Marbache sector near Pont-à-Mousson. Brannon's ambulance company was stationed there near the Moselle River at Millery where it established a dressing station at Atton for the upcoming battle. The Division engaged in a major attack on Metz in early November as part of the AEF Second Army and suffered numerous casualties. Brannon and his fellow medics were kept very busy as their troops advanced under fire into German positions. This proved to be their last battle of the war. On November 11 an armistice took effect ending the combat.

After the armistice, in a brief report submitted in Mayenne, France, by Lieutenant Brannon on January 3, 1919, he said he had been "in and about" the village of Jezainville, near Pont-à-Mousson, on duty with the 365th Ambulance Company for a month from November 18 to December 17, 1918.[3] His unit returned to the United States in February 1919 and he was discharged near his home in July 1919 at Camp Zachary Taylor, Kentucky. Brannon was recognized for his service and listed in the Kentucky Medical Association Honor Roll of Louisville physicians serving in the military.[4]

Career

Dr. Brannon returned to his wife Octavia in Louisville in 1919. She had lived there with his family at 1712 West Chestnut Street during his army service. Octavia Brannon was a public school teacher who had been born in Missouri.

For more than 50 years Brannon practiced medicine in several cities in Kentucky. In the early 1920s, he and Octavia moved to Paducah on the Ohio River in the far southwest corner of the state, where Kentucky joins Illinois and Missouri. He had a medical practice there at 507 South Street. By the mid–1920s he had returned to his birthplace, Louisville. By 1930 he was a widower and lived again with his family at 1712 West Chestnut Street. He had a medical office at 503 South 10th Street in downtown Louisville. He later had an office on 18th Street.

In 1934, at age 50, he was admitted to the U.S. National Home for Disabled Volunteer Soldiers (referred to as the Soldiers' Home) in Dayton, Ohio, 150 miles northeast of Louisville. Veterans who became ill, including African Americans, had been treated there since shortly after the Civil War. The cause of his illness was not noted, but by 1940 he was practicing medicine again, this time in Harlan in southeastern Kentucky in Appalachia. He lived downtown at 241 North Main Street. Harlan was well known at the time for its railroad, rapid growth and busy coal mining industry. Its population grew almost tenfold from 1910 to 1940, from 657 people to its peak of 5,122. Undoubtedly there was a need for a physician for the local African Americans. In the 1940s industry slowed there and the population began to shrink. It continued to shrink every decade. That probably motivated Dr. Brannon to relocate to Northern Kentucky.

By the 1950s he had moved from Harlan to Covington, just across the Ohio River from Cincinnati, Ohio. There, sometime between 1951 and 1954, Dr. Brannon met and married a widow named Estella Shannon. He and Estella lived at 1404 Russell Street, less than mile from his medical office at 1014 Greenup. According to Ted Harris, a retired engineer in Covington, there were several African American physicians in Covington then and they all lived in the same neighborhood. It was a nice middle class section of the city where many educators also lived. When Dr. Brannon came to Covington he joined Dr. James E. Randolph in his practice for a number of years. They shared office space on the first floor of their building on Greenup Street. Brannon is remembered by people who knew him in Covington as light skinned (mulatto) and of average size about 5'7" or 5'8" in height.

In the 1950s, segregation was still practiced in Kentucky, and the African American children of Covington attended the city's black school. African American doctors were not allowed to become members of the local Kenton County or Northern Kentucky medical societies, nor were they allowed to practice in hospitals in Kentucky. They were forced to use hospitals in Cincinnati to care for their more seriously ill patients, which Dr. Brannon and others did. His associate Dr. Randolph became the first African American physician to gain privileges at Covington's St. Elizabeth Hospital in the 1960s, something Dr. Brannon had been unable to do.

Brannon was a Baptist and there were three Baptist churches in Covington. He is listed in a printed program in September 1952 as delivering a talk to the Ninth Street Baptist Church Senior Choir during a week-long celebration of the 21st anniversary of its pastor.

His wife Estella died suddenly on May 8, 1960, at Saint Elizabeth Hospital at the age of 73.[5] After her death he remained in Covington five more years, retiring in 1965 at the age of 81. He then moved to Cincinnati where he lived at 953 Church Hill Avenue. He married again in the mid–1960s in Cincinnati. When he died in 1970 at the age of 87,[6] his third wife, Clysta B. Brannon, a public school teacher, survived him. His obituary reported other survivors including a son, Lloyd Brannon, one of his sisters, Hattie Taylor, and his brother, Charles Brannon. Services for him were held in his hometown of Louisville.[7] Brannon had served his nation in war and the African American community throughout his life.

Notes

1. Todd L. Savitt, *Race and Medicine in Nineteenth- and Early-Twentieth- Century America* (Kent, OH: Kent State University Press, 2007) 191–199.
2. Emmett J. Scott, *The American Negro in the World War*, Chapter 11, 142–143.
3. RG -120, Records of the American Expeditionary Forces (World War 1), 92nd Division, 317th Sanitary Train, National Archives, College Park, MD.
4. "The War Service of the Medical Profession," *The*

Journal of the American Medical Association (JAMA), June 1, 1918, Vol. 70, No. 22, 1672.
5. Estella Brannon, Kentucky Death Index 1911–2000, ancestry.com.
6. Dr. Alvin Poweleit, *Our Northern Kentucky Negro Doctors*, www.nkyviews.com/Other/pdf/NK_Negro_Doctors (accessed February 23, 2015).
7. "Obituary, Dr. Horace Brannon," *The Post & Times Star*, October 22, 1970, 27K.

Harvey L. BROWN

9 December 1876–12 January 1960
Leonard Medical School, 1905

Roots and Education

Harvey Brown was born in Terry, Mississippi, only 17 miles south of the state capital in Jackson. As a youngster he began working in the town's livery stable. He returned to that job for many years to afford school, all the way through medical school.[1] He graduated from Jackson College in Laurel, Mississippi, and went on to graduate from Leonard Medical School in 1905. He returned to Mississippi to practice. The 1910 U.S. Census lists him as head of household living on Front Street in Laurel, Mississippi.

Early in his medical career he was summoned to a home and delivered what appeared to be a stillborn baby. Amazingly, he revived the child with mouth-to-mouth resuscitation.[2]

Military Service

After practicing for 12 years in Laurel, at the age of 41 Dr. Brown joined the U.S. Army Medical Reserve Corps and reported for training on August 7, 1917. He was one of the oldest doctors in camp at Fort Des Moines. On November 3, 1917, he was sent to Camp Funston, Kansas. By August 27, 1918, he was in France and commanding officer of the 366th Ambulance Company of the 317th Sanitary (Medical) Train, 92nd Division. One of his initial reports to the division surgeon, 92nd Division covered sanitation and gives us some insight into wartime conditions.

"Report that one room of the building occupied by Ambulance Co. #366 is occupied by French prisoners. It has been found that these men are infested with lice, and they are otherwise very filthy.

"The water supply for Ambulance Co. #366 and the French prisoners are in the kitchen of the company, and it is impossible to keep the men separated under such conditions.

"Request that immediate steps be taken to remove these prisoners so that the room might be properly fumigated."[3]

His September 8, 1918, report on the monthly physical inspections includes mention that the men are generally in very good condition with "bodies clean, feet in very good condition and teeth fair." That report includes "one case of acute Gastritis, a case of chronic gonorrhea and two old cases of syphilis."

Lieutenant Brown adjusted well to military life and was promoted. By October 31,

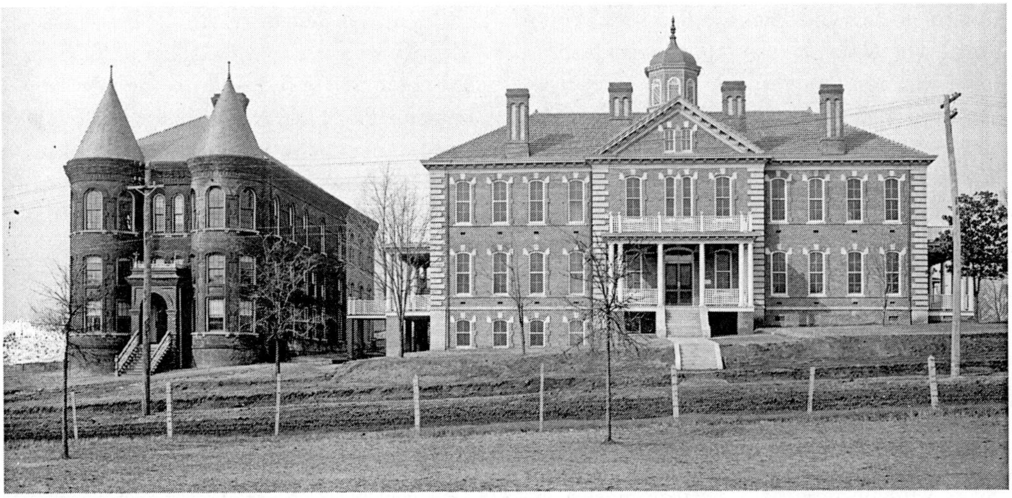

Leonard Medical College, Shaw University, 1912 (courtesy State Archives of North Carolina).

1918, he signed off this report as "Captain" Brown, the "condition of Billet is Good, but very crowded, one Adrian (French) barrack for 123 men with supplies and office." The war ended 11 days later on November 11. In January 24, 1919, Captain Brown's weekly personnel report for his ambulance company still lists 120 enlisted men reporting to him. After returning to the United States in early 1919, he was discharged on April 10, 1919.

Career

Dr. Brown returned to his medical practice in Laurel and reopened his office on Front Street. The town, 140 miles north of New Orleans, had been established as a lumber town and it was served by a main railroad. It had a large cotton mill, a large African American population, and flourished in the 1920s, but, like so much of the country in the 1930s, was hit by the Great Depression. Through it all Dr. Brown was "humble, unassuming, gentle, tolerant and kind," according to Dr. Henry Knaive, another local physician.

By 1933, he was involved with a number of local businessmen to improve the lives of the citizens. He was busy with his civic programs, his practice and his membership in the American Legion, but he also attended the Jackson College Alumni Club. The *Chicago Defender* reported on the 1936 business meeting of the planning group that included Dr. Brown, enjoyed a "tasty repast," and the singing of dear old "Jackson Fair," the school song.[4] The *Defender* also reported on his October vacation that year. He went by train to St. Louis and then drove with friends on to Cleveland, Ohio, for a meeting of the American Legion.[5]

In the late 1940s, he helped a group of local African American veterans organize American Legion Post 210.[6]

In 1954, Dr. Brown was in New Orleans, Louisiana, attending a civic club meeting at a tavern in suburban Gretna when the air conditioning unit exploded. He was taken to the Veterans Hospital were he was treated for "multiple fractures of an arm and leg." He spent some time in the hospital before returning to Laurel.[7]

When Dr. Brown died at the age of 83 he was buried in Nora Davis Cemetery in Laurel. His second cousin Hazel T. Jones of Jackson made the arrangements. Brown willed his medical journal and personal books to the Oak Park Vocational High School. Thirty years after his death, Annette Swinney, a close personal friend, described him simply as "a beautiful man."[8]

NOTES

1. Cleveland Payne, "The Service of Harvey Brown," *Laurel Leader Call*, August 26, 1994, 6-A.
2. *Ibid.*
3. RG 120, Records of the American Expeditionary Forces (World War 1), 92nd Division, 317th Sanitary Train, National Archives, College Park, MD.
4. "Jackson College Alumni Club Meets," *Pittsburgh Courier*, May 21, 1936, A8.
5. "Laurel, Miss," *Chicago Defender*, October 3, 1936, 10.
6. Cleveland Payne, "Oak Park in the Military," *Laurel Leader-Call*, June 30, 2002, C-1.
7. "Three Hurt When Air Conditioning Explodes in Tavern," *Lake Charles American-Press*, June 15, 1954, 25.
8. Cleveland Payne, "Oak Park in the Military," *Laurel Leader-Call*, June 30, 2002, C-1.

Vanderbilt BROWN

25 May 1886–25 April 1921
Boston College of Physicians and Surgeons, 1912

Roots and Education

Vanderbilt Brown was born in Danville, Virginia, to Thomas Brown and Maria Jones (also listed as Voust). Nothing is known of his early life until he graduated from Biddle University in Charlotte, North Carolina, in 1907. He went on to earn his master's degree in 1916.[1] He then traveled to Boston, Massachusetts, where he enrolled in the College of Physicians & Surgeons. He received his medical degree there in 1912. His records there cited a certificate "showing equivalent education" for his early education.[2]

After graduation, he was awarded an official appointment as an intern at the Kansas City Hospital, but he was also invited to intern at Tuskegee Institute Hospital and took that option. In 1913 he worked at Tuskegee under Dr. John A. Kenney.[3] Following his internship, Brown practiced medicine back in North Carolina, first in Durham and then in Charlotte. In May 1917 he was one of the city's seven African American men who applied for officers' training camp at Fort Des Moines. Charlotte's Mayor

McNinch examined them and pronounced all seven, "fine specimens of physical manhood." He judged them well equipped mentally and morally to be commissioned officers.[4]

In 1914, the West Virginia State Board of Health recognized his North Carolina license to practice medicine and granted him reciprocity.[5] He later established a practice in Charleston, West Virginia.

Military Service

In June of 1917, he was back in his hometown of Danville, Virginia. When he volunteered for service in the Army Medical Corps he used his mother's home there as his address. From there he reported to the Fort Des Moines' Medical Officers Training Camp (MOTC) on August 17 at the age of 30. He was in training camp for 79 days before moving on to Camp Funston, Kansas. There Lieutenant Brown was assigned to the 365th Field Hospital of the 92nd Division's 317th Sanitary (Medical) Train and sailed for France in 1918.

Brown's military career mirrored his medical practice, in constant motion. By the end of August 1918, he was reassigned to the 365th Ambulance Company. This was about the time influenza struck. There was little that could be done for those who contracted the disease except provide warmth, rest, and a gentle diet, and hope that their patients did not develop pneumonia. This was a very frustrating and well-documented epidemic. Tests were run, laboratory and clinical findings compared mortality rates, and a host of articles were written.[6] The patient just had to be lucky to survive.

In early September, he was transferred to the 366th Infantry. At this time, the 366th was moved by railroad, with other units of the 92nd Division, to Le Chemin. After arriving there early on the morning of September 23, the 366th was marched overland from St. Dié to Granges. Conditions were harsh and the march was hard on the men and disastrous to the horses and mules (whose carcasses lay strewn along the roads). They arrived at the Meuse-Argonne on September 25, 1918. The 366th was in a support position there until the end of the month when they were moved to Ste. Menehould. Along the way, the physicians were responsible for sanitary arrangements, waste disposal, and good water.[7]

From the Argonne Forest, the 366th was moved to the Marbache sector with the newly formed AEF Second Army in early October. The 366th fought in the front lines in the Metz offensive of late October and early November. It sustained numerous casualties including 43 men killed, seven missing in action, and nearly 200 gassed and wounded.[8]

He was still with the 366th when the war ended. Before his discharge, Brown had a last duty station at Camp Lee, Virginia, caring for wounded men. His mother came to see him, and interestingly he was able to secure an allotment by claiming her as a dependent parent during the months of April and May of 1919.

Career

By the end of 1919, Dr. Brown settled in Charleston, West Virginia. In addition to his medical practice, he had an active social life. In 1920 the *Washington Bee* reported, "Dr. Vanderbilt Brown of Charleston, WV, attended the Howard-Lincoln game. He will visit New York before returning home."[9]

Dr. Brown's life was cut short in 1921. He was single and living at his new home at 177 Dickinson Street in Charleston, when he died of a gunshot wound. The circumstances of the shooting are unknown. A promising life ended prematurely. He is buried where he was born, in Danville, Virginia.

NOTES

1. Biddle University General Catalog, 1913–14.
2. "Vanderbilt Brown," Directory of Deceased American Physicians, 1804–1929, ancestry.com.
3. *The New York Age*, September 12, 1912, 2.
4. "Seven Colored Men Ask to Be Officers," *Charlotte News*, May 31, 1917, 2.
5. West Virginia Biennial Report, State Board of Health, June 1913–1914, 14.
6. Carol R. Byerly, PhD, Public Health Reports 2010; 125 (Suppl 3): 82–91, ncbi.nim.nih.gov.
7. Emmett J. Scott, *Scott's Official History of the American Negro in the World War*, Chicago: Homewood Press, 1919, 142–145.
8. W. Allison Sweeney, *The American Negro in the Great World War* (G.G. Sapp, 1919), reprinted 1969 by Negro Universities Press, New York, 213–214.
9. "The Week in Society," *Washington Bee*, December 11, 1920, 5.

Arthur Davis BROWNE

16 December 1887–23 May 1974
Leonard Medical School, 1912

Roots and Education

Arthur Davis Browne was born in Salisbury, North Carolina, to Anderson and Nancy Rankin Browne.[1] Salisbury is the county seat of Rowan County and records gathered by the Genealogical Society of Rowan County for 1880 report Browne's grandmother was a washerwoman and his father worked in a chewing tobacco factory. The other local industry was liquor production. They were poor people who became even poorer in the late 1800s. With the introduction of cigarettes, the local chewing tobacco industry collapsed. The liquor distilleries went away when prohibition was passed by the state in 1908.[2]

The Browne family was certainly in Salisbury at the time of the 1906 Salisbury Lynching. Claude A. Clegg, III, professor of history at Indiana University, described it:

> On August 6, 1906, three African American men—Nease and John Gillespie and Jack Dillingham—were lynched in Salisbury, North Carolina. These mob murders were ostensibly precipitated by the axe murder a month earlier of a local white family for whom the men had worked. Following the abduction of the men from the local jail and their midnight hanging before an audience that some estimated to be in the thousands, one of the lynchers was arrested and prosecuted for his role in the mob executions. He was the first lyncher convicted in North Carolina history.[3]

The number of lynchings in North Carolina diminished greatly over the four decades following the Salisbury murders due at least in part to law enforcement's willingness to prosecute. Despite these incidents, the Browne family stayed in Salisbury.

Browne was educated first in the Salisbury public school system and then at Livingstone College. Livingstone began as a place for training ministers for the African Methodist Episcopal Zion Church. It was organized to instruct students in grammar school through collegiate and theological levels of education. The grammar school qualified students for the normal course designed for teacher training. It continues to exist today as a historical black coeducational liberal arts college.[4]

Browne graduated with an A.B. degree from Livingstone College and enrolled in medical school at Shaw University's Leonard Medical School in Raleigh, North Carolina. He entered at a time when Leonard was struggling to improve its program and lengthen its terms. Laboratories were upgraded, microscopes purchased, admission standards raised, and in 1911, a modern hospital was built. Dr. Browne was awarded his medical degree in 1912. After graduating from Leonard, Dr. Browne went to Atlanta, Georgia, and established a medical practice in 1914.

Local Raleigh physicians worked hard and donated their hard-earned money to upgrade Leonard, but it wasn't enough to meet standards.[5] In the succeeding years, Leonard's program was reduced to the equivalent of a two-year pre-med curriculum, and by 1918, the school closed.

In 1917 Dr. Browne was single and living at 226 Lambert Street, Atlanta.[6] When America entered the First World War, he volunteered. His World War I draft registration card described him as short and stout. Twenty-five years later, his World War II draft registration card in 1942 was more specific. He was 5'2" and weighed 135 pounds.

Military Service

Browne received a commission as a first lieutenant in the Medical Reserve Corps. He arrived at Fort Des Moines on August 16, 1917, for training at the army's first Medical Officers Training Camp (MOTC) for African American doctors. He completed 80 days of training on November 3, 1917, and was sent to Camp Dix, New Jersey.

He was assigned as a medical officer with the 350th Field Artillery Regiment of the 92nd Division. Two of the division's artillery regiments and a machine gun battalion were training at Camp Dix in preparation for service in France. He served overseas with his artillery unit and following the end of the war he returned with it to the United States in February 1919.

During October and November 1918 his

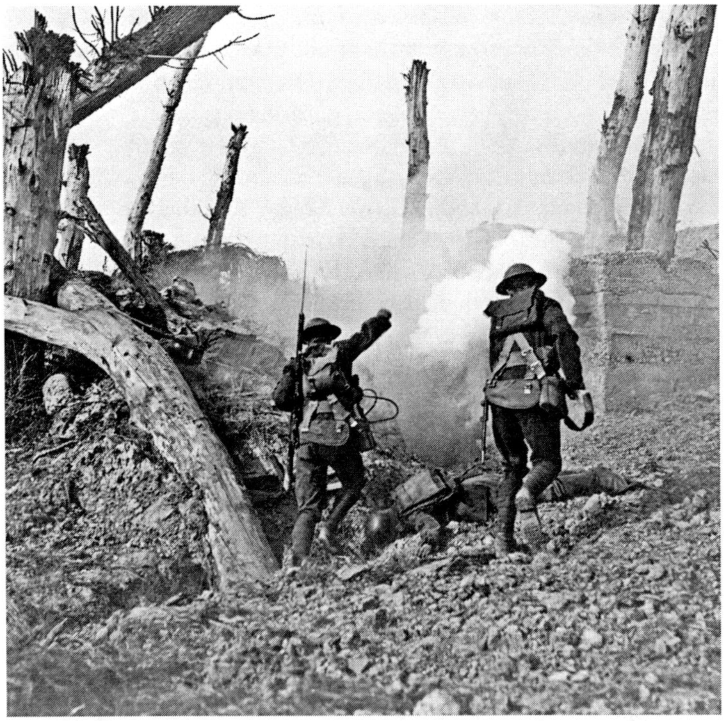

Two U.S. troops run past German remains to bunker (National Archives).

unit was engaged in major combat operations, supporting a large attack on Metz by elements of the AEF Second Army.

Colonel Allen J. Greer commended the artillery brigade in General Orders N. 31, November 7, 1918: "From the outset of the 92nd's organization, it was a problem to get together an artillery brigade that would be thoroughly efficient and dependable. It was doubted whether this first artillery brigade made up of Negro soldiers would be sufficiently trained in artillery to make an effective fighting unit. During the training period and afterward on the battlefield, General Sherburne frequently expressed the opinion that his artillerymen were the equal of any in the American Expeditionary Forces. The high degree of efficiency was evidenced by the accuracy and effectiveness of their barrages and bombardments as laid down by these Negro gunners."

Browne did not have to endure the frontline carnage of the infantry, but he would have treated his share of illnesses like influenza and pneumonia, as well as combat injuries and gassings resulting from air attacks and German artillery.

Career

When he returned from France in February 1919, Browne was sent to Camp Meade, Maryland, and discharged on April 11. His mother and stepfather, John A. Cooke, lived close by in Philadelphia. A news report said he returned to their home on April 15, and went immediately to New York to see some "very dear friends." Apparently he enjoyed himself in New York because six weeks later his parents reported him missing.[7]

By 1920, he was in Baltimore, Maryland, and then made his way to Salisbury (a different city with the same name as his birthplace) in Wicomico County, on Maryland's Eastern Shore. There he opened a general practice. This Salisbury would become his home for the rest of his life. By 1921 he was married in Philadelphia to Ernestine W. Derritt of Staunton, Virginia.

In 1930, according to the U.S. Census, he and his wife lived in West Salisbury at 907 Main Street. Her mother and father lived with them. His wife was a teacher, and her father was also a public school teacher. Browne's 1942 World War II Draft registration card lists his address as 115 Willow Street, Salisbury, Maryland. And by the 1950s he was living at 600 Isabella Street near Cypress Street in Salisbury, where he had a medical office in his home.

While living in Salisbury, Dr. Browne was a member of the Methodist Episcopal Church and a member of many civic and fraternal organizations, such as the Elks, the IOOF, the Knights of Pythias, and the Masons. In September 1954, Dr. Browne and his wife were recognized by The Salisbury Kiwanis Club for being among 100 families on the Eastern Shore to care for 118 underprivileged tenement children from New York City by inviting them "for 330 weeks of sunshine and fresh air, for giving of yourself and offering your love."[8]

The doctor's 1934 biographical sketch says, "Among his activities it may be noted—editing the first Negro newspaper published on the Eastern Shore, and organizing the Wicomico County Federation of Colored Health and Welfare Clubs in Wicomico County. Public Health lectures in this county and lower Delaware, and contributing articles to various medical publications."[9]

An unusual news item about Dr. Browne appeared in a Baltimore paper in 1941 entitled "Parole of Doctor, 3 Others Favored." It said that Dr. Browne, 52, a Salisbury physician, was given a year's sentence in the house of correction in September 1940 on a charge of receiving stolen goods. He had paid $5 for a physician's medical bag and contents, which were offered to him by a local man. Testimony at the trial indicated he readily turned over the bag when approached by authorities and said he knew the value of the materials received and he had planned to give them up when the correct owner claimed them. The article went on to describe Dr. Browne as a humanitarian, a physician for 28 years and a leading figure in the civic life of Salisbury where he practiced since 1921. Parole officers speaking in his defense reported that among his many activities to aid African Americans he led the drive to establish a nursery school and a public library in the community and much of his medical practice was without remuneration. Wicomico County judges and other officials of the county and Salisbury signed petitions asking for his parole. The Governor eventually granted it.[10]

The local Salisbury newspaper carried several more stories about Dr. Browne during the 1950s and 1960s. An amusing article in January 1957 read "Physician Is Fined on Dog Charge" for failing to have his dog, a brown mongrel, inoculated. He had a run-in with the local dogcatcher about his dog running loose and chasing cars and was fined $5 and costs.[11]

Another news article in 1966 reported a "Fire Quelled at Doctor's Office." On June 20, firemen were called to a fire at Dr. Browne's office at 600 West Isabella Street. The fire was contained to one room and was believed to have started from an electrical short circuit in an electric fan. Ten men were on the scene for an hour extinguishing the blaze.[12]

Life for African American physicians was challenging, but men like Dr. Browne persisted and were well liked within their communities. Ernestine and Arthur Browne were married for many years. They died in May 1974 within three days of one another. They are buried together at the Culpeper National Cemetery in Culpeper, Virginia.[13]

The couple left no children, but many grateful patients and friends remembered them.

Notes

1. "Arthur D. Browne, MD," *Biography-Business*, Compiled by the City of Salisbury, 1935, 56.
2. James S. Brawley, *The Rowan Story 1753–1953* (Salisbury, MD: Rowan Print Co., 1953) 264–266.
3. www.journalofamericanhistory.org (accessed August 26, 2013).
4. www.rowancountync.gov (accessed August 26, 2013).
5. Todd L. Savitt, *Race and Medicine in Nineteenth- and Early-Twentieth-Century America* (Kent, OH: Kent State University Press, 2007) 154–168.
6. World War I Draft Registration Card, 1917, ancestry.com.
7. "Parents Start Search for Dr. Arthur D. Browne," *Chicago Defender*, May 31, 1919, 15.
8. "Kiwanis Display Ad," *The Salisbury Times*, September 13, 1954.
9. Brawley, *The Rowan Story,* 207.
10. "Parole of Doctor, 3 Others Favored," *DC-American*, February 1, 1941, 24.
11. "Physician Fined," *The Salisbury Times*, January 25, 1957, 8.
12. *Ibid.*, June 21, 1966, 12.
13. Brawley, *The Rowan Story*, 207.

Samuel Simon BRUINGTON

3 August 1892–4 November 1932
Howard Medical College, 1908

Roots and Education

Bruington was born in California and raised in Georgetown, South Carolina. He was the son of Reverend S. P. and Mary N. Bruington. After graduating from the State College in Orangeburg, South Carolina, he earned his medical degree at the Howard University Medical School in Washington, D.C., in 1904. He then returned to South Carolina and in June 1905, passed the examination of the South Carolina State Board of Medical Examiners and received his medical license.[1] He remained in Georgetown practicing medicine until the First World War.[2]

Georgetown, South Carolina, is a small coastal city about 35 miles south of the resort area known as Myrtle Beach. In those years the town had a nascent timber industry, built around a sawmill, a river network, and its working harbor. The industry was successful and grew, adding a paper mill. While there, Bruington became a member of the National Medical Association (NMA). On August 27, 1914, at a general session of the NMA meeting in Raleigh, North Carolina, he presented a medical paper entitled "What Is Pellagra?"[3] Pellagra was common in the South in those years and was originally thought to be a disease, but the condition proved to be caused by a vitamin deficiency.

It appears the doctor may have had an entrepreneurial spirit because he once had a business venture in Georgetown. He was one of two African Americans who during 1916–17 leased a downtown theatre at 701 Front Street called the Peerless Theatre.[4] The exact reason for this venture is unclear, and the lease was later rescinded.

Military Service

When America entered the First World War in 1917, Bruington volunteered and was commissioned as a first lieutenant in the Army Medical Reserve Corps. He was sent to Fort Des Moines in October 1917 and completed 36 days of training.[5] He was then assigned to the 92nd Division's 317th Sanitary (Medical) Train at Camp Funston at Fort Riley, Kansas. A memorandum dated December 26, 1917, indicated that during a medical examination at the Fort Riley Base Hospital he was found to be suffering from sub-acute bronchitis but with no evidence of pulmonary tuberculosis. Lieutenant Bruington was attached to the 92nd Division's 367th Ambulance Company from early 1918 until May 1918.[6] On May 28, 1918, he was honorably discharged from the army for physical disability, thus his seven months of active military service during the war took place within the United States.[7] Although his obituary stated he served overseas, his unit did not depart for France until June 1918, after his release from service.

Career

By February 1919, Dr. Bruington had relocated to Newark, New Jersey, where he lived and worked for the next 14 years.[8] He became a successful and popular physician there and was a member of the Medical Society of New Jersey.[9] A newspaper report from May 16, 1919, described him as a "popular soldier-doctor" who was master of ceremonies at a quarterly meeting of a fraternal organization in Newark called the American Woodmen.[10] He became a member of the Essex County Medical Society, the Essex County Anatomical and Pathological Society and several fraternal organizations including the Masons. He was active with the NAACP.[11]

He met his wife, Alma Shaw, in Newark. She was from nearby New York City and formerly from Charleston, South Carolina. They had four children, one of whom was named Samuel Jr. Dr. Bruington and his wife were members of the St. James AME Church on Union Street in Newark where he served as a Trustee and Steward. His home and his medical office were both located at 115 Spruce Street, where he enjoyed a large and loyal clientele.

In August 1924, Bruington was a speaker at an Independent Colored Voters Association meeting supporting the Senate candidacy of the Honorable Hamilton F. Kean, a long time Republican.[12] It is apparent the doctor participated actively in community affairs that extended well beyond his medical practice.

It was doubly sad when he died at only 50 years of age in 1932 following a mastoid operation at the Newark Eye, Ear, Nose and Throat Hospital. His last child, a daughter, was born only one day before his death. He left a widow, four young children, and a sister, Mrs. Pricilla Gasque of Newark. Dr. Bruington was a popular and community-oriented man, and his memorial service was described as one of the best-attended funerals ever held in his church.[13]

NOTES

1. South Carolina State Board of Medical Examiners, Records of Licenses By Examination, 1894–1969, Microfilmed by SC Dept. of Archives & History, 1985.
2. "Doctor Said He Wouldn't Live Longer, and He Didn't," *Afro-American*, November 19, 1932, 5.
3. "Minutes of the NMA Meeting, General Session,

August 24, 1914, Raleigh, NC," *Journal of the National Medical Association (JNMA)*, October–December 1914, Vol. 6, No. 4, 244.
4. "Princess Theatre," Georgetown, SC, http://www.scmovietheatres.com/geo_all.html (accessed February 20, 2015).
5. Table of Medical Reserve Corps—Colored—Receiving Instruction, Medical Training Camp, Fort Des Moines, Iowa, RG-112, Records of the Surgeon General, National Archives, College Park, MD.
6. RG-120, Records of the 317th Sanitary Train, 92d Division, National Archives, College Park, MD.
7. "The Official Roster of South Carolina Soldiers, Sailors and Marines in the World War, 1917–18," Vol. 2, 1230, South Carolina Department of Archives & History.
8. "Newark N.J.," *The New York Age*, February 22, 1919.
9. AMA Deceased Physicians Masterfile 1906–1969, Box 141, U.S. National Library of Medicine, National Institutes of Health, Bethesda, MD.
10. "Newark Nuggets," *Chicago Defender*, May 17, 1919, 2.
11. "Obituary, Dr. S. S. Bruington," *New York Times*, November 6, 1932, 38.
12. "'Kean for Senator' Movement Sweeping New Jersey," *Pittsburgh Courier*, August 9, 1924, 14.
13. "Doctor Said He Wouldn't Live Longer, and He Didn't," *Afro-American*, November 19, 1932, 5.

William Henry BRYANT

25 December 1886–10 April 1964
Meharry Medical College, 1915

Roots and Education

William H. Bryant was born on Christmas Day to Fisher and Martha (Ruffin) Bryant in Wilson in Wayne County, North Carolina. His father was a laborer. His paternal grandmother was Mary Jane Bryant. He attended the local public school at Wilson and then studied for four years at Saint Augustine's School in Raleigh. Saint Augustine's had been founded in 1867 following the Civil War by the Episcopal Church to educate freemen. Bryant went north to Boston (North Carolina) High School for two years. Four years later in 1911, he earned his B.S. degree at North Carolina A & M College in Greensboro. It was a land grant school and was renamed A & T College in 1915.

Young Bryant worked hard to earn money to continue his education with jobs in the Pullman railroad service and in hotel work in the North during vacations. His Pullman work gave him the opportunity to see much of the United States and Mexico. He then enrolled at Leonard Medical School of Shaw University in Raleigh where he studied for two years. He transferred to Meharry Medical College in Nashville where he was a football player and a popular student.[1]

Dr. Bryant graduated from Meharry in 1915. The Meharry newspaper reported in January 1916 that he had passed the North Carolina State Board in 1915 and earned his medical license.[2] He practiced in Henderson, North Carolina, for two years.

Henderson had a new (1911) Jubilee Hospital. Prior to the hospital's establishment, Henderson's African Americans had to travel 40 miles for hospital care. In those days the trip was a long one over rough roads. Dr. John Adam Compton donated the land for the building, and the women of the Presbyterian Church collected funds to make construction possible. One wing of the hospital was devoted to tubercular patients and a nurses training department was added. The building was in use until 1950.[3]

When America entered the First World War in 1917, Dr. Bryant registered for the draft in June. His registration shows he was 30 years old, married to Victoria and lived at 712 Vaughan Street in Henderson.[4]

Military Service

Bryant was among 43 physicians from Meharry who volunteered to serve as physicians in the army. He received a commission as a first lieutenant in the army's Medical Reserve Corps and was ordered to Fort Des Moines for training at the African American Medical Officers Training Camp (MOTC). He arrived September 21, 1917, and completed 44 days of military training.

As was the case with many of his fellow graduates, he was assigned to the 92nd Division's 317th Sanitary (Medical) Train at Camp Funston, Kansas.[5] He was then assigned to its 367th Ambulance Company, commanded by another MOTC graduate, Captain Ulysses G. B. Martin. From Camp Funston he went to France in June 1918. His ambulance company included five physicians and a large complement of enlisted medical personnel to triage, treat and evacuate wounded personnel.

When soldiers were not involved in active combat operations, the physicians attended to the general health of the officers and men and

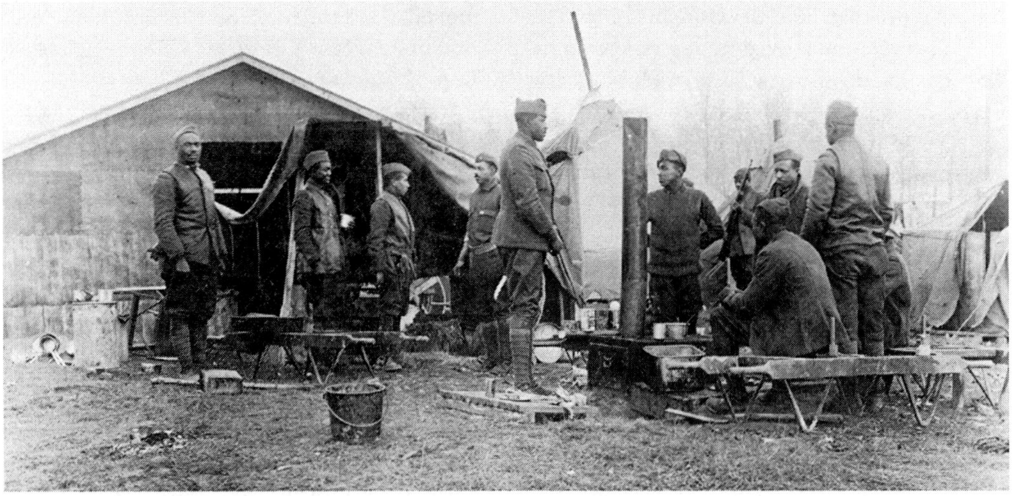

Troops at field kitchen of the 317th Supply Train at Belleville near Pont-à-Mousson (National Archives).

trained the enlisted medics. They often worked in infirmaries established to care for troops suffering from disease or injury. Tuberculosis, pneumonia, influenza, and venereal disease were commonly treated. Field conditions with poor sanitation were a constant preoccupation of all medical personnel. Maintaining combat readiness was not an easy matter given conditions in the trenches and dugouts. The cold and damp weather conditions in France caused much illness. Constant troop movement was very challenging to all medical personnel.[6]

In November 1918, his unit participated in a major offensive at Metz as part of the AEF Second Army. The division suffered 1,511 casualties of all kinds.[7] He served honorably with the same unit throughout the war and returned to the United States in February 1919.[8]

Career

After his discharge in the spring of 1919, Dr. Bryant established a general practice in Goldsboro, North Carolina, only about 25 miles south of his birthplace in Wilson. He and his wife Victoria lived at 415 School Street.[9] He became deeply involved in the Goldsboro community. At the high school's closing exercises in 1921 he gave prizes for the two best essays on sanitation.[10] In June 1928, he and two other doctors conducted physical examination clinics for school children in nearby Mt. Olive, under the auspices of the Health Committee of the Council of Negro Organization. Also that same month he attended the state medical meeting in Henderson.[11]

Life was not all work. In 1923 the *Chicago Defender* reported on his fishing and hunting trip with the Reverend Foster at Morehead City, and in October 1929 he and another friend, Dr. C. Holt, and family attended a football game at his alma mater in Greensboro.[12]

Daughter Wilhelmina was born in 1925, and the family moved to 309 Price Street.[13] Dr. Bryant had a farm about three miles west of Goldsboro and in August 1930 the newspaper reported he carried in samples of the first open cotton for the season in a double handful of open bolls, showing "Old King Cotton at His Best."[14]

In September 1930, when a local welfare league was established in Goldsboro, Dr. Bryant was elected vice president. The group met twice a month at Dillard High School.[15] He was also an active member of the local Episcopal Church.

Throughout his life, Bryant continued his medical education with the National Medical Association (NMA). In 1955, at the 60th NMA Convention in Los Angeles, he was one of 199 physicians to receive an award for 40 years or more of service in the medical profession.[16]

Dr. Bryant died at the age of 77 while visiting in Pacoima, California. He was buried at the Los Angeles National Cemetery. He hadn't moved more than 26 miles from his birthplace in Wilson, but he moved a long way from his early roots as the son of a laborer. He is remembered for his lifelong effort to improve the health and welfare of the African American community of Goldsboro.

NOTES

1. Arthur Bunyan Caldwell, *History of the American Negro and His Institutions, North Carolina Edition*, Vol. IV (Atlanta, 1921) 265–266.
2. "List of Those Who Have Passed State Boards, Class of 1915," *The Meharry News*, Vol. 14, No. 3, January 1916, 5.
3. "Jubilee Hospital," Contributions of Vance County People of Color, 394.
4. U.S. World War 1 Draft Registration Card, Vance County, North Carolina, ancestry.com.
5. Table of Medical Reserve Corps—Colored—Receiving Instruction, Medical Training Camp, Fort Des Moines, Iowa, RG-112, Records of the Army Surgeon General, National Archives, College Park, MD.
6. U.S. Army Medical Department, Office of Medical History, Vol. VIII Field Operations, Chapter IV, Medical Service of the Division in Combat (Washington, D.C.: GPO, 1925) history.amedd.army.mil (accessed April 23, 2015).
7. W. Allison Sweeney, *History of the American Negro in the Great War* (New York: Negro Universities Pressm 1969) 201.
8. RG-120, Records of Combat Divisions 1918–1919, 92nd Division, 317th Sanitary Train, U.S. National Archives, College Park, MD.
9. 1920 U.S. Federal Census.
10. "City Colored High School," *Goldsboro Daily Argus*, May 21, 1921, 1.
11. "Raleigh News—Goldsboro, NC," *Afro-American*, June 23, 1928, 19.
12. "Goldsboro, NC," *Pittsburgh Courier*, October 5, 1929, 5.
13. 1930 U.S. Federal Census.
14. "North Carolina: Goldsboro, NC," *Chicago Defender*, August 23, 1930, 17.
15. "Goldsboro, NC," *Pittsburgh Courier*, Sept 20, 1930, A3.
16. "Forty Year Practitioners," *Journal of the National Medical Association (JNMA)*, November 1955, Vol. 47, No. 6, 412.

Charles Conrad BUFORD

26 January 1891–20 March 1960
Meharry Medical College, 1916

Roots and Education

Buford was a Kentuckian through and through. His grandfather Felix G. Buford was a Kentucky farmer in south central Kentucky at Tracy in Barren County, not far from the Tennessee border. The 1880 U.S. Census recorded he had ten children. His father Gilbert (Gilly) Buford worked on Felix's farm.[1] By 1900, Gilbert moved the family to South Union close to Bowling Green, Kentucky. Charles (Charley) Buford was the oldest son.[2]

Young Buford graduated from Bowling Green Academy in 1912. The school had opened in 1902 with 57 students in the Colored Cumberland Presbyterian Church in Bowling Green. Its mission statement read, "The object of this school is threefold (1) education in general of all negro children, especially in Kentucky, who desire the advantage of a first-class institution at reasonable rates; (2) education along special lines which shall fit our young men to fill more efficiently the pulpits of our churches; (3) to develop the negro youth into good Christian citizens by educating the head, heart and hand." The school's attendance grew to more than 150 students before it closed in 1933.[3]

After graduating from the academy and working, Buford entered Meharry Medical College in Nashville at 21 years of age. His family connections to the Baptist Church probably helped guide him there.[4] Buford graduated from Meharry in 1916 and returned to Bowling Green to practice medicine. When he registered for the World War I draft in June 1917, he was unmarried and living in downtown Bowling Green at 319 Main Avenue.[5]

Military Service

Meharry Medical College conducted the most successful military recruitment campaign among its medical graduates. Buford was one of nearly 50 physicians and dentists who volunteered to serve. He was commissioned as a first lieutenant in the Army Medical Reserve Corps and arrived at the Medical Officers Training Camp (MOTC) on September 25, 1917. After 48 days of training, Lieutenant Buford was sent to Camp Funston at Fort Riley, Kansas, where he joined the 317th Sanitary (Medical) Train of the 92nd Division.[6] He was assigned to the 367th Ambulance Company and served with that unit throughout the war.

Captain Ulysses G. B. Martin, a fellow MOTC graduate, ably led the ambulance company. Lieutenant Buford also served with Lieutenant William H. Bryant, another MOTC grad.[7] They saw significant combat service and cared for many sick and wounded soldiers in the U.S. and in France in 1918–19. The primary job of the ambulance company in combat was to treat and evacuate the wounded from dressing stations on the front line to triage field hospitals, thence to evacuation and base hospitals as needed. They often traveled at night to avoid exposure to enemy artillery fire and aerial attack by German airplanes. The physicians treated serious casualties with wounds from artillery, mortars, machine guns and gas. The German artillery fire included high explosive shells with shrapnel and chemicals, such as phosgene and mustard gas.

Following the armistice on November 11, the 92nd Division returned to the United States in February 1919, and Buford was sent to Camp Zachary Taylor in Louisville, Kentucky, where he was discharged June 12, 1919.

Career

Dr. Buford settled in Lexington, Kentucky, where he established a practice downtown at 118½ South Mill Street. He initially lived at 418 North Upper Street with an uncle, James J. McCutchen, who was Pastor of a local Baptist church.[8] Buford married Roberta, a local teacher who had been born in Ohio in 1893. Their son, Charles C. Buford, Jr., was born in 1921. By 1925 the family had moved to 406 North Upper Street and his medical practice was now located at 269 East Second Street, where it remained for the next 41 years. The ensuing years were busy, productive years for the family. By 1930 they moved into a beautiful home at 423 North Upper Street.

News reports of happenings in Lexington in the late 1920s and 30s reveal Dr. Buford's active participation in a wide variety of civic and professional activities including the Blue Grass Medical Society, the African American medical society in Lexington. It was part of the State Medical Society, which in turn was part of the National Medical Association. The members met regularly to discuss professional medical issues and they dealt with community health matters.[9]

Dr. Buford was a prominent member of Lexington's African American society and was listed among the distinguished guests at the finale of the Lexington Fair in 1929.[10] The Lexington Fair was the premiere Negro summer attraction in the region. It was one of the largest in the South and attracted more than 5,000 people, with many from neighboring states of Tennessee, Ohio, Indiana, and Illinois.

At the Kentucky State Medical Society three-day meeting in 1931 in Lexington, Dr. Buford conducted several educational sessions (called surgical clinics) at Saint Joseph Hospital. Subjects included anesthetics, tularemia, and surgery.[11] His interest in his craft is further evident as he attended many medical society meetings including a trip to Louisville in 1932 during the Falls City Medical Society meeting.[12]

In addition to medicine, Dr. Buford was active with the Boy Scouts. Initially, he had a son of scouting age. In 1936 he was one of a group of nine Scout leaders who went to Ohio to attend a training course with other leaders from Ohio, Kentucky, and West Virginia.[13] His interest in Scouting continued for many years and in December 1950 he was one of 24 Boy Scout leaders who took part in the National Scout Health and Safety Service under the direction of Fred Maise of New York. He and several other leaders were awarded Certificates of Completion.[14]

In January 1937 one of his close associates, Dr. Obed Cooley of Lexington, died. Buford was a pallbearer at the funeral services for his good friend who had been a physician in Lexington for 25 years.[15] His involvement in the medical community included his election as president of the Blue Grass Medical Society. When the terrible big flood of 1937 struck Lexington, he worked hard to organize the response to the local community's need to help refugees.[16]

Dr. Buford did make time for fun. In early October 1937, he and his wife went to Frankfort with friends and colleagues where they attended the football game at Kentucky State College for Negroes.[17]

Dr. Buford always maintained an interest in veteran's affairs. In December 1937 he joined the R.E. Hathaway Post No. 3593—Veterans of Foreign Wars for Colored Veterans.[18] Years later he was described as a member of a rather elite group of African American men who were the first members of the Post.[19] In

May 1940 he was a featured speaker at Memorial Day services at African Cemetery No. 2, which is the earliest recorded cemetery in Lexington to be organized, owned and managed by African Americans. It contains more than 5,000 graves.

Family was important to Dr. Buford. His father died in 1921, but his mother survived for many more years. In 1950 Dr. Buford and his mother attended a service for his aunt Ida Belle Webb in Glasgow, Kentucky. When she died of a stroke on January 5, 1950, more than five hundred people attended her service at Pleasant Union Baptist Church.[20]

Dr. Buford's commitment to his profession remained steadfast. In 1952, at the 52nd annual meeting of the Blue Grass State Medical Association at Kentucky State College in Frankfort, Dr. Buford was elected its president.[21] In 1954 he was appointed to the post of state vice president for Kentucky of the National Medical Association.[22]

The city directories for Lexington from 1921 to 1956 contain many entries for Dr. Buford and his wife Roberta. Son Charles is also listed, as a student in 1939 and as a "checker" in 1940. C. C. Buford, Jr., followed his father into the medical profession and moved to New Jersey where he practiced in Trenton.[23] When Dr. Buford, Sr., died at the age of 69, he was buried nearby in the Ewing Cemetery in Mercer County, New Jersey. His son joined him there in 1983, 23 years later, when he died at the age of 62.[24]

NOTES

1. 1880 U.S. Federal Census.
2. 1900 U.S. Federal Census.
3. Notable Kentucky African Americans Database, Bowling Green Academy, University of Kentucky Libraries. http://nkaa.uky.edu/record.php?note_id=367 (accessed June 12, 2012).
4. Meharry Medical College Archives (accessed July 17, 2012).
5. World War I Draft Registration Cards (1917–1918).
6. Table of Medical Reserve Corps—Colored- Receiving Instruction, Medical Training Camp, Fort Des Moines, Iowa, RG-112, Records of the Army Surgeon General, National Archives, College Park, MD.
7. Record Group 120, Records of the AEF World War I, 92d Division, 317th Sanitary Train, National Archives, College Park, MD.
8. 1920 U.S. Census.
9. "Lexington, KY," *New Journal and Guide* (1916–2003), April 9, 1927, 8.
10. "Thousands Attend Lexington Fair on Louisville Day: The Menelek Club Covers Itself with Glory," *The Pittsburgh Courier*, September 7, 1929, 2.
11. "Kentucky State Medical Society Holds Annual Convention," *Chicago Defender*, June 6, 1931, 11.
12. "Kentucky State News: Louisville News," *Chicago Defender*, September 17, 1932, 23 .
13. "Lexington, KY," *Chicago Defender*, June 13, 1936, 20.
14. "Lexington," *Chicago Defender*, December 2, 1950, 22.
15. "Kentucky State News, Lexington," *Chicago Defender*, January 30, 1937, 13.
16. "Kentucky State News, Lexington," *Chicago Defender*, February 13, 1937, 23.
17. "Kentucky State News, Lexington," *Chicago Defender*, October 9, 1937, 23.
18. "Kentucky State News, Lexington," *Chicago Defender*, December 18, 1937, 20.
19. Notable Kentucky African Americans Database, R.E. Hathaway Post No. 3593 (Lexington, KY), University of Kentucky Libraries. http://nkaa.uky.edu/all.php?sort_by=R.
20. "Glasgow," *Chicago Defender*, January 21, 1950, 22.
21. "Blue Grass Medics Hold Meet," *Atlanta Daily World*, June 22, 1950, 3.
22. "NMA Activities," *Journal of the National Medical Association (JNMA)*, March 1954, Vol. 46, No. 2, 146.
23. *Ibid.*, 145.
24. Find-A-Grave, findagrave.com, Buford, New Jersey.

John David CARR

11 April 1885–5 September 1928
University of West Tennessee, 1910

Roots and Education

John Carr was born to William E. and Ruth J. Carr in Danville, Virginia. His father was a Presbyterian minister. His mother, a native of Washington, D.C., was a teacher at the Presbyterian school he attended.

After his early education at his mother's school, he left Danville to study medicine at the University of West Tennessee's College of Medicine and Surgery in Memphis, and graduated in 1910. The university could only offer basic course work. It had no endowment and received no financial support from either the state or any religious denomination. Students received clinical experience at the city's Negro Baptist Hospital. Dr. Carr was licensed in Tennessee (1910) and West Virginia in 1915. He practiced at various places before the First World War—his hometown of Danville (1910), then Lexington, Kentucky (1911), Cleveland, Ohio (1914) and Knoxville, Tennessee (1917).[1]

Military Service

Carr volunteered for the Army Medical Reserve Corps and received his orders on August 9, 1917. On September 20, 1917, at the age of 32, he reported to Des Moines for training camp. He was there for 45 days, and went on to Camp Funston, Kansas, headquarters for the 317th Sanitary (Medical) Train, 92nd Division. On November 15, he was assigned to the 365th Ambulance Company. On December 31, 1917, Major David B. Downing, commanding officer of the train, assigned Carr and McLaughlin as assistants to Rufus Vass to cover the infirmary. All three had trained together at Fort Des Moines.

By January 31, 1918, Carr had the added responsibilities of auditing expenditures of the ambulance company's funds.

On June 10, 1918, the 317th Sanitary Train left Camp Funston by train for Camp Upton, New York. This was the last stop on the trip to France. On June 19, 1918, they embarked from Hoboken, New Jersey, on the steamship *Great Northern* heading for duty with the American Expeditionary Forces. The trip was uneventful, but sanitary conditions aboard ship were only fair and ventilation was poor. There were four cases of pneumonia contracted aboard ship during the voyage.

The ship arrived at the port of Brest, France, on June 25, 1918. Troops were quartered at the terrible Pontanezen Barracks. Every American who came through this place described these old Napoleonic barracks as dank, dark, cold and filthy. "Sanitary arrangements were very bad, and there was no provision for waste disposal. Camp orders required the kitchen waste and human waste to be dumped in a common pile about 100 yards in rear of camp. It being practically impossible to combat the fly menace."[2]

On July 5, 1918, the Ambulance Section (including Carr's 365th) arrived at the Bourbonne-les-Bains training area. Majors Downing and Simmons appear to have had problems with Carr. On July 31, 1918, Downing submitted a memorandum stating it was the "opinion based on reports of written examinations in military, surgical and medical subjects" that despite Downing's continual reminders "his work was not satisfactory but he has failed to improve."[3]

On August 6, 1918, Carr (and another of his classmates from Fort Des Moines, Lieutenant Edward Bates) were sent to headquarters for examination of competency.[4]

Things were going downhill quickly for Carr. On August 18, 1918, Major Edward B. Simmons reported to his commanding officer Lieutenant Colonel Downing that Carr was "lazy and inefficient in every way." Several other doctors who had graduated from Fort Des Moines (Dana Baldwin, Herndon White and Oliver Landry) were also having trouble with military life, but more likely with Downing. Downing sent a memo to headquarters again on August 27, 1918, saying White, Carr and Baldwin "have not the adaptability for service in the Sanitary Train."[5]

On August 28, Carr was "relieved from further duty with the 92nd Division" and recommended for duty at the Casual Camp Blois. Camp Blois would most certainly not have been regarded as a desirable assignment. Blois, a city of about 25,000 people at the time, was a rear echelon base hospital center and classification camp for replacements. It was a very large casual camp for soldiers not assigned to regular units. Officers and men were held pending their return to duty or to America. It was a place where a large part of the military was transient and support activity was principally directed to serving a floating population. It was impossible to establish personal friendships as many soldiers stayed only a few days.[6] Carr was ultimately returned home and honorably discharged.

Lieutenant Colonel Downing and Major Simmons were white. Downing was a career military officer. Simmons was a reservist. They had likely never met an educated African American, let alone had any reporting to them. Certainly racism has to be considered as a factor in their inability to deal with some of the doctors in their unit.

Career

After the war, Dr. Carr returned to Tennessee and settled in Memphis. According to the 1920 U.S. Census, he and his wife Lillian were living in a rented duplex home at 823 Mississippi Boulevard. In 1923 his medical office is listed in the local phone directory at 140 South 4th Street. By 1925, his office has moved to the center of the city's black business district at 316 Beale Avenue and in 1927 his office was across the street at 321 Beale Avenue.

Beale Street at this time in history has been described as prosperous and at night "the area took on a carnival atmosphere, with gambling, drinking, prostitution, murder and voodoo, thriving alongside nightclubs, theaters, restaurants, stores, pawnshops and hot music. The Monarch Club was known as 'The Castle of Missing Men' because its gunshot victims could be quickly disposed of at the undertaker's, which shared their back alley."[7] Carr's business was likely especially busy during evening hours.

Unfortunately, Dr. Carr died at his office at age 43 on September 5, 1928, of acute dilation of the heart (a heart attack). It was noted on his death certificate that excessive smoking and overwork were contributing factors to his demise. His body was returned to his mother Ruth's birthplace, Washington, D.C., for burial.

NOTES

1. Directory of Deceased American Physicians, 1804–1929, AMA, National Library of Medicine, Bethesda, MD.
2. "Headquarters, 317th Military Train, 92nd Division, Medical—History," Unclassified/Declassified Holdings of the National Archives, Box 15, College Park, MD.
3. "Headquarters, 317th Sanitary Train, 92nd Division Reports," Unclassified/Declassified Holdings of the National Archives, Box 210, College Park, MD.
4. *Ibid.*
5. *Ibid.*
6. *Service with Fighting Men: An Account of the Work of the YMCA,* Vol. 2, 112, www.books.google.com (accessed January 9, 2013).
7. http://historic-memphis.com/memphis-historic/beale/bealestreet.html (accessed October 18, 2014).

Raymond Holmes CARTER

28 May 1881–19 January 1976
Leonard Medical School, 1907

Roots and Education

Carter was born to Dr. Edward Randolph and Obedia Cecile (Brown) Carter. His father "was just about the most famous and effective black minister during the days of struggle that showed the entire world of Negro worth in Atlanta."[1] His father came to Atlanta from Athens as a shoemaker and continued his trade while attending Atlanta Baptist College. He became pastor of Friendship Baptist Church and stayed in that position for 58 years. He and Obedia had five children. Raymond and his brother Edward Jr., would become physicians. The parents lived long enough to celebrate their 64th wedding anniversary in 1940.

Carter received his early education at his father's alma mater, Atlanta University, which he attended until 1892. Then he entered Atlanta Baptist College. These institutions were merged later and became Morehouse College. Raymond received his A.B. degree in 1903. His father was secretary of Morehouse for 23 years.

Carter continued his education at Leonard Medical School in North Carolina and received his medical degree in 1907. He returned to Atlanta, and for a year and a half he was resident physician at Fairhaven Infirmary, Atlanta. In December 1910, he was elected assistant secretary of the Georgia State Association of Colored Physicians, Dentists and Pharmacists and served in that capacity until 1912, when he was elected secretary. He would be involved with that organization for the rest of his life.[2]

On December 27, 1910, Carter married Manie W. Cohron, daughter of Emmett Cohron of St. Joseph, Missouri. She had been a student at Spelman College in Atlanta. In September 1912, he saw potential in the growing town of Newnan, Georgia, about 40 miles from Atlanta, so the couple moved there, and he opened a practice.[3]

Military Service

In 1917, at the age of 36, Dr. Carter volunteered for the Army Medical Reserve Corps. He reported for basic training on August 17 at the Medical Officers Training Camp at Fort Des Moines. After 79 days of training, he was assigned to the medical detachment of the 366th Infantry Regiment at Camp Dodge, Iowa. He served in France with those men.

His medical detachment was responsible for maintaining the health of the 3,500 soldiers

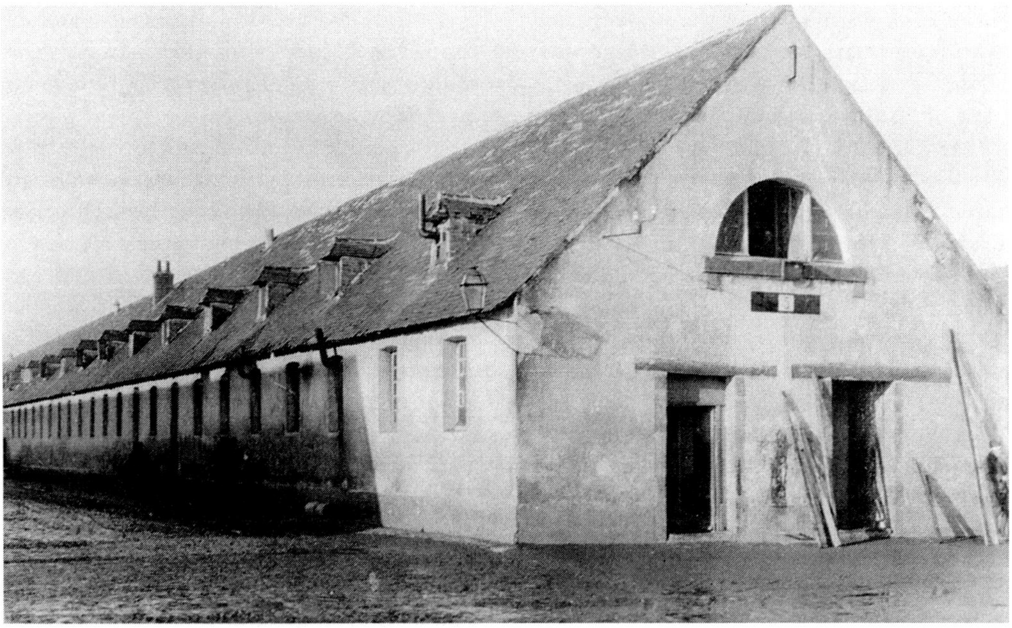

Old stone Pontanezen barracks, Brest, France (National Archives).

in the regiment. It had seven officers and more than 100 enlisted men caring for the sick and wounded. By the end of the war the regiment had suffered 225 wounded, 12 deaths from wounds, and 20 killed in action. Most of the casualties occurred in the final days of fighting on November 10–11.[4] Carter remembered the harsh conditions many years later in 1936 when he spoke to high school students in Atlanta. He told them if war does not actually kill, it maims thousands of soldiers for life, and he spoke of the strain of restless days and nights the doctors experienced caring for wounded soldiers.[5]

His good friend, Dr. Homer E. Nash spoke at Carter's funeral in 1976 at the Friendship Baptist in Atlanta about their time in France during World War I. "I was a captain in a field hospital near the battle lines in France in 1918 while Dr. Carter served as a captain and medical officer with the forces out in the lines." In the audience during the funeral was attorney Thomas J. Henry, who was injured by German gas in a battle that also injured Dr. Carter.[6]

Career

After the war, Dr. Carter took a postgraduate program at Harvard University in ear, eye, nose and throat treatments. Then, for a short time, he was chief of the eye, ear, nose and throat section of the U.S. Veterans Hospital #91 at Tuskegee, Alabama.

The Carters moved back to Atlanta, and in 1929, he was appointed to the hospital staff of Morehouse College. For a number of years they lived in his father's home on Tatnall Street, SW, until the area was torn down as a part of urban renewal. The Carters then moved to 517 Collier Ridge Drive, NW, and remained there the rest of their lives.

Dr. Carter was always active in the Boy Scouts of America. In 1934, he was president of Atlanta's "Scouters Club" and involved in planning its summer camp and leaders training.[7] By 1936, he was "Colored Commissioner of the Boy Scouts of America."[8] In 1953, he was one of the very few recipients of the Scouts' Silver Beaver Award.[9] It is one of the highest awards of the Boy Scouts of America. Recipients are registered adult leaders who have made an impact on the lives of youth through service given to the council. It is given to those who implement the Scouting program and perform community service through hard work, self-sacrifice, dedication, and many years of service.

Carter was quoted in the *Atlanta Daily World*'s February 23, 1938, front-page story about Georgia's defeat of an anti-lynching bill, "Use of Ballot and Money Will Help Negro Offset Defeat." He told reporter William Fowlkes, Jr., "Mississippi's beginning the passage of an anti-lynch law is indicative of the tendency of the South to wake up to handling the problem herself. The ballot and money are what we need."[10]

He was also quite a thespian. In 1936, he dressed in his World War I uniform, complete with brown khaki, leather boots, and bullet belts and presented a vivid description of the horrors of World War I to the night school twelfth graders. He told of his experience as a medical officer near "no man's land" in France. He showed the arms every soldier carried. And, he concluded everyone "should strive to promote peace."[11]

Another performance came in 1941 when Dr. Carter played the lead in *The Family Upstairs* in Sale Hall Chapel as a fundraiser for the Morehouse Auxiliary. The cast also included college faculty and students.[12] The plot is Joe Heller's (played by Dr. Carter) wife's anxiety to get daughter Louise married. Joe's ambition is to get son Willie to work. The comedy was well received and a good fundraiser for Morehouse.

Carter was active in medical, civic, educational and religious circles throughout his life. In 1940, he was secretary of the Child Welfare Association and involved in its important research studies.[13] He also volunteered at the West Side Health Center. Started by the Urban League as a comprehensive health service, it made medical care "easily accessible to the Negro population and was staffed by competent Negro personnel."[14] Dr. Carter continued to work with the center as it expanded from primarily dealing with venereal disease to clinics in ringworm, prenatal care and tuberculosis.

When a medical clinic was opened to care for the African Americans of Mayfield, Georgia, Dr. Carter was there as the ear, eyes, nose and throat specialist. Much of this expansion was with help from Atlanta's Hungry Club. The Hungry Club at the Butler Street YMCA began as a forum for political discussions and expanded to include promotion of voter registration, health issues and a variety of community programs.

When the national organization of Omega Psi Phi fraternity held its National Negro Achievement Week Program in 1946, Dr. Carter headed the Atlanta chapter at the weeklong activities.[15]

In 1951, Dr. Carter moderated a program for the Georgia Division of the American Cancer Society at Atlanta's Hungry Club.[16] In 1954, his medical presentations addressed another area of medicine when he presented a paper on "Psychosomatic Disorders" at the Georgia State Medical Association.[17] In 1956, he led the discussion of arthritis by a panel of experts at the Atlanta Medical Association.[18]

Throughout the 1950s Dr. Carter received a number of honors. In 1950, he was elected president of the Georgia Medical Association of Physicians and Pharmacists. In 1953, Morehouse College recognized Carter for his long and distinguished service to the college since his graduation in 1903.[19] This service included annual health lectures to incoming freshmen. His lifelong membership in the National Medical Association (NMA) was recognized in 1955 at NMA's 60th Convention when he was cited as "one of 199 physicians who received an award for 40 years or more of service to the medical profession."[20]

The Carters' son R. H. Carter, Jr., followed his father's medical profession and in the 1950s advertised his services in the *Atlanta Daily World* for "fitting of glasses, treatment of eye disease, eye examinations and filling prescriptions for glasses and hearing aids."[21]

The Carters worshiped at same church his father had pastored for 62 years, Friendship Baptist Church in Atlanta. In 1955, he taught a class to the men of the church. It focused on the Sermon on the Mount.

When Manie Carter died in 1963 her funeral rites were held at the Friendship Baptist Church. The good doctor died in 1976 at the age of 94, "leaving behind four children, and a host of people who looked upon him as a great human being,"[22] His funeral was at his father's church with most of Atlanta's African American medical community in attendance. The Morehouse Glee Club sang. Dr. Hugh Gloster, president of Morehouse College, and a student there when Dr. Carter was its medical officer, spoke of Dr. Carter as being "born into a Morehouse Family."[23]

Pastor William V. Guy spoke of Dr. Carter as "a man we are thankful for; a man from which we all have a lot to learn: A life so richly more lived, we can take joy in what he left behind."[24]

He and Manie are buried in South View Cemetery in Atlanta.

NOTES

1. Arthur Bunyan Caldwell, Editor, *History of the American Negro and His Institutions, Georgia Edition* (Atlanda: A. B. Caldwell Publishing Co., 1917) 322–23.
2. *Ibid.*
3. *Ibid.*
4. 92d Division, Summary of Operations in the World War, Prepared by the American Battle Monuments Commission (Washington, D.C.: GPO, 1944) http://www.history.army.mil/topics/afam/92div.htm (accessed April 22, 2015).
5. "Dr. R. Carter Is Guest Speaker at E.P. Johnson," *Atlanta Daily World*, November 15, 1936, 6.
6. George M. Coleman, "Atlantans Honor Dr. Carter as a 'Good Doctor Man,'" *Atlanta Daily World*, January 25, 1976, 1.
7. "Scouters' Club Will Meet This Evening," *Atlanta Daily World*, June 19, 1934, 1.
8. "Scouts Will Honor Pioneer Worker at Cemetery," *Atlanta Daily World*, January 18, 1936, 1.
9. *Ibid.*, "Dr. R. H. Carter Is Brotherhood Speaker Sunday," February 12, 1953, 1.
10. "Use of Ballot and Money Will Help Negro Offset Defeat," *Atlanta Daily World*, February 3, 1938, 1.
11. *Ibid.*, "Dr. R. Carter Is Guest Speaker at E.P. Johnson," November 15, 1936, 6.
12. "The Family Upstairs' to Be Presented," *Atlanta Daily World*, May 17, 1941, 3.
13. *Ibid.*, "Child Welfare Association Plans Important Social Research Study," June 4, 1940, 2.
14. *Ibid.*, "West Side Health Center to Observe 5th Anniversary," June 5, 1949, 1.
15. "Omegas End Achievement Week Activities," *Atlanta Daily World*, November 10, 1946, 1.
16. *Ibid.*, "War on Cancer to Be Discussed at Hungry Club," March 21, 1951, 1.
17. *Ibid.*, "Modern Medical Lore Interests State Doctors...," May 6, 1954, 1.
18. "Arthritis to Be Topic of Medic Forum," *Atlanta Daily World*, February 23, 1956, 1.
19. *Ibid.*, "Carter Cited by M'house Alumni," June 13, 1953, 1.
20. "The Forty Year Practitioners," *Journal of the National Medical Association*, November 1955, Vol. 47, 412.
21. "Display Ad 4," *Atlanta Daily World*, June 16, 1957, 2.
22. Coleman, George M. "Atlantans Honor Dr. Carter as a 'Good Doctor Man,'" *Atlanta Daily World*, January 25, 1976, 1.
23. *Ibid.*
24. *Ibid.*

Daniel W. CRAWFORD

1874–10 December 1937
Knoxville Medical College, 1905

Roots and Education

Nothing could be found about Daniel Crawford's family or early life. He first appears in records when he enters school in Knoxville, Tennessee, in 1901.

In 1895, there were less than 400 African American physicians in the United States. Several small independent medical colleges were opened before 1900. Knoxville College's Medical Department was established in 1895 by a "group of local white physicians who were more interested in making money than furthering the school's mission of educating black Christian physicians." The college closed the medical school on campus in 1900, but the same faculty reopened it off campus.[1] Daniel Crawford was a student at the school. He chopped wood, painted furniture and took on odd jobs to pay his way through school. He finally received his medical degree in 1905 and stayed in Knoxville to practice medicine. In 1909 and 1910, Dr. Crawford had joined the school's faculty. In 1909, Abraham Flexner visited the school as part of his survey for the American Medical Association. His scathing report of the medical education provided at Knoxville certainly contributed to its closing in 1910.[2]

The Knoxville College Hospital stayed open for a while. In 1911, Dr. Crawford assisted at "quite a successful surgical operation.... A tumor weighing ... 25 pounds was removed.... This growth involved every vital organ in the pelvic and abdominal cavity." The patient made it through the surgery and was reported doing well.[3]

Military Service

Crawford volunteered for service in the First World War and reported for basic training at Fort Des Moines Medical Officers Training Camp (MOTC) on Sept 29, 1917. He was there for 52 days before he was transferred to Camp Funston and then to France with the 92nd Division's 367th Field Hospital.

In trench warfare, field hospitals were located from 10 to 15 kilometers (6 to 8 miles) behind the front, or further back to be beyond range of ordinary shellfire. The distance and the buildings varied greatly. Whenever possible, existing buildings were used. Convenient roads and availability of water and fuel had to be considered, too.[4]

By November 1918, Lieutenant Crawford was transferred to command the medical detachment of the 325th Field Signal Battalion. The Signal Battalions were responsible for the communications network and had to adapt to the conditions of trench warfare. The repair teams sustained many casualties, however, due to heavy concentrations of poison gas. While the enemy repeatedly knocked the division's telephones and radios out of action, the earth telegraphy stations remained in operation.

In general, from division headquarters forward, telephone lines ran to each infantry battalion as well as between adjoining battalions. Wires were strung on short (four-foot) stakes or run along the trench walls. The major trunk lines were placed in special shallow trenches (known as *carniveaux*) or buried several feet underground to provide protection from enemy shelling and from foot and vehicle traffic.

First Lieutenant Crawford's unit was the only black signal unit to serve in World War I. When he joined them in late September, they were headed for the Argonne. A platoon of the 325th, supporting the 368th Infantry, saw action during the battle. In addition to their signal duties, several platoon members volunteered to take a German machine gun nest encountered while scouting a location for a new command post. One of these signalmen, Corporal Charles S. Boykin, was killed during this engagement, which ultimately succeeded in capturing the enemy position.[5] Crawford was promoted to captain before the war's end.

Career

After World War I, Dr. Crawford returned to Knoxville and his general practice. He was a member of the National Medical Association, the national organization for African American physicians. In August 1920, he attended the annual meeting in Atlanta, Georgia. In addition to hearing presentations on medical treatments coming from the war experience, he likely renewed the acquaintances he made while in the Army Medical Corps.

In 1921 he left Knoxville to take a yearlong course in eyes, ear, nose and throat treatments at the University of Illinois. After completing this, his local phone book listing included this specialty. He practiced at 101½ West Vine Avenue.[6] During his years of practice in Knoxville, Dr. Crawford was active in the local African American medical and surgical society, eventually serving as its president.

He moved to Oklahoma after the 1921 Tulsa race riots. He opened an office at 205½ North Greenwood Street and immediately became active in the Tulsa Negro Business League. The next year, he was elected vice president. Fellow army veteran and physician George I. Lythcott was also active in the organization.[7]

In 1925, Tim Owsley, columnist for the *Chicago Defender*, described Dr. Crawford's home on Greenwood in Tulsa as "one of the finest homes in the city."[8] That year, he was president of the Tulsa local chapter of the National Negro Business League. He secured Governor M. E. Trapp as a speaker to welcome the group to Tulsa. He was also in charge of the entertainment features of the meeting set for August 19–21. Among other events, Dr. Crawford planned "a mammoth parade to show off the agricultural and industrial resources of the State of Oklahoma."[9]

By 1926, Dr. Crawford had completed a residency at Hubbard Memorial Clinic in Tulsa, and passed the exam for his Oklahoma medical license.

When 67 African American physicians attended the Oklahoma Medical, Dental and Pharmaceutical Association's annual meeting in Tulsa, Dr. Crawford led a very popular session on socialized medicine.[10]

At some time in the 1920s he married Settie, a local real estate agent. The two adopted a son, William Woods. In the 1920s the city business directory listed his "Optician" office address as 205½ Greenwood. His practice must have been successful because by the 1930 Census, the family included a maid in their home at 1436 North Greenwood Street.

Dr. Crawford was active in a variety of community organizations. In 1931, he chaired the management committee of the Greenwood branch of the YMCA and was appointed ex-officio member of the cabinet of the whole city's YMCA, the first black man to hold such a position.[11] During 1931, he was involved in the construction of a hospital for the black community. Using his position as master of the victory lodge of the A.F. and A.M. Masons and with his community and medical contacts, Dr. Crawford worked hard to make this a reality.[12] In 1932, Tulsa Municipal Hospital Number Two opened at 603 East Pine to serve the African American community.[13]

Early in 1936, Dr. Crawford spent four weeks in the hospital following a major operation.[14] Crawford had worked hard and had a successful medical career serving the city's African American Community before "a gloom was cast over Tulsa, Oklahoma, when death claimed Dr. D. W. Crawford"[15] in 1937. He died at the age of 63 in a Veterans Administration facility in Muskogee, Oklahoma.

NOTES

1. Ncbi.nlm.nih.gov/pubmed/11740123 (accessed March 2, 2015).
2. *Ibid.*, "Knoxville Medical College," 251 (accessed March 2, 2015).
3. "Items of Race Interest," *Indianapolis Freeman*, June 17, 1911, 2.
4. U.S. Army Medical Department, Office of Medical History, Vol. VIII, Field Operations, Chapter IV, Medical Services of the Division in Combat (Washington, D.C.: GPO, 1925) history.amedd.army.mil (accessed April 23, 2015).
5. http://www.history.army.mil/books/30-17/S_5.htm (accessed July 21, 2014).
6. James N. Simms, Simms Blue Book and National Negro Business and Professional Directory, 1923 (Cleveland, OH: Gordon Publishing Company, 1977) 278–279.
7. "Tulsa, Okla.," *Chicago Defender*, February 9, 1924, 17.
8. "The Georgias," *Chicago Defender*, November 28, 1925, 7.
9. "Gov. Trapp of Okla. to Make Welcome Address," *The New York Age*, July 3, 1925, 1.
10. "Oklahoma Medics in 30th Meet at Tulsa," *Chicago Defender*, May 22, 1937, 5.
11. "Tulsa Man Is YMCA Ex-Officio Member," *Afro-American*, January 10, 1931, 16.
12. "Tulsa to Erect a Negro Hospital," *Philadelphia Tribune*, October 8, 15.
13. http://tcmsok.org/tcms-history/tulsa-hospital-histories/a-history-of-tulsa-hospitals-1900-1968 (accessed July 29, 2014).
14. "Farnham Reported Slightly Improved," *Woodland Daily Democrat*, March 3, 1936, 1.
15. "World's Flashlight," *The* (Wichita, KS) *Negro Star*, January 14, 1938, 4.

Arthur Leo CURTIS

26 July 1889–28 June 1936
Howard Medical College, 1912

Roots and Education

Arthur Leo Curtis was born in Chicago, Illinois, to Namahyoka Sockume of Delaware Indian extraction.[1] His father Dr. Austin M. Curtis was a well-educated and respected surgeon. His father had received three degrees (including one in dental science) from Lincoln University in 1888 and then his medical degree from Northwestern in 1891. He was house surgeon at Provident Hospital in Chicago for a year before taking the position of chief surgeon at Freedmen's Hospital and moving the family to Washington, D.C. Arthur was in the sixth grade.[2]

After attending public school in Chicago and Washington, D.C., Arthur was privileged to be able to attend an excellent integrated residential preparatory school, Williston Seminary (renamed Williston Academy in 1925) in Easthampton, Massachusetts. The school offered a four-year college preparatory program and had a student body of 202 men. Graduates were accepted at all the best colleges and universities, including among them Amherst, Cornell, Dartmouth, Harvard, Pennsylvania, Tufts, Williams, Yale, and Princeton. They also entered schools of medicine, law, engineering and science. He entered the school as a sophomore level in 1905 and graduated three years later in 1908. He enrolled in the Classical course, emphasizing Latin and Greek, and he earned honors for his academic performance. He wrote his senior thesis (still on file in Williston archives) discussing problems and opportunities posed by immigration into the U.S.[3] There were 38 men in his graduating class. While there he enjoyed history and played intramural sports including track, baseball, football and, despite his five-foot height, basketball.[4] He also won the Amherst Cup for best individual debater from the Adelphi and Gamma Sigma Debating Societies.[5] According to the 1908 yearbook, young Curtis was nicknamed "Buck" by his classmates. He was proud of his prep school and in 1928, 20 years after his graduation, he wrote from his office at 1717 U Street, NW, in Washington, D.C., to Professor Morse, the Williston Alumni Secretary. He spoke of his warm feelings for the school and of his plans to return that June for his 20th reunion saying "I shall bring with me not only my wife and father, but my check book to do my bit toward the new building program of the School."[6] The school, founded in 1841, is still in operation today.

From Williston, Arthur Curtis went directly to Howard University in Washington, D.C., and again he joined the basketball team. With his help, Howard basketball went from a bit player to national champion. And all without a gymnasium! The team's goal in the 1911 season was to defeat the best New York teams. This was the season that came to be known as the "Birth of Black Basketball." The wildest game was against the New York All-Stars. Final score: Howard 69, All-Stars 14. Howard went on to win the 1911 championship among the best black teams in the country.[7] Curtis was awarded his medical degree from Howard's medical school in 1912.

After a year of internship at Freedmen's Hospital, he opened his private practice in the District at 1939 13th Street, NW, and then later at 1717 U Street, NW. During this time, Curtis also was an instructor in surgery, diagnosis and anesthesia at Howard University and was a visiting surgeon at Freedmen's Hospital.[8]

He was a member of the Congregational Church and became the local examiner for Standard Life Insurance. He was also a member of the NAACP, Odd Fellows (its examining physician), the National Medical Association (NMA), and the Medico-Chirurgical Society of Washington, D.C.

The first American Medical Association was formed in May of 1847 and it was initially closed to African Americans. The Medical Society of the District of Columbia organized in 1817 and chartered in 1819 did not admit African Americans. The Medico-Chirurgical Society of Washington, D.C., was chartered in 1895 for African American medical professionals when it became apparent that discrimination would not soon end. The National Medical Association was founded the same year.[9]

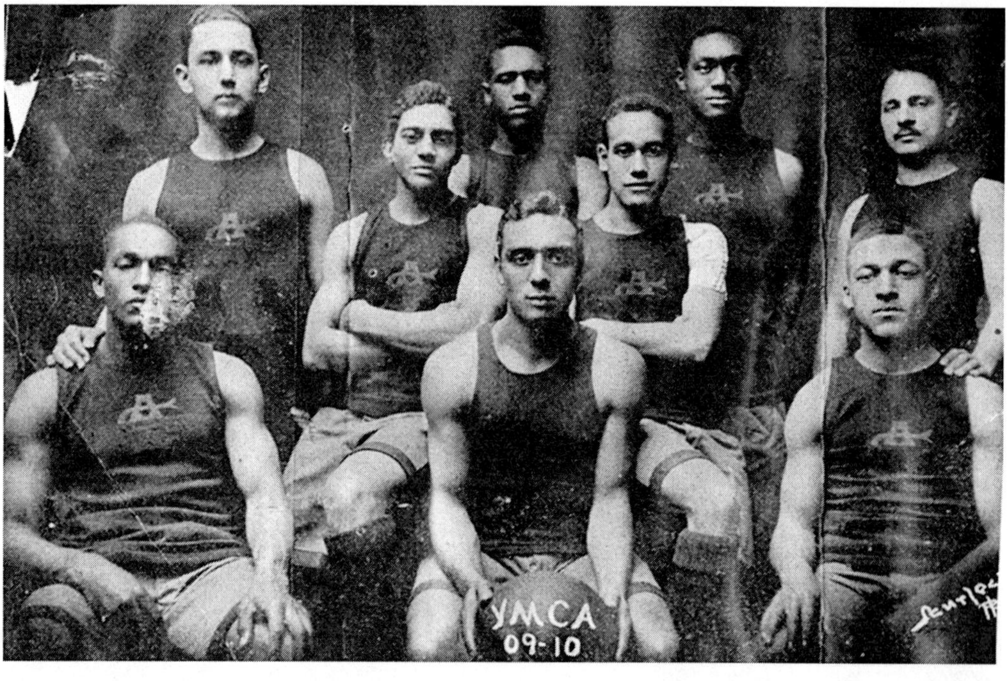

Arthur L. Curtis (top row, left) with 1910 YMCA basketball team (courtesy National Museum of American History Archives, Smithsonian Institution, and Moorland-Spingarn Research Center, Howard University).

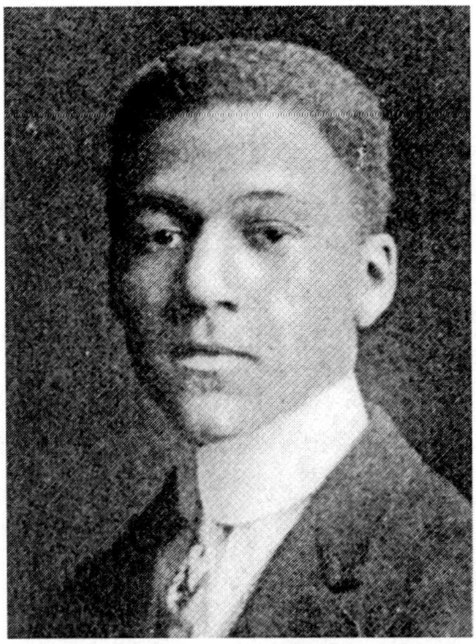

Arthur L. Curtis, graduation 1908, Williston Seminary (courtesy Williston Northampton School).

On March 18, 1916, his father, one of the foremost African American surgeons, had performed abdominal surgery on his own son, Dr. Arthur Curtis. The *Savannah Tribune*'s coverage of the event includes "Dr. Curtis [the father, Austin M.], in his long practice, has accomplished some of the rarest feats in surgery, but in successfully handling this operation upon his own son, he has established a new record in this community."[10]

On June 16, 1916, Dr. Curtis married Helen Neola Gordon of Washington, D.C. They purchased "an elegant home at U Street, NW, and [were] prominent in the social life of the city."[11] There would be no children.

Military Service

On June 5, 1917, Dr. Curtis registered for the draft. Two of his brothers also volunteered to serve and all were commissioned first lieutenants. His brother Maurice was a physician with the Medical Reserve Corps, and brother Merrill was an officer with the 349th Field Artillery.

Curtis trained from August 20 to November 3, 1917, at the Fort Des Moines' Medical Officer's Training Camp, and from there he was sent to Camp Meade, Maryland. He was assigned to duty with the 368th Infantry Regiment and worked as the assistant regimental surgeon in the regimental infirmary. On December 4, 1917, he wrote from Camp Meade to Dr. Joseph Sawyer at his prep school alma mater, Williston Seminary, saying he had spent 10 weeks in Des Moines, Iowa, "training enlisted hospital corps men" before coming to Camp Meade. In a postscript to his letter he wrote, "P.S. I might add Doctor, that my Father and Mother take considerable pride in the knowledge that they have three sons, and all three are in the service of their country as commissioned officers of the Army."[12]

He served with this detachment of the 92nd Division until August 1918. The next month, he was reassigned to the division's 367th Field Hospital, where he remained until war's end in November 1918. His unit was there to assist the 366th Field Hospital, where Louis T. Wright, a fellow MOTC graduate, was in charge of the main surgical unit for the division. The two were set up in an old French Adrian Barracks building on the east bank of the Moselle River at Millery. There was space for 200 patients. It became the primary 92nd Division triage hospital. Operating teams with an x-ray machine were located there.[13]

Curtis and others in his medical unit treated the horrific wounds of trench warfare largely caused by artillery (gas and shrapnel) and machine guns. Army reports tell of the carnage he and other doctors encountered, and the lightening spread of the influenza pandemic that would reach its height just before the great Meuse-Argonne offensive in September 1918.

Following his return to the United States in early 1919, Curtis was discharged on March 9, 1919.

Career

Back in Washington, D.C., after the war, Dr. Curtis returned to his medical practice. He was proud of his military service and ever after he was helpful to wounded veterans. In 1922 Dr. Curtis returned to France for further medical study at the University of Paris. In 1923 he addressed the Association of Former Interns of Freedmen's Hospital on "Hardships of European Post-Graduate Study." In 1925 he was a clinical instructor in surgery at the Howard

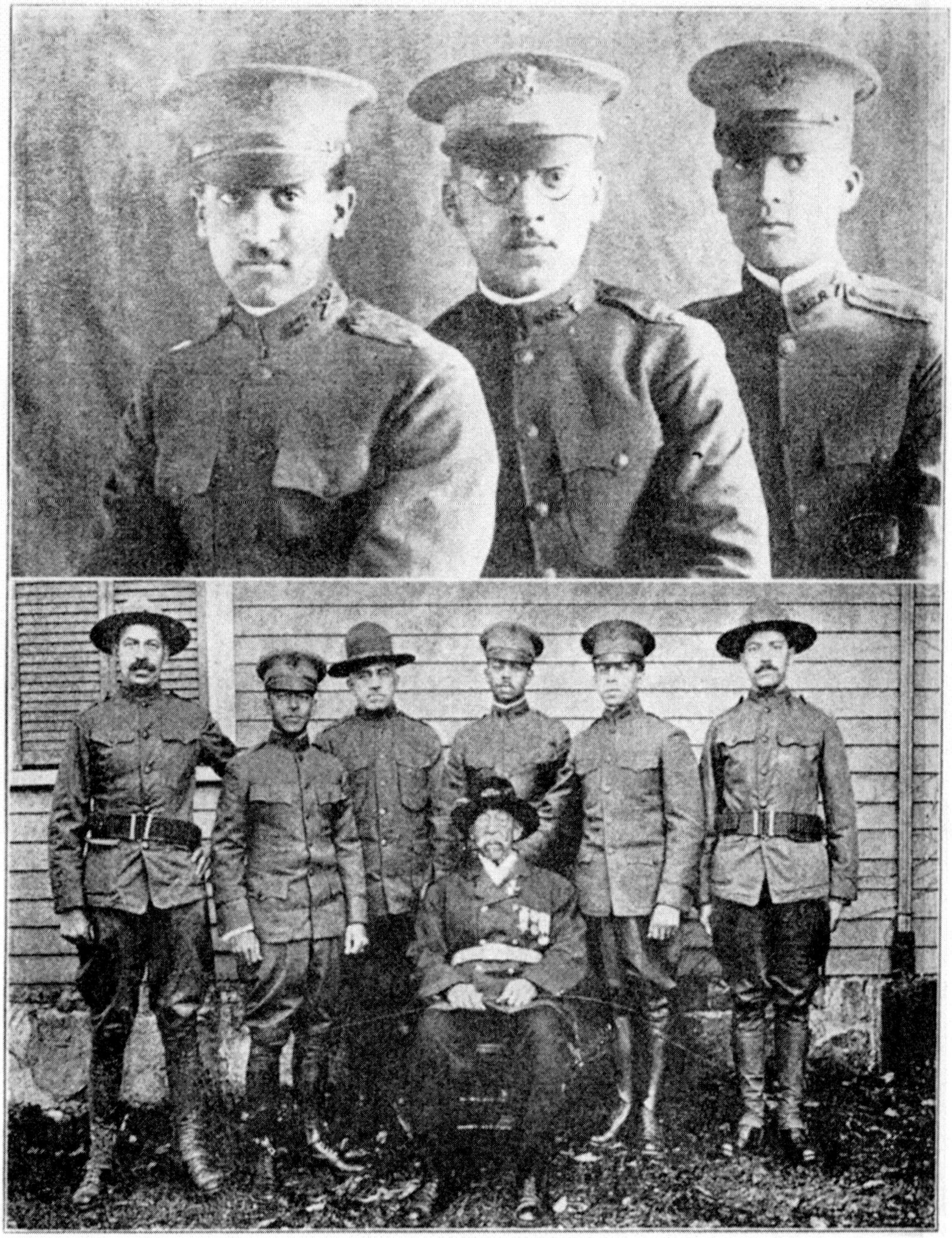

Above—The Curtis brothers, three sons of Dr. and Mrs. A. M. Curtis, Washington, D. C., commissioned as Officers in United States Army. *Left to Right*—A. Maurice Curtis, Medical Reserve Corps; Arthur L. Curtis, 368th Medical Corps; Merrill H. Curtis, 349th Field Artillery, all First Lieutenants.

Below—The Gould family of fighters. Seated in front is Wm. B. Gould of East Dedham, Mass., a veteran of the Civil War. Standing are his six sons who have also served their country. *Left to Right*—Lawrence W. Gould, 1st Lt. James E. Gould, Major Wm. B. Gould, Jr., Lt Herbert R. Gould, 1st Lt. Ernest M Gould, and Frederick C. Gould

The Curtis family in World War I (Emmett J. Scott, *Scott's Official History of the American Negro in World War I*, 1919).

University School of Medicine and a visiting surgeon at the Freedmen's Hospital. He was also an associated surgeon in the Curtis Private Surgical Sanitarium. Whatever the hardships of European post-graduate study he had encountered, he returned to France to study again in 1926.

In 1924, despite Curtis' service to the nation, racial housing discrimination was enforced against his wife, Helen Curtis, as she attempted to purchase a residence in Washington, D.C., on S Street, NW, in a white neighborhood. The celebrated case went to court and was decided with the District Court of Appeals holding that the "color line" could legally be drawn in restricting the sale of real estate, and that "white property owners who fear an invasion of colored residents could bind themselves not to transfer property to colored persons."[14] The District of Columbia court still reflected fears held in the south and elsewhere.

Curtis's political connections were obvious because in 1925, Dr. Curtis was named to the Medical Aid Committee for the inaugural parade of Republican president Coolidge.[15]

Father and son joined forces for a demonstration surgery at the Pennsylvania state medics annual meeting in 1929. Curtis administered a spinal anesthetic for this thyroidectomy, and his father performed the surgery. The news coverage of the event describes his father as having been the "subject of national renown for the past 35 years and is known throughout the nation as one of the 'fathers of surgery.'"[16]

When his mother (Namah G. Curtis) died in 1935, her obituary mentions that her physician husband and children survived her. Three of their sons would go on to practice medicine.[17]

Dr. Curtis' focus was always on following in his father's greatness in the field of medicine, which he did successfully until he fell ill and died in Castle Point, New York, at the age of 46, succumbing to chronic pulmonary tuberculosis. He is buried with his brother Merrill in the World War I section of Arlington National Cemetery—Section 4, Site 2986-B.

Notes

1. Arthur Bunyan Caldwell, *History of the American Negro and His Institutions*, Washington, D.C. Edition, Vol. VI (Atlanta, 1922) 55.
2. R. W. Logan and M. R. Winston, *Dictionary of American Negro Biography* (New York: Norton, 1927) 141.
3. Copy of Curtis' original handwritten thesis entitled "The Immigration Problem" provided by Richard Teller, Archivist & Asst. Librarian, Williston, May 18, 2015.
4. The Williston Northampton School Archives, Easthampton, Massachusetts, by Richard Teller, Archivist & Asst. Librarian.
5. "Son of A. M. Curtis," *Washington Bee*, March 23, 1917, Vol. 26, Issue 43, 8.
6. Copy of Letter dated April 30, 1928, from Dr. Arthur L. Curtis to Professor Sidney N. Morse provided by Richard Teller, Archivist & Asst. Librarian, Williston, May 18, 2015.
7. Hoopedianba.com (accessed October 2, 2013).
8. "Son of A. M. Curtis," *Washington Bee*, March 23, 1917, Vol. 26, Issue 43, 56.
9. http://www.aaregistry.org/historic_events/view/first-black-medical-society-founded (accessed November 16, 2012).
10. "Interesting News Nation's Capitol, Dr. Curtis Performs Successful Operation on Son," *Savannah Tribune*, Mar, 18, 1916, Vol. 31, Issue 19, 1.
11. Arthur Bunyan Caldwell, *History of the American Negro and His Institutions*, 56.
12. Copy of Letter dated Dec. 4th, 1917, from 1st Lieut. Arthur L. Curtis to Dr. Joseph Sawyer provided by Richard Teller, Archivist & Asst. Librarian, Williston Seminary.
13. U.S. Army Medical Department, Office of Medical History, Vol. VIII, Field Operations, Chapter IV, Medical Services of the Division in Combat (Washington, D.C.: GPO, 1925) history.amedd.army.mil (accessed April 23, 2015).
14. "'Color-Line' in Transfers Held Legal," *Pittsburgh Courier*, June 14, 1924, 1.
15. "Committees Named for Inaugural," *The Washington Post* (1923–1954); March 1, 1925, S9.
16. "State Medics Hold Constructive Sessions Here," *Pittsburgh Courier*, June 22, 1929, 9.
17. "Mrs. N. Curtis, Wife of Dr. Curtis, Dies Suddenly," *The New York Age*, Nov. 30, 1935, 1.

William T. Darnell

15 April 1883–28 May 1951
Jenner Medical College, 1908

Roots and Education

J. Turner Darnell was one of the best-known horse trainers in Ohio. From his farm in Wilmington, he was credited with having developed some of the best "steppers" to ever perform in the state. He owned some fast horses, too. "Ebony Todd" was said to have done a furlong in 18 seconds. He also trained racehorses for other owners and was known to always "deliver the goods." As a youth he attended grammar school in Wilmington and then worked in a grocery store and later opened his own restaurant before getting into training horses as a full-time career. He married Eliza

Jane Thompson and soon three children had joined the family—William T., Ethel May and Vernon. Only Vernon continued with horses.[1] J.T. was an active Republican and served as a delegate to district party conventions. He was a prominent member of the Masonic, Odd Fellows and Knights of Pythias lodges.

But this story is not about the father. It's about his oldest son William T. Darnell. He was born in Wilmington, Ohio, on April 15, 1883. By 1900, William was 17, and his father moved the family to Union, Ohio. The town is located in the northern corner of the Miami Valley near the Stillwater River. At that time it was an agricultural community with a small downtown. William attended public school.

In the 1880s and 1890s, Chicago was home to as many as 18 medical schools including Jenner Medical College. The school had been incorporated in 1893 as a commercial enterprise and a night school.[2] Advertisements for the "oldest and best night school in existence" ran around the Midwest. The idea was a young man could work during the day and earn his medical degree at night. "Hundreds of Graduates are prepared to tell you of their success."[3] William Darnell went to Chicago and graduated from Jenner with a medical degree in 1908. One year later the school closed. Dr. Darnell stayed another year in Chicago as an intern at the Booker T. Washington hospital. Then he decided to travel to Mexico and practice there for a year. He was not happy with the politics or the weather there so he returned to Ohio.[4]

In late September 1910, Dr. Darnell was quietly married in Xenia, Ohio, to Beatrice M. Ross.[5] Beatrice was born in Missouri in 1889 and had advanced her education through two years of college, which was uncommon at the time. The couple moved into a house on Main Street where he set up his medical practice. It is likely that she helped manage his office.

In 1911, the *Xenia Daily Gazette* reports of a shooting where Dr. Darnell "was summoned and dressed Robinson's injuries."[6] At another time, the newspaper reported him treating a bad dog bite.

Then in 1912, their daughter Juanita was born. The "Colored Society" column then reported Dr. Darnell improved his residence on the corner of Main and Columbus streets, likely making room for his new daughter.[7]

The *Xenia Gazette* also covered the 1916 story of him reviving a veteran of the Spanish American War who had been stricken with heart trouble and fallen to the ground unconscious on East Market Street.[8]

When prominent Chicagoans Mr. and Mrs. Charles E. McGooden came to Wilmington to attend a funeral, they stopped as guests of Dr. Darnell who then took them to see Dayton and Columbus.[9] He and Beatrice seemed to enjoy entertaining.

In 1916, the *Gazette* covered his community activities. One was to serve as assistant to Dr. H. R. Hawkins with the beautiful baby contest held in conjunction with the Farmers' Fall Festival.[10]

On July 10, 1917, the *Gazette* reported Dr. Darnell had passed his examination and qualified for service as a first lieutenant in the U.S. Army Medical Reserve Corps and expected to be called at any time.[11] The next month the *Gazette* reported on a surprise affair at the doctor's home on East Main Street, arranged by the Maple Leaf Club. There were a number of impromptu speeches including one by Colonel Charles Young, a leading African American military hero who had been expected to lead the 92nd Division but was declared too old. Colonel Young spoke about "things that help make a true soldier."[12]

Military Service

At the age of 34 on August 31, 1917, Dr. Darnell reported to Fort Des Moines for training at the army's Medical Officers Training Camp. He was then assigned to the 317th Sanitary (Medical) Train at Camp Funston, Kansas. Before leaving for France in mid–1918, he was assigned to the medical detachment of the 349th Machine Gun Battalion. After its arrival in France, his battalion entered the St. Dié sector for a time of intensive combat training. On September 2, it repulsed an enemy raid at La Fontenelle. It was held in reserve during the first phase of the Meuse-Argonne offensive.

On October 10, the entire 92nd Division

moved to Pont-à-Mousson. By November 1, 1918, Lieutenant Darnell, still with the 317th Sanitary Train, was now Captain Darnell and in charge of surgery. On November 10, as the fighting was ending, the division advanced, capturing 710 prisoners. It inflicted many casualties on the Germans but also saw a number of its own men dead and wounded.[13] Following the November 11 armistice, Captain Darnell remained overseas until February 22, 1919, when his unit boarded the *Aquitania*, an English vessel, for the return trip to the United States. In March, the *Gazette* reports Captain Darnell arrived safely in New York. He was stationed briefly at Camp Upton on Long Island before being honorably discharged on April 5 and heading home.[14]

Career

By summer of 1919, Dr. and Mrs. Darnell were invited by a citizens group of Middletown, Ohio, to relocate there. The *Xenia Gazette* reported, "his friends and acquaintances here regret their leaving but hope that they will prosper."[15]

The couple moved to nearby Middletown and bought the home that they would inhabit for the rest of their lives at 601 Yankee Road. The doctor opened an office at 812 South Main Street. Over the years he built an excellent practice from his office on Main Street. He would also serve on the staff of the Middletown Hospital.

Dr. Darnell took an interest in politics. In 1924, he joined a group of African American leaders of the community to form the Butler County Colored Voters' League. The league promoted greater participation in all elections, especially presidential. Every section of the county was represented. All candidates were up for discussion.[16] In 1928, Dr. Darnell was elected president of the group.[17]

In 1935, elections for the Middletown city commission took a twist. It was the first time a minister, a black man and a woman had ever run for city office. The black man was Dr. W. T. Darnell. It was also the first time 13 citizens had taken out petitions to run for four posts. Darnell managed to gather 566 votes. The leading incumbent garnered 6,251 votes, and all four posts went to white men. The town was clearly not ready for change.[18]

Dr. Darnell was active in the Buckeye State Medical, Dental and Pharmaceutical Association, serving as its medical corresponding secretary in 1939. He was also a long-standing member of the National Medical Association. He believed in the "Big Brothers Club," whose members he entertained at a luncheon in 1927.[19]

And, he never forgot his military experience. In 1925, Captain Darnell was named chairman of the executive committee that organized the Ohio Reunion of the Association of Colored Ex-Service Men of the 92nd and 93rd Divisions.[20]

Dr. Darnell died at Middletown Hospital of coronary thrombosis (heart attack) on May 28, 1951. He was 68 years of age. After his death, Beatrice continued to live in their home on Yankee Road for a number of years before moving to Montgomery, Illinois, where she died in 1987 at the age of 98.

John Quincy Adams said, "If your actions inspire others to dream more, learn more, do more and become more, you are a leader." Dr. William T. Darnell led his troops and his community by example. He left a significant legacy to Middletown, Ohio.

Notes

1. Albert J. Brown, History of Clinton County, Ohio (Indianapolis, IN: B. F. Bowen & Company, 1915) 394.
2. Winton U. Solberg, *Reforming Medical Education: The University of Illinois College of Medicine* (Urbana: University of Illinois Press, 2009) 20.
3. Ad in *Milwaukee Journal*, August 21, 1909, 4.
4. Albert J. Brown, History of Clinton County, Ohio, 394.
5. "Personals," *Chicago Defender*, October 1, 1910, 4.
6. "Old Man Shot Without Provocation," *Xenia Daily Gazette*, April 19, 1911, 8.
7. *Ibid.*, "Colored Society," October 17, 1912, 5.
8. *Ibid.*, August 21, 1916, 17.
9. "Prominent Chicagoans Touring Ohio," *Chicago Defender*, July 17, 1915, 1.
10. "Xenia Blossoms Forth," *Xenia Daily Gazette*, October 14, 1916, 8.
11. *Ibid.*, July 10, 1917, 8.
12. "Colored News," *Xenia Daily Gazette*, August 18, 1917, 17.
13. http://www.wattpad.com/19066-history-of-the-american-negro-in-the-great-world?p=92 (accessed October 1, 2013).
14. *Ibid.*
15. "East End News," *Xenia Evening Gazette*, September 11, 1919, 3.
16. "Colored Voters to Rally Friday," *The Journal News*, October 15, 1924, 1.

17. *Ibid.*, "Colored Voters League Formed," September 28, 1928, 17.
18. "Incumbents Win by Wide Margin," *The Journal News*, November 6, 1935, 15.
19. "Colored News," *Hamilton Daily News*, April 16, 1927, 15.
20. *Ibid.*, "Former Xenian to Head Association, November 21, 1925, 3.

Julian DAWSON

20 March 1888–14 May 1955
Northwestern University, 1914

Roots and Education

Dawson was born in Albany, Georgia. He was one of seven children (Patti Lee, Wallace, William, Julian, Janie May, Blanch, and Lillian) born to Levi and Rebecca Gill Dawson. His father was a barber and his mother a seamstress.[1]

After graduating from Fisk University in Nashville in 1910 (with honors and in three years[2]), he attended Northwestern University Medical School in Chicago and graduated in 1914. He then entered general practice in Jacksonville, Illinois. A short time later, and still single, he moved his practice to Galesburg, Illinois, to 1089 Grand Avenue. He was a member of the Congregational Church, the Masons, and the Alpha Phi Alpha fraternity.[3]

Military Service

Dawson volunteered for the U.S. Army's Medical Officers Reserve Corps in 1916. He was called to active service in August 1917. He finished at the head of his Medical Officers Training Camp class at Fort Des Moines, and was promoted to captain (on the recommendation of the camp commander, Lieutenant Colonel Bingham). He was assigned as regimental surgeon, 365th Infantry Regiment of the 92nd Division. On November 29, 1917, during his leave before serving in France in 1918, he married Aline. They would have four children (Julian Jr., Alice R., Ira, and Irma).[4]

It was not until 1944 that the *Chicago Defender* newspaper wrote of Dawson's First World War service with the headline "Dawson Won Acclaim as Both Doctor and Soldier." The article reads:

> A front-line French station hospital buried on the reverse side of a mountain on the St. Dié sector shook and shivered as German shells fell on its well-protected shell-proof roof, during a bitter battle of the last World War.
>
> Inside stocky-built Capt. Julian Dawson, brilliant chief medical officer of the 365th Infantry, braced himself as his dugout trembled; and calmly—though rapidly—continued surgery on the worst cases which were brought in from the firing line.
>
> Captain Dawson didn't have to accept his dangerous assignment. As regimental surgeon, he could have stayed back at headquarters. But the surgeon of the second battalion, which was bearing the brunt of the attack, had been wounded. And up there fighting was the captain's own brother, Lieutenant William Dawson, now congressman of the Illinois First district.[5]

After serving in numerous campaigns in France with the 92nd Division, Dawson returned to the United States and was discharged in 1919. He joined the famous "Old Eighth" Infantry, Illinois National Guard, in 1922.

Throughout his life, Dr. Dawson continued to serve with the Illinois National Guard. He was promoted to lieutenant colonel and assigned as the commanding officer of the 184th Field Artillery from 1940 until the unit was

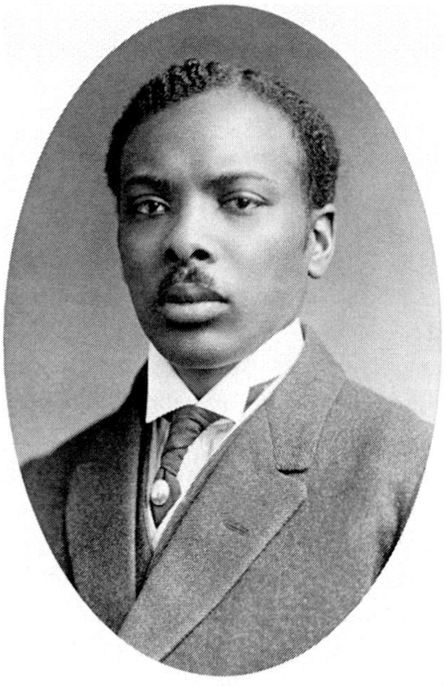

Julian Dawson, graduation 1914, Northwestern University Medical School (courtesy Galter Health Sciences Library Special Collections, Feinberg School of Medicine, Northwestern University, Chicago, Illinois).

called into federal service in 1941. The *Chicago Defender* reported a shake up in the "Old Eighth" and Dawson was retired with the rank of brigadier general. He wanted very much to take the unit into service during World War II, but he was not in good health, suffering a cardiac condition. Much to his dismay, Lieutenant Colonel Randall took the unit into service.[6]

Career

Early in his career, Dr. Dawson was appointed a junior surgeon on staff at Provident Hospital, but by 1923, he decided he needed more post-graduate work to advance at the hospital.[7] He pursued his post-graduate work in Vienna, Austria. Dawson credited his wife Aline for making this possible. "I sent my Army base pay home regularly. When I returned, I found my wife had saved every penny of it. This was my nest egg and enabled me to arrange finances so I could go abroad in 1923." The Dawsons traveled to the University of Zuweisen in Vienna, Austria, with two small children. Julian Jr. was three and Alice was 10½ months. Aline gave birth to their third child three weeks after arriving in Vienna.[8]

Dr. Dawson returned to the surgical staff of Cook County's Provident Hospital. He was not afraid to try new methods. In 1928, a *Chicago Defender* article was headlined "Patient Dies But Surgeons Restore Life." In the midst of an emergency case on the ruptured stomach of William Coffey, the patient stopped breathing and his heart ceased to beat. "The surgeons (Dr. Dawson with Dr. McDonald assisting) injected adrenalin chloride and strychnine. Within two minutes Coffey's heart began to beat." Ultimately, the patient was expected to make a full recovery.[9] Heroics and his effective and efficient work were rewarded with rapid advancement. He rose from a member of the outpatient department to senior medical staff and director of the department. He was named senior attending surgeon in 1936.[10] Dr. Dawson ultimately received a Rosenwald Fund fellowship and continued his studies.

In 1951, due to ill health, Dr. Dawson retired from the active staff and was named "Emeritus, Senior Attending Surgeon."

Provident continues today as a community teaching hospital in Southside Chicago. Its emergency room is the third busiest in the city, serving more than 50,000 persons a year.

In 1952, Dr. Dawson was driving himself on Main Street in St. Joseph, Missouri, when he suffered a heart attack. By the time the fire department resuscitator squad arrived, he was on his way to the hospital in an ambulance.[11] He was back home in Chicago after a short stay.

On May 14, 1955, the *Chicago Defender* reported that final rites were held in Chicago for Brigadier General Julian Dawson (retired) former commander of the 184th Field Artillery Regiment of the Illinois National Guard. He died at his home at the age of 68. His wife Aline, four children and eight grandchildren survived him.[12]

Julian Dawson was a highly respected medical and military man. He rose to the top of both professions in the Chicago area. He spent his life studying, finding new and better ways to help his fellow man. In the last years of his life, his poor health forced him to retire from both careers. His military connection was the one he missed most.

Notes

1. 1900 U.S. Federal Census.
2. Brooks, "Dawson Won Acclaim as Both Doctor and Soldier," *Chicago Defender*, May 13, 1944, 10.
3. John L. Thompson, *History and Views of Colored Officers Training Camp for 1917 at Fort Des Moines, Iowa* (Des Moines: The Bystander, 1917) 44.
4. 1930 U.S. Federal Census.
5. Brooks, "Dawson Won Acclaim as Both Doctor and Soldier," *Chicago Defender*, May 13, 1944, 10.
6. "Shake Up Old Eighth on Induction Eve," *Chicago Defender*, January 11, 1941, 1.
7. *Ibid.*
8. *Ibid.*
9. "Patient Dies but Surgeons Restore Life," *Chicago Defender, March* 3, 1928, 10.
10. *Ibid.*
11. "Doctor Leaves Hospital After Heart Attack," *News-Palladium*, July 18, 1942, 3.
12. Colin, "Rep. Dawson's Brother Dies," *Chicago Defender*, May 14, 1955, 1.

Oscar Wilson DEVAUGHN

14 November 1883–11 June 1942
Meharry Medical College, 1915

Roots and Education

DeVaughn was born in Douglasville, Georgia, to Sandy DeVaughn. By the age of 16, he lived with his sister and brother-in-law in Cold Water, Calhoun County, Alabama. He was in his 20s when he began his college career at Morris Brown College in Atlanta, Georgia. It is a historically black college affiliated with the African Methodist Episcopal Church. He went on to Meharry Medical School and graduated in 1915. Dr. DeVaughn passed the Georgia state boards the same year and opened medical practices in Greenville and Manchester, Georgia. By the time he volunteered for service in the U.S. Army Medical Reserve Corps, Dr. DeVaughn had married Eugenia and moved to Oakland, California. The couple resided at 1608 Seventh Street.

Military Service

First Lieutenant DeVaughn was 30 years old when he reported for basic training on August 27, 1917, at the U.S. Army's Medical Officers Training Camp (MOTC) at Fort Des Moines. He was there for 68 days before his transfer to Camp Meade, Maryland. He was one of eight MOTC graduates sent to Camp Meade for further training and to provide care for the African American troops of the 368th Infantry Regiment and 351st Field Artillery stationed there.

He served there for six months until June 27, 1918, when he was honorably discharged with a physical disability and sent home.

Career

Dr. DeVaughn returned to Oakland, California, and passed his license to practice medicine. He and his wife Eugenia lived at 2809 Stanton Street in Berkeley when his license was revoked on July 8, 1930. In 1931, the judgment was set aside and he resumed his practice.

During the 1930s, many poor and black women resorted to self-induced abortions, but these had a high rate of infection and hemorrhage. The Depression years make vivid the relationship between economics and reproduction. Women had abortions on a massive scale. "Women reported having no complications after their abortions in 91 percent of those performed by doctors."[1]

Abortion was illegal so doctors would extract oaths of secrecy from patients seeking an abortion or seeking help after a botched abortion attempt. Relatively few doctors were charged under the abortion laws, but prosecutors went after cases where the patient was killed or seriously injured. When abortion providers were convicted, they could be fined or face periods of incarceration.[2] Dr. DeVaughn was one of these doctors.

In March of 1934, William Fernandez sued Dr. DeVaughn and his partner Dr. Busch for $150,000. Fernandez claimed the doctors were negligent in treating his wife. She died after the two doctors treated her for five days for blood poisoning.[3] The case was ultimately dismissed. In the article on the suit, the *Plain Dealer* newspaper referred to Dr. DeVaughn and Dr. Busch as "prominent in their professions and in the social and civic life of the bay cities."[4]

In the late spring of 1934, Dr. DeVaughn was back in court. This time he was convicted of criminal abortion and subordination of perjury of witness May Perata. He was found guilty and on June 27, sent to San Quentin prison for an indeterminate sentence. He was there for seven years.

During his incarceration his wife Eugenia stayed in Alameda, adjacent to West Oakland, and she took in four boarders at their home at 1228 Eighth Street. When he was paroled on June 2, 1941, he and Eugenia moved up the street to 1234. They were there when he registered for the World War II draft early in 1942. At the time, he was 57, and worked at the West Oakland Pharmacy. He was still on parole when he died later that year.

NOTES

1. Leslie J. Reagan, *When Abortion Was a Crime* (Google eBook, Berkeley: University of California Press, 1996) 138.
2. Jeanne Flavin, *Race Criminals, Our Bodies, Our Crimes: The Policing of Women's Reproduction in America* (Google eBook), 14.
3. "Asks 150 for Wife's Death," *Plaindealer*, March 16, 1934, 2.
4. *Ibid.*

Edgar Arthur DRAPER

12 May 1886–17 November 1956
University of Pennsylvania, 1912

Roots and Education

Edgar Draper was born to Justina (Jessie) and Joseph W. Draper in Philadelphia, Pennsylvania. His father was a hotel waiter. There were three other children in the family, Bertha, Frederica and William. All the children were baptized in the Crucifixion Episcopal Church. The family lived at 2109 West Fitzwater Street. After completing elementary school, Edgar graduated from the city's Central High School in 1906. Central was established for exceptionally gifted students and granted a collegiate degree. He went on to the University of Pennsylvania for two years and then on to its medical school.[1]

In 1912, he graduated second in his class from Perelman School of Medicine at the University of Pennsylvania. This is the oldest and widely regarded as one of the top medical schools in the United States.[2] He then interned at Mercy-Douglass Hospital from 1912 to 1914.

After graduation Dr. Draper appeared to be looking for a city for his practice in the mid–Atlantic. He tried Baltimore, Maryland, and Williamsburg, Virginia, before settling in Cape May, New Jersey. Cape May claims to be America's first seaside resort. The National Park Service reports, "Cape May has one of the largest collections of late 19th century frame buildings left in the United States."[3]

By the early 1900s, Cape May was easily accessible by train from Philadelphia. It and nearby Whitestown had significant year-round black populations and were summer destinations for those living in Philadelphia, Baltimore and Washington, D.C., so it was likely not unfamiliar to Dr. Draper. In 1914, he became the first African American doctor in Cape May County.[4]

His medical practice was so well received that the following year he was invited to be the toastmaster at a dinner honoring Dr. William Edward Burghardt DuBois, co-founder of the NAACP and one of the most influential African Americans before World War I. DuBois was an occasional summer visitor to Cape May for several years. This event was held at the Hotel Dale, located at the corner of Lafayette and Jefferson streets. It was considered an important hotel then, especially for the African American community, at a time when segregation still prevailed.[5]

Military Service

In August of 1917, at the age of 30, Dr. Draper enlisted for service in the U.S. Army Medical Reserve Corps. He was commissioned a first lieutenant and reported for duty at the Medical Officers Training Camp in Fort Des Moines on September 8, 1917. On November 3 he was sent to Camp Funston, Kansas, with the 317th Sanitary Train of the 92nd Division, where he was assigned to the 367th Ambulance Company.

After arriving in France in July 1918, the 367th had no ambulances for several months and wasn't engaged in combat until late in the war, thus the duties of those assigned to this unit were more clinical. Draper and his medics were concerned with maintaining the health and readiness of the soldiers and oversaw the sanitary arrangements, waste disposal and the water supply. Much of the available fresh water near the battlefields of France had been contaminated with a gas-forming bacillus so the medical units attached to the sanitary trains were taught how to test and treat water with hypo chloride of lime to make it potable.[6] These were not inconsequential responsibilities. It was also not always easy as the men were not accustomed to the taste of chlorinated water so considerable encouragement and patience was required to get them to drink the treated water.[7]

Draper served with the 367th Ambulance Company until shortly before the end of the war when he was transferred to the 367th Field Hospital in November 1918, where his duties involved caring for wounded and sick soldiers being transported to debarkation locations and then home to the United States. Draper reported to Dr. Louis T. Wright who was in charge of the surgical wards. Wright described an incident in which a misunderstanding occurred regarding treatment for an officer's finger injury, which Draper had not dressed as directed. Upon inquiry he concluded that Draper had received conflicting instructions and had actually done his best.[8]

When Draper returned to the United States after the war, he was honorably discharged on March 21, 1919.

Career

He married twice, first to Pauline Gaskins, by whom he had a daughter, Audrey. This first marriage ended in divorce. On March 9, 1929, he married Katherine Ellen Shumate. They were together for the rest of his life. They had no children. For several years his mother Justina and sister Frederica lived with the couple at the house at 811 Jefferson Street in Cape May.

In the 1920s African-Americans comprised about 30 percent of Cape May's population and owned nearly 60 businesses in the town's central district.[9]

Dr. Draper was a skilled diagnostician. This plus his "outstanding personality and character were such as to overcome the prejudices of that time and to give him patients of all income levels.... He is best remembered for his devotion to those, both black and white who were in the lowest income brackets."[10] In addition to his medical practice, he was a member of St. Simon Cyrenean P.E. Church in Philadelphia, the American Legion, the Masons and the La Malta Social Club.

Dr. Draper had practiced in Cape May for more than 30 years when he died of a cerebral hemorrhage at the age of 68 in Cape May's Burdette Tomlin Memorial Hospital. His funeral took place at St. Simon's Church with the Reverend J. Logan, Sr., officiating. He is buried in Eden Cemetery in Collingdale, Pennsylvania, with a military headstone. After his death his wife Katherine moved to Washington, D.C., where she lived at 123 Randolph Place.

On August 12, 1971, 15 years after his death, Dr. Draper was honored when an extension of Washington Street was dedicated to him. A plaque commemorating his service to the community is still there.[11]

Notes

1. Edgar Arthur Draper, MD, *The Cape May County Magazine of History and Genealogy*, June 1971, 467.
2. http://en.wikipedia.org/wiki/Perelman_School_of_Medicine_at_the_University_of_Pennsylvania (accessed October 21, 2014).
3. http://en.wikipedia.org/wiki/Cape_May_Historic_District (accessed October 22, 2014).
4. http://www.shorenewstoday.com/snt/news/index.php/cape-may/history/30083-bizarre-history-of-cape-may-g-african-americans-made-important-contributions-to-cape-may.html (accessed October 22, 2014).
5. *Ibid.*
6. "Medical History of the 92nd Division," Office of the Surgeon General, Washington, D.C., Record 314.7–2, National Archives, College Park, MD.
7. *Ibid.*
8. Wright, Louis T. "*I Remember*" (unpublished autobiographical typescript) Moorland-Spingarn Research Center, Howard University, Washington, D.C., Undated, 89–90.
9. http://www.capemay.com/Editorial/march08/afroamericanhistory.html (accessed October 22, 2014).
10. "Edgar Arthur Draper, MD," *The Cape May County Magazine of History and Genealogy*, 468.
11. *Ibid.*

William Holmes DYER

29 August 1886–21 January 1958
University of Illinois, 1916

Roots and Education

"Billie" Dyer was one of seven children born to Alfred and Laura Ward Dyer. His paternal grandmother was the daughter of a Cherokee Indian and a white woman who came to Illinois from North Carolina. His grandfather Aaron Dyer was a slave who migrated to Springfield, Illinois, via the Underground Railroad.[1] Billie's father, Alfred, made his living tending furnaces and working at the lumber

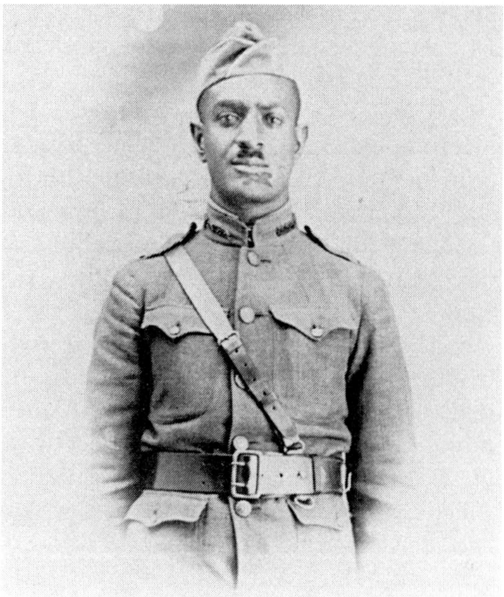

Lieutenant William H. Dyer (courtesy Schomburg Center for Research in Black Culture, New York Public Library, Astor, Lenox and Tilden Foundations).

company. Alfred also ran the Sunday school of the town's African Methodist Episcopal Church. Billie's mother was born a slave to the wife of a Union general.[2] She would not talk about her childhood. She was the one who always expected more of Billie.

Billie's brightness was recognized by John Hartz who was white and four years his senior. The two became friends, and when John Hartz went off to college, he wrote Billie every week. At the age of 21, John Hartz took a job with the railroad and he soon lost his life in a tragic rail accident. John's father, Captain David Hartz, knew of the friendship and after his son's death, took to counseling and supporting Billie toward his lifelong goal of becoming a surgeon.[3]

It wasn't until 1910 that Billie enrolled at Lincoln College in his hometown of Lincoln, Illinois. At the age of 24, he was one of the older freshmen. In his biography of Dr. Dyer, author Clif Cleaveland says, "I presumed that Billie had had to work for several years to afford collegiate study."[4] Dyer went on to the University of Illinois College of Medicine in Chicago, and graduated at the age of 30 in 1916.[5] From there he went to Kansas City where he interned at the Old General Hospital. He completed his internship in 1917, just as America entered into the First World War.

Military Service

Dr. Dyer lived at 315 Nebraska Avenue in Kansas City, Kansas, when he volunteered and was commissioned as a first lieutenant in the Army Medical Reserve Corps. When Lieutenant Dyer left his hometown of Lincoln for military training at Fort Des Moines, Iowa, three hundred people saw him off at the railroad station. He arrived at the Medical Officers Training Camp on September 24, 1917. After completing his training on November 11, he was assigned as a medical officer to the 92nd Division's 317th Ammunition Train at Camp Funston, Kansas.

Before leaving for France he reconnected with Bessie Bradley of Alton, Illinois. The two had met during his internship in Kansas City. In June 1918, the two were secretly married.[6] She was a teacher and artist. The marriage

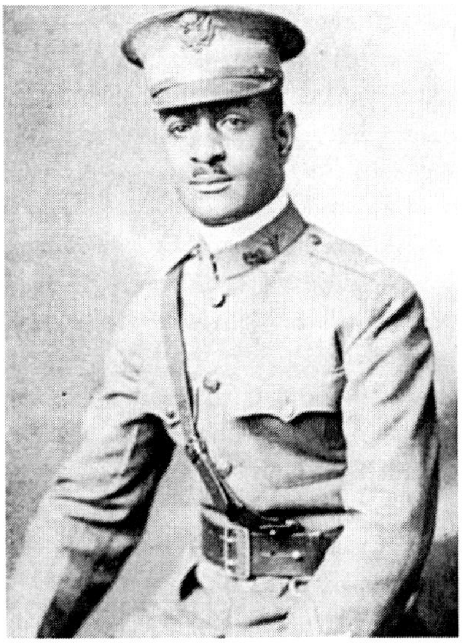

Lieutenant William H. Dyer (courtesy Dyer grand-niece Priscilla Florence and D. Leigh Henson, PhD, Missouri State University).

would last 40 years, until his death in 1958. There would be no children.

Dyer served with the ammunition train throughout the war. He wrote a lengthy personal memoir of his war experience to his wife. It can be found at the Lincoln Public Library in Lincoln, Illinois. Library director Richard Sumrall reported real estate agent Jim Woods found the diary in Dallas, Texas. Mr. Woods realized the significance of the document and forwarded it to the Lincoln Public Library.

On June 15, 1918, Lieutenant Dyer wrote of boarding the old German passenger vessel, the *Covington*, at Hoboken, New Jersey. There was a crew of about 800, and the *Covington* carried nearly 5,000 troops past the Statue of Liberty and on to France. On June 16, Lieutenant Dyer received his first assignment, physical inspections of some 600 men. The troops were safely deposited in France, but the Germans sank the *Covington* on its return voyage.

On August 23, 1918, Dyer wrote of the convoy's trip from Bruyères to Raon L'Étape. "No headlights were allowed as they travelled at night on these muddy roads. All along the roadside and in the woods were graves of brave French soldiers who in 1914 had met the German assault and died. Houses with roofs blown off or completely demolished stood along the roadside giving the whole country the appearance of desolation and destruction."

At the outset of the great Meuse-Argonne campaign, Dyer wrote on September 25, 1918, "The old woods ... trembled as if by earthquake, the flashes of cannon lighting up the inside of our eyes and our ears were deafened." At the hospital, Lieutenant Dyer saw "a stream of ambulances bringing wounded soldiers." The dead "were also being brought back, on trucks, piled like cordwood and dripping blood."

Still later, Lieutenant Dyer wrote of the deprivations the African Americans suffered. When they moved up to Ste. Menehould in the Argonne Forest region where the greatest American battle of World War I occurred, "no accommodations here, not even water to drink or cook with. Mud everywhere, over shoe tops. While camped in this wet filthy woods many of our boys became ill from the dampness, cold and exposure; thereby, causing me much worry and work, caring for them."[7]

Although the war ended on November 11, Lieutenant Dyer's medical team didn't get a break. On December 15, he was awakened to administer medical care to those who survived the collision of a passenger train and a train full of French soldiers on their way home. He and his medical team set up an aid-station and worked all night caring for the survivors.[8]

The following months were busy caring for the soldiers sick from exposure to constant cold and wet. He too was ill with influenza for a week and later was very ill before leaving with his unit for Le Mans.[9] During the journey, he found he was "having difficulty walking.... He took off his boots and discovered his feet were frozen." On February 22, 1919, the 317th finally boarded the *Aquitania* for the trip home.[10]

Career

Dr. Dyer returned to Kansas City and established his medical practice. For many years, his office was located at 434 Quindaro Boulevard in Kansas City, Kansas. He initially returned to the staff of the Old General Hospital. During his 40 years practicing medicine in Kansas City, he was a pioneer and worked on the staffs of Bethany, Douglass, St. Margaret's and Providence hospitals. For many years he also worked as a surgeon for the Santa Fe Railroad and the Kansas City Kansas Police Department.

In 1953, he was honored by his home city of Lincoln, Illinois, at its centennial celebration as one of its "Ten Most Distinguished Men." He was the only African American. In 1955 the Alumni Association of Lincoln College honored him for his achievements and meritorious service. In 1956, at the age of 70, the mayor of Kansas City, Paul F. Mitchum, commended Dr. Dyer for handling most of the police cases involving African Americans. The mayor accused many other physicians, who received $82.50 a month to be on the police surgeon rosters, as shirking their duties.[11]

By the mid–1950s, the workload was having its toll on Dr. Dyer. He wrote from Kansas City to Hugh Hartz, brother of his childhood friend John and son of his mentor Captain David Hartz. "In the last four months I have been put on the staffs of three of the major hospitals in our city. I thought at first it was an honor but with the increase in activities, which such appointments entail, my work has increased twofold. Since it is the first time one of my race has had such appointments, I have been

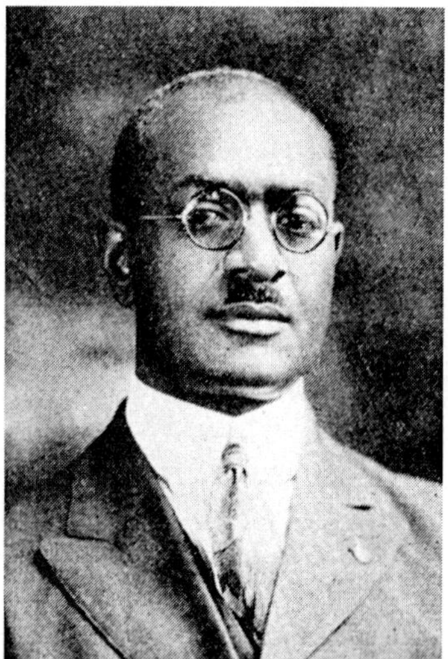

Dr. William H. Dyer (national pictorial, members of the National Medical Association, 1925, courtesy Kansas City Public Library).

working diligently to make good, thereby keeping those doors open."[12]

Two years later, Dr. Dyer died of a heart attack. His body was found in his wrecked car near his office. "There was 15 inches of snow on the day he died. Seven people died of heart attacks in the metropolitan area after shoveling snow that day. For Dr. Dyer to drive from his home and almost make it to his office took much effort and determination. It would not be surprising to me if he had to shovel himself out of the snow drift(s) as he traveled to work. That same effort and determination is probably part of the reason he had such a noteworthy medical career in this community."[13]

His body was returned to his hometown of Lincoln for burial. His wife Bessie joined him there the following year. Dyer's contribution to the welfare of the local African American community was extremely significant for nearly 40 years.

Over the longer term, Dyer's pioneering work in Kansas City helped pave the way for future generations of African American doctors. The quality of his work and his temperament convinced some skeptical white physicians that African Americans were qualified to serve alongside them in local hospitals.

NOTES

1. William Maxwell, *Billie Dyer and Other Stories* (A Plume Book, 1993) 6.
2. *Ibid.*, 10.
3. *Ibid.*, 15.
4. Clif Cleaveland, M.D., *That Democracy Might Reign: The Story of Billie Dyer, Healers & Heroes* (American College of Physicians, 2004) 20.
5. AMA Deceased Physicians card, National Library of Medicine, Bethesda, MD.
6. Cleaveland, *That Democracy Might Reign*, 22.
7. William Maxwell, *Billie Dyer and Other Stories* (New York: Knopf, 1993) 24.
8. Cleaveland, *That Democracy Might Reign*, 27.
9. *Ibid.*, 28.
10. Maxwell, *Billie Dyer and Other Stories*, 28–29.
11. "Mayor Mitchum Cites Police Emergency Statistics," *The Kansas City Star* (Kansas City, Missouri), July 5, 1956, 27.
12. *Ibid.*, 30–31.
13. Email to the authors from Georgia Murphy, Kansas Collection Librarian, Kansas City Kansas Public Library, September 22, 2010.

William Wesley FELDER

5 June 1887–22 December 1931
University of West Tennessee, 1914

Roots and Education

This son of a farmer hailed from Davis Station in Clarendon County, South Carolina, hardly more than a crossroad in an agricultural area between Summerton and Manning. It is much the same as it was a hundred years ago. Four country roads converge from various odd angles at Davis Station. In 2013, a large cotton gin was still in operation there, and men gathered before and after work at an open-air raw wooden "refreshment" stand, coffee in the morning, stronger drink in the evening. Today the enormous bales of cotton are wrapped in colorful yellow and blue plastic sheets in preparation for transport by truck. In the past, there was a rail spur to haul the cotton bales away.

Felder was the sixth of eight children of Henry and Jane Felder. The family likely attended the Laurel Hill AME Methodist Church at 2032 M. W. Rickenbaker Road in Davis Station. It is still there and serving the needs of that community as a church and now the only store. There was no school in Davis Station when young Felder lived there so his parents would have had to find a way to get him to Summerton to attend school, or more likely, he walked the five miles. It took a lawsuit in the early 1940s to get the county to provide busing to the school. Even then, there was no bus for the children of Davis Station area to the Summerton school.[1]

Felder's higher education began when he was fortunate to attend Allen University, a historically African American college, founded by the African Methodist Episcopal Church in 1870. The school was first named Payne Institute in honor of Bishop Daniel Alexander Payne, a native South Carolinian and founder of Wilberforce University. Payne was the driving force behind the quest for an educated clergy and laity in the African Methodist Episcopal Church. The university was relocated to Columbia, South Carolina, in 1880 and renamed Allen University. Today it is located on Harden Street and is still an active private university.[2]

Felder graduated from Allen and made his way to Memphis, Tennessee, to attend medical school at the University of West Tennessee. It was founded in 1900 by physician, journalist and educator Dr. Myles Vanderhorst Lynk. It had departments of medicine, law, dentistry, pharmacy, and nursing. Dr. Fanny Kneeland, one of the first women to practice medicine in Memphis, was a member of the faculty. The Jane Terrell Baptist Hospital provided clinical training. Lynk became the first black physician in Jackson, Tennessee, and founded the first medical journal published by an African American, *The Medical and Surgical Observer*, which was published monthly from 1892 to 1894. He also published a literary magazine from 1898 to 1900. Lynk was a cofounder of the National Medical Association for African American physicians in 1895.[3] When his school closed in 1924, it had issued 216 medical degrees.

When Felder graduated in 1914, he returned to South Carolina. He took his medical licensing exam in June 1914 and failed. It was not unusual for graduates of any of the smaller private African American medical schools to fail the exams. The schools simply did not offer the labs, materials or hospital experience of the more established schools. In November, he took the exam again, passed, and was awarded his medical license by the State Board of Medical Examiners.[4]

That same year, he moved to Sumter, South Carolina, and opened his medical practice. He had returned to less than 30 miles from where he was born. He married a young woman named Maude. She had been born on December 28, 1899, in North Carolina. In 1915, she gave birth to their only daughter, Marie Felder.

Dr. Felder became an active member of the Sumter community. As early as March 1915, he was one of four local African American physicians who presented a program on Sanitation and Health to 400 local citizens.[5] Two years later in 1917, as America entered the First World War, Dr. and Mrs. Felder were settled in Sumter at 354 Manning Avenue where he was a member of the Mt. Pisgah AME Church.[6] His name was listed among 19 leading African American citizens, including three physicians, who met with other patriotic citizens at the Lincoln School on April 16 to assert their loyalty to the United States and pledge their allegiance to the flag.[7]

Military Service

He responded to the national call for African American physicians to join in the war effort and received a commission as a first lieutenant in the U.S. Army Medical Reserve Corps. He was sent to Fort Des Moines for military training in August 1917.[8] Lieutenant Felder completed his training in November and received orders to report to the 92nd Division's 317th Sanitary Train at Camp Funston, Kansas, where he was assigned to the 366th Ambulance Company. He was one of that unit's four medical officers. The other physicians were Captain Charles H. Garvin (commanding officer), Lieutenant Harvey L. Brown, and Lieutenant Romeo A. Johnson.[9] In January 1918, while stationed at Camp Funston, Felder, with many other soldiers, was confined for a time in a medical detention camp established to prevent the spread of disease. The camp, made up of tents, was very cold. There was little for the men to do. When the contagion danger finally passed, he was returned to duty on January 24. Then in April Felder fell ill for two weeks and was confined to quarters from April 8 to April 22 before being returned to duty. Unit records of the division show a number of its physicians fell ill for brief periods during their service in Kansas and in France.

He was shipped to France where his ambulance company supported combat operations of the 92nd Division from September to November 1918. Ambulance companies were established to care for and transport ill and injured soldiers. Each of the four infantry regiments in the division had an ambulance company and a field hospital. Each ambulance company consisted of 12 ambulances and was staffed with several physicians and medical support troops. The "ambulance" of the First World War bore no similarity to those 100 years later. Many were animal drawn. They, and motorized ambulances, traveled over muddy rutted roads that were usually full of other similar vehicles moving supplies to battle lines.

In combat situations these doctors treated and transported wounded and gassed soldiers from aid stations to field hospitals where they were triaged. Soldiers who were unable to walk were carried or transported on litters to the ambulances. At triage hospitals, they were treated and some were returned to their units, while others were sent from field hospitals to other rear hospitals for more treatment.

In non-combat situations, the ambulance companies established infirmaries to care for troops suffering from disease and injury. Tuberculosis, pneumonia, influenza, and venereal disease were commonly treated. As the war progressed and gas casualties were more prevalent, soldiers were taken to specialized hospitals that focused on respiratory and eye problems, and skin burns, caused by the various different kinds of gas used by the Germans.

Field conditions had poor sanitation systems and were a constant preoccupation of all the medical personnel. Maintaining combat readiness was not an easy matter given conditions in the trenches and dugouts. The water supply and food supplies were a constant source of concern. The cold and damp weather conditions in France caused much illness and constant troop movements were very challenging to all the medical personnel.

During the war, Dr. Felder witnessed and treated battle trauma, injury and disease on a much grander scale than he had or would ever see again. His experiences during his year and a half in the army accelerated his learning and advanced his skills significantly, much to the benefit of the citizens of Sumter. He arrived back in the U.S. on February 24, 1919, and was honorably discharged on March 19, 1919, to resume his practice.[10]

Career

The 1920 U.S. Census shows the family rented a house at 532 Dingle Street in downtown Sumter. Dr. Felder became active in the state Palmetto Medical, Dental and Pharmaceutical Association. This group was one of the first late 19th-century professional societies founded by African American medical professionals for socializing and sharing information on new medical discoveries and technologies. The various chapters throughout the state held monthly meetings and all met annually in April for a three-day conference. On May 1, 1920, he attended the 25th Session of the Palmetto Medical Association in Sumter, held at the Shiloh Baptist Church. The meeting was attended by 115 medical professionals from cities around the state. His presentation was entitled "Medical Service at the Front."[11]

The following ten years must have been good ones for the doctor and his family. By 1930, he, Maude and Marie (now a teenager) lived in a nice home he owned at 516 West Oakland Avenue in Sumter.

Sadly, he died the following year in December 1931 of uremia (advanced kidney disease) at age 41. Had dialysis machines or kidney transplants been available in those years, he might have enjoyed a long, productive life.

Dr. Felder was buried at Walker Cemetery on West Oakland Avenue, only a few blocks from where he lived. He rested beneath a veteran's headstone provided by the U.S. Army.[12] In 1967, his remains were moved to Arlington National Cemetery in Arlington, Virginia, where he now rests in section 44, grave 4, with his wife Maude, who survived him by 40 years. She passed away on September 25, 1972.

Their daughter Marie married a veteran of the Second World War, Charles Francis Dunston. They too now rest together at the Arlington National Cemetery.

NOTES

1. Sharron Haley, "Another Page in History Has Turned," *Clarendon Citizen*, January 30, 2012.
2. http://www.allenuniversity.edu/about-us/allens-legacy (accessed January 2, 2013).
3. http://tennesseeencyclopedia.net/entry.php?rec=818 (accessed January 2, 2013).
4. South Carolina State Board of Medical Examiners, Records of Licenses by Examination, 1894–1969, microfilmed by SC Dept. of Archives & History, 1985.
5. "Much Interest in Health," *The Watchman and Southron Newspaper*, Sumter, South Carolina, March 31, 1915, Library of Congress, Washington, D.C., Chronicling America online collection.
6. John L. Thompson, *History and Views of Colored Officers Training Camp for 1917 at Fort Des Moines, Iowa* (Des Moines: The Bystander, 1917) 50.
7. "Notice," *The Watchman and Southron Newspaper*, Sumter, SC, April 18, 1917.
8. Table of Medical Reserve Corps—Colored—Receiving Instruction, Medical Training Camp, Fort Des Moines, Iowa, RG-112, Records of the Army Surgeon General, National Archives, College Park, MD.
9. "Roster of Officers, 92nd Division, 1 November 1918, RG-120," Records of the American Expeditionary Forces (World War I), Box 6, National Archives, College Park, MD.
10. "The Official Roster of the South Carolina Sol-

diers, Sailors and Marines in the World War, 1917–1918," Vol. 2, p. 1328, South Carolina Dept. of Archives & History.

11. "Palmetto Medical Association," *The Watchman and Southron Newspaper*, Sumter, SC, May 1, 1920.

12. "U.S. Headstone Applications for Military Veterans, 1925–1963," ancestry.com.

Charles Sumner FISHER

25 January 1882–25 August 1920
Leonard Medical School, 1908

Roots and Education

Charles Sumner Fisher was born January 25, 1882, in Eufaula in Barbour County, Alabama. His parents, Warren Fisher and Flora Cooper, were married on May 15, 1873, in Eufaula. They had several children and the family later moved from Eufaula to Birmingham where Dr. Fisher's father was employed as a "common laborer."

In 1902, at age 20, Fisher graduated from the Normal School of Knoxville College in Tennessee.[1] Then, in 1908, he graduated from Leonard Medical College at Shaw University in Raleigh, North Carolina. Built in 1881, Leonard was established when medical schools were professionalizing. It was the first medical school for African Americans in the United States to offer a four-year curriculum, as well as the first four-year medical school in North Carolina.[2] Although the medical school is now closed, Leonard Hall is still part of Shaw University. Upon his graduation from medical school, Dr. Fisher married Ruth C. Keene on May 9, 1908, in Raleigh. Ruth was born in North Carolina in 1884 and was the daughter of Louisa Walden.

According to the 1909 Burlington, North Carolina, city directory, Dr. Fisher practiced medicine there from his office at 317 Worth Street. Lisa Kobrin, reference librarian at the May Memorial Library in Burlington, found "this was also the business address for a prominent local black minister and tinsmith named Spencer Thomas and his son Samuel Thomas." Cities in North Carolina and South Carolina that needed medical doctors often contacted Leonard Medical School in order to attract young physicians, and that is likely the case with Dr. Fisher. Burlington was then a growing industrial city about 60 miles west of Raleigh with textile and other mills.

In 1909, the couple's first daughter, Flora Louisa, named for Charles's mother, Flora, and Ruth's mother, Louisa, was born. A second daughter, Ada, was born several years later.

By 1912, Dr. Fisher had moved his family and his practice to Maxton, North Carolina.[3] It is likely Dr. Fisher responded to a need for a doctor and the opportunity that presented. Maxton is located in the southeastern part of the state close to the border with South Carolina. He was a member of the United Presbyterian Church, as well as the Knights of Pythias and Masons.[4] From Maxton he volunteered in 1917 for service in the First World War.[5]

Military Service

In 1917, at the age of 35, Dr. Fisher, along with a number of other graduates of Leonard Medical School, reported to Fort Des Moines for basic training at the Medical Officers Training Camp (MOTC). He was a first lieutenant and arrived on September 17, 1917. In his closing report on the camp, Lieutenant Colonel Bingham included Fisher in a list of 11 graduates singled out "on account of their exceptional ability and qualifications, their ability to command men and loyalty to their superiors." Bingham further recommended he "be promoted to the grade of captaincy."

Captain Fisher was sent to Camp Dix, New Jersey, on November 3, 1917, as the senior medical officer of the 349th Field Artillery of the 92nd division. The monthly rosters of the officers of the 92nd Division show him serving with that unit in France throughout the war.[6] After returning to the United States in early 1919, Fisher was honorably discharged from the army at Fort Oglethorpe, Georgia, on April 26, 1919.

Career

Following the war, Fisher and his family moved to Henderson in Vance County, North Carolina. In 1920 his college reported they were living at 311 Clark Street and he was a practicing physician.[7] Army records list their address as 320 Clark Street.[8] A February 12, 1920, U.S. Census report lists Charles Fisher as a patient at the Camp Sevier Public Health

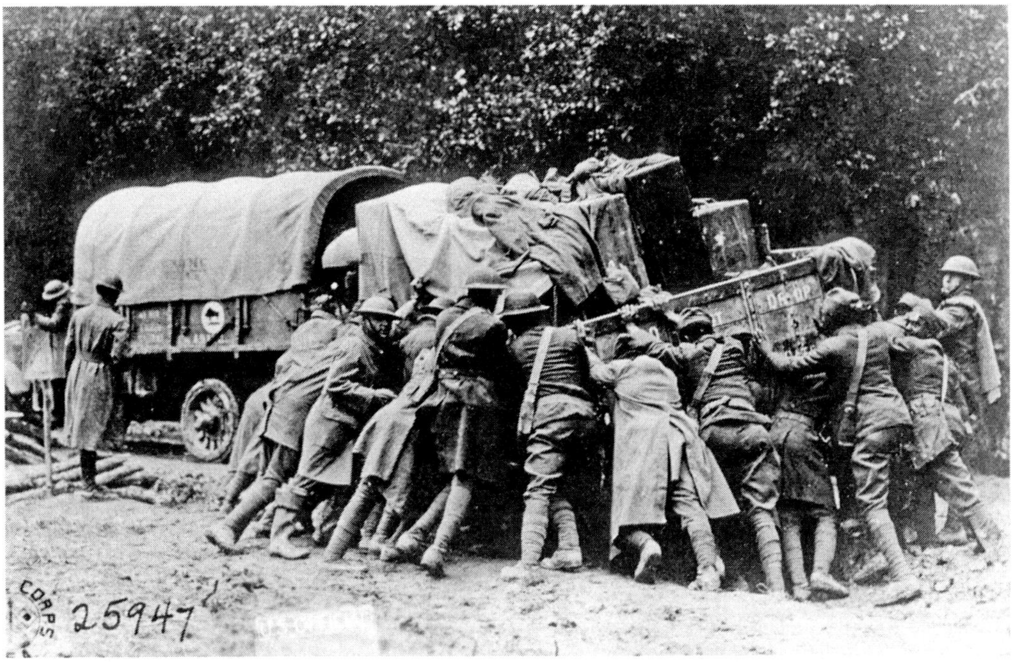

The 92nd Division en route to Meuse-Argonne, September 1918 (National Archives).

Hospital in Greenville, South Carolina. It was a former army hospital that had become the U.S. Public Health Hospital No. 26 in April 1919. It had been established to provide care primarily for influenza and tuberculosis patients.

Unfortunately, Dr. Fisher died there on August 25, 1920, leaving a widow, Ruth Celeste Fisher, and two children, Ada and Louise. He was only 38 years old when he passed. His parents outlived him. His mother died the following year in Birmingham and his father died there two years later in December 1923.

With Dr. Fisher's untimely death the African American community lost the services of a patriot and an educated and skilled medical practitioner. Marriage records for Vance County, North Carolina, show his widow, Ruth C. Fisher, was remarried two years later on August 14, 1922, to an attorney named Richard B. Horner of Washington, D.C.

Notes

1. *Knoxville College Bulletin*, Quarterly, Series 18, No. 3, June 1920, Catalogue 1919–1920, Alumni Index, FISHER, Charles S., Normal '02; M.D., 311 Clark Street, Henderson, North Carolina.
2. http://www.nps.gov/history/NR/travel/raleigh/Leo.htm (accessed December 26, 2012).
3. *Shaw University 1912 Annual Catalog of Officers and Students of Leonard Medical School*, p. 40, Special Collections of the University of North Carolina, Wilson Library, Chapel Hill, NC.
4. John L. Thompson, *History and Views of Colored Officers Training Camp for 1917 at Fort Des Moines, Iowa* (Des Moines: The Bystander, 1917) 50.
5. Colored Medical Officers Assigned, *Philadelphia Tribune*, December 1, 1917, 4.
6. RG 120–92d Division AEF, Roster of Officers of the 92nd Division, Box 6, National Archives, College Park, MD.
7. *Knoxville College Bulletin*, June 1920.
8. Fisher, Charles Sumner, World War I Military Service Card, North Carolina State Archives, Raleigh, NC.

Patterson Tilford FRAZER Jr.

15 October 1889–30 March 1947
Meharry Medical College, 1913

Roots and Education

Frazer was born in Allensville, Kentucky, to Henry and Sarah Campbell Frazer. Both of his parents were from Allensville, a tiny rural town in southwestern Kentucky near the Tennessee border. It was tobacco-farming country. His father was a tenant farmer. Patterson was named for his uncle, Patterson T. Frazer, Sr. Until around 1900, he lived at home with his parents and seven siblings.

At the age of 12, he had the good fortune to be sent to Hopkinsville, Kentucky, to attend school. Hopkinsville is a small city in Christian County, 30 miles west of his birthplace. It was notable during the Civil War because Christian County was the birthplace of Jefferson Davis, president of the Confederate States of America. The city was contested during the war and changed hands at least half a dozen times, occupied in turn by Confederate and Union forces. In December 1864, Confederate troops captured the town and burned the Christian County Courthouse which had been used by the Union army as barracks. A skirmish between Union and Confederate forces took place in the field opposite Western State Hospital near the end of the war.[1]

At one time after the Civil War, Hopkinsville was a place of more than 200 thriving black-owned businesses run by doctors, lawyers, realtors and pharmacists. Some black churches sat corner-to-corner with nearly 25 clubs and juke joints, including the Chesterfield Lounge, which was frequented by Al Capone. Today, many of these places are tucked away, rundown or extinct.[2]

Patterson Frazer attended the Hopkinsville Male and Female College. It was owned by Baptist associations and had six teachers. The school operated between 1883 and 1915. Located on five acres of land, it was an elementary and high school that could house up to 50 boarders. Frazer lived with his Uncle Patterson's family at 947 Vine Street. His uncle was president and principal of the school.[3]

After graduating from Hopkinsville, Frazer enrolled at the Meharry Medical College, 60 miles south in Nashville, Tennessee. Meharry had its meager beginning from an endowment of $30,000 from the five Meharry bothers. The school grew into a most respected institution with some remarkable leadership. Dr. F.A. Stewart, a Fisk and Harvard graduate, became the first black head of the Department of Surgery. Robert F. Boyd, one of the founders of the National Medical Association and its first president, followed him.[4] Other leading African American physicians graduated from Meharry and continued support of the institution after graduation. Patterson Frazer earned his medical degree in 1913.

Dr. Frazer returned to Kentucky, and in 1915, he opened his medical practice in the small town of Cadiz, about 20 miles west of Hopkinsville.

Military Service

When America entered the First World War in 1917, Dr. Frazier left his practice and volunteered. He listed his address as his father's home at 104½ East Sixth Street in Hopkinsville.[5] Frazier was commissioned as a first lieutenant in the Medical Reserve Corps and went to Fort Des Moines, Iowa, to the Medical Officers Training Camp (MOTC). He was trained until November 11, 1917, when he was sent to Camp Funston at Fort Riley, Kansas. He was assigned to the 317th Sanitary (Medical) Train of the 92nd Division.[6] He was then attached to the 368th Ambulance Company and served with them for six months.

On January 5, 1918, Lieutenant Frazier was put on sick leave. He did not report for duty again until January 26. On April 30, 1918, his name appears with seven other physicians on a Report of Surplus Officers. It appears these officers were available for reassignment to other units as needed. On May 20, he was given orders of separation from service. By the end of the month, on May 31, 1918, he appears in a memorandum from the commanding officer of the 317th Sanitary Train, Lieutenant Colonel Downing, addressed to the division's personnel officer. It lists six medical and dental officers as "surplus officers," including Frazer.[7] Despite the fact that he volunteered, it appears he was not healthy enough for military duty in France. He was honorably discharged from the army in June 1918 following nine months of active service.

Career

After Dr. Frazer returned from his military service, he opened a medical practice in Hopkinsville. Hopkinsville city directories from 1922 through 1935 trace Dr. Frazer's residences and offices during that period. In the 1926 directory, the city's population is estimated to be almost 15,000 people and growing.

There were 26 physicians in the directory. During the 1920s and early 1930s his office was at 104½ East Sixth Street, located near the city's Thomas & Gaither Colored Hospital at 109½ East Seventh Street. The ½ on the address indicates it was located on the second floor or rear of a building.

By 1935, his office had moved to 510 South Virginia Street. His residence in the 1920s was at 424 Cypress Street. In 1928 he is listed there with his wife Katie. The marriage foundered, and by 1930 Katie is shown living alone at that address.

On August 14, 1930, he married Miss Lue Bernice Clark in Chicago, Illinois. They lived at 921 Hayes Street in Hopkinsville.[8] The couple did not have children.

They were still there when Dr. Frazer passed away at the age of 57 on March 30, 1947. He died after having been ill for 11 days with influenza and pneumonia.[9] His 42-year-old wife Bernice survived him and remained in their home in Hopkinsville.

Dr. Frazer had enjoyed a productive and successful career as member of the African American community there for more than 25 years. He is remembered as the town doctor and for Frazer's Natatorium (an indoor swimming pool) which he helped fund for the community in the 1930s. It was a rare to have such a facility for any African American community at that time in history.[10]

NOTES

1. http://en.wikipedia.org/wiki/Hopkinsville,_Kentucky (accessed October 13, 2012).
2. http://www.kentuckynewera.com/web/news/article_47fbaf00-00a5-11e3-b5e6-001a4bcf887a.html (accessed September 19, 2013).
3. "Notable Kentucky African Americans Database," of Kentucky Libraries, www.uky.edu/Libraries/nkaa (accessed July 31, 2012).
4. "*A Century of Black Surgeons: The USA Experience*," Book Reviews, *Journal of the National Medical Association (JNMA)* Vol. 79, November 12, 1987, 1305.
5. *Ibid.*
6. Table of Medical Reserve Corps—Colored—Receiving Instruction, Medical Training Camp, Fort Des Moines, Iowa, RG-112, Records of the Army Surgeon General, National Archives, College Park, MD.
7. Record Group 120, Records of the 92nd Division, 317th Sanitary Train, National Archives, College Park, MD.
8. "*Caron's Hopkinsville, Kentucky, City Directory*," U.S. City Directories, ancestry.com.
9. "Dr. Patterson T Frazer," Kentucky Death Records, 1852–1953, ancestry.com.
10. "Notable Kentucky African Americans Database," University of Kentucky Libraries, www.uky.edu/Libraries/nkaa (accessed July 31, 2012).

Charles Herbert GARVIN

27 October 1890–17 July 1968
Howard Medical College, 1915

Roots and Education

Garvin was born in Jacksonville, Florida, to Charles Edward and Theresa (De Corcey) Garvin. His father was a letter carrier. He received his early education in the public schools of Jacksonville and for one year in New York City. He attended Atlanta University Academy, 1904–1908, and went on to undergraduate school at Howard University in 1911. His leadership skill was recognized early and in 1912 he was elected president of the Alpha Phi Alpha fraternity at its fourth annual convention held in Ann Arbor, Michigan. The prestigious African American fraternity had 12 active chapters at universities.[1] He stayed at Howard for medical school and graduated at the top of his class in obstetrics in 1915. He went on to intern at Freedmen's Hospital in Washington, D.C.,[2] where he was promoted to assistant visiting surgeon.[3]

Fresh from his internship at Freedmen's Hospital, Dr. Garvin entered practice in Cleve-

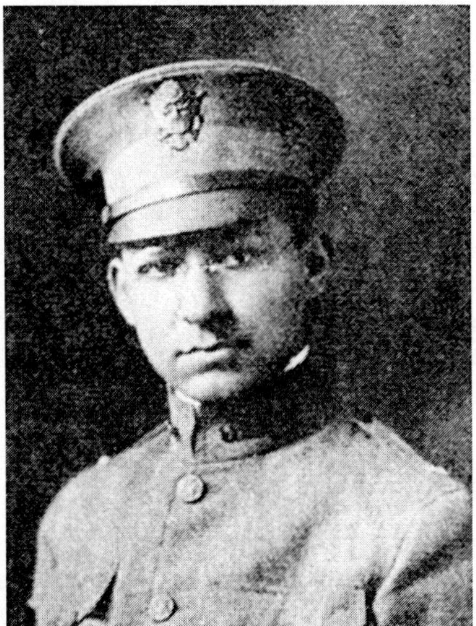

Lieutenant Charles H. Garvin (Emmett J. Scott, *Scott's Official History of the American Negro in World War I*, 1919).

land, Ohio, in October 1916. During this period, hundreds of thousands of black migrants poured into Cleveland seeking industrial jobs in this port city. Nevertheless, it was no promised land for black physicians. They came to build practices and found they were not even considered for hospital staff appointments. Their operations and surgical procedures were carried out in their homes by improvised methods.[4]

Dr. Garvin made a habit of attending clinics of the world-famous Dr. George W. Crile (founder of the Cleveland Clinic and discoverer of adrenalin) at the old Lakeside Hospital of Western University. He spoke up during those clinics and his status among the physicians of Cleveland grew. His friendships with those at the clinics led to his appointment to the staff of the Genito-Urinary Department at Lakeside Hospital.

Military Service

Garvin volunteered for military service in October 1916, more than six months before America even entered World War I. Soon after the United States declared war in April 1917, he reported for duty at Fort Des Moines on August 21, 1917. His leadership abilities were quickly recognized at the MOTC Training Camp. On October 21, 1917, camp commander Lieutenant Colonel Bingham recommended Garvin be one of 12 first lieutenants promoted to the rank of captain "on account of their exceptional ability and qualifications, their ability to command men and loyalty to their superiors, be promoted to the grade of captaincy." Garvin would not receive his promotion until after he returned to the United States at the end of the war.

First Lieutenant Garvin served 11 months in France. Initially he was battalion surgeon of the First Battalion, 367th Infantry, 92nd Division. Then in September of 1918, he was promoted to commanding officer of the 368th Ambulance Company.[5] In addition to his surgical duties, he was in charge of everything about the company—the medics, the wagoners, the company funds, waste disposal, and the kitchen. Garvin's company had at least some ambulances that were animal drawn. That required care for the animals by their wagoners, as well as maintenance for their motorized vehicles.

Garvin showed no tolerance for slackers. When Jasper Cherry disobeyed an order to take his ambulance out on the night of November 18, he was demoted to private. When there were problems in the kitchen with vice cook Walter Frost, Private Lyle Harbin was moved into his position.[6] He had the same lack of tolerance to the "insidious propaganda" from General Pershing who made so many negative reports about black soldiers. Garvin responded with a letter describing the "superior performance, in the face of adversity, of African American soldiers and officers who served in the war." The letter was published nationally in black newspapers in 1931.[7]

The companies usually operated in shifts with some in reserve while others were active. In quiet sectors, where the action was limited, more forward medical care could be provided because the numbers requiring it were small and manageable. In active sectors, the number of casualties was greater and the need for triage and movement to the rear was more demanding. Patients were stabilized and moved back for care to the divisional triage or field hospital. Influenza and coughing cases could be isolated to prevent pneumonia.[8]

After his division returned to America in 1919, he was discharged after serving his country for a year and a half.

Career

Dr. Garvin returned to Cleveland and resumed his growing practice. He was invited to join the faculty of Western Reserve University Medical School.[9] On June 30, 1920, he married Rosalind West who had majored in education at Howard University. The Garvins became heralded civic leaders of the African American community. They had two sons, Charles and Harry.

By the mid–1920s, a younger African American leadership group was emerging. "New Negro" leaders such as lawyer Harry Davis and physician Charles Garvin tried to transcend the factionalism that had divided black leaders in the past. They believed in racial pride and solidarity, but not at the expense of equal rights

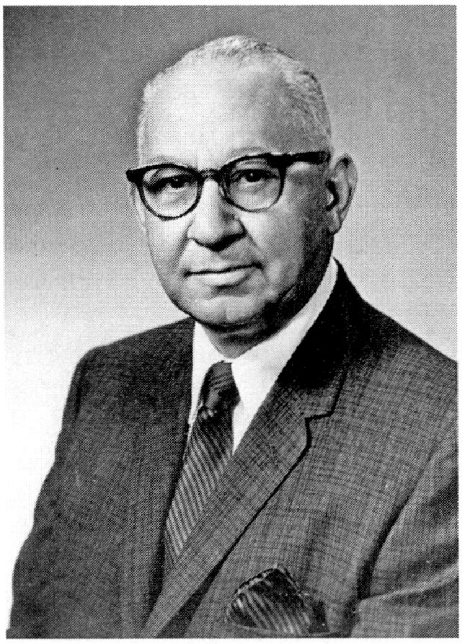

Dr. Charles H. Garvin (courtesy Western Reserve Historical Society, Cleveland, Ohio).

for black Clevelanders. The postwar era also brought changes to local institutions. Black churches were not able to deal with all the problems created by the huge influx of migrants. The Garvins were involved in the Negro Welfare Association that helped newcomers find jobs and housing. The Cleveland branch of the NAACP would soon be led by the "New Negroes" and expand its membership to 1,600 by 1922. The NAACP fought the rising tide of racism in the city by bringing suits against restaurants and theaters that excluded blacks, or intervening behind the scenes to get white businessmen to end discriminatory practices.[10]

Dr. and Mrs. Garvin pioneered integrated housing during a period of intense racial separation in the city. When he had gained financial stability, he determined to build a house on Wade Park Avenue in an exclusive all-white neighborhood near Western Reserve University. African Americans in Cleveland were concentrated in the Black Belt, near the center of the city. When neighbors found out an African American was building on Wade Park Avenue, they tried to cut off his financing. That didn't work. The first bomb was thrown shortly after the family moved in. Later a second bomb was thrown through a window but did not explode. Dr. Garvin picked it up and threw it back out of the window. When detonated later by the police, the bomb proved to be powerful enough to have destroyed the house. Time passed and the family came to dwell in peace. There was a gardener, but the flowerbeds and arrangements for the house were the work of Dr. Garvin.

In 1925, he and fellow U.S. Army Medical Corps veterans Dr. Linnell L. Rodgers and Dr. James A. Owen gathered another seven African American physicians in the Cleveland area and formed the Cleveland Medical Reading Club to keep abreast of programs and advances in medicine. Later in his career he would be a member of the Cleveland Academy of Medicine, the American Venereal Disease Society and the Cleveland Medical Association. He was published in the *Ohio State Medical Journal* as well as the journals of the National and American Medical Associations.[11] His 1935 article in the November issue of the *Journal of the National Medical Association* (NMA) highlighted the research of many African American physicians who had not been recognized for their work. He also stated the astonishing fact that there "are nearly 4,000 Negro doctors in the United States."[12]

In his article about neglected fields of research in a 1920 NMA journal article, he said, "The Negro doctor, under the spell of needed research, inspired and self-reliant, is determined to speak authoritatively about the diseases to which his folk are heirs."[13] The NMA journal in 1935 included a tribute to him with the titles of 26 articles written over 47 years, 17 in his field of urology. His interest in medicine extended beyond his practice to research and writing, especially tracing the history of African Americans in medicine. He amassed an important collection of books on the black experience and also completed a manuscript (as yet unpublished) and wrote several articles on the subject. His account of the history of Cleveland's African Americans in medicine was published in 1939 in the *Women's Voice*, a national women's magazine.[14]

Dr. Garvin was an active supporter of African American business enterprises in Cleveland. He was one of the founders of the Dunbar Life Insurance Co. He helped organize Quincy Savings and Loan and served as a director and board chairman. He was a trustee of the Urban League of Greater Cleveland, the Cleveland branch of the NAACP, and the Cleveland Public Library. He was also national president of the prestigious Alpha Phi Alpha fraternity.[15]

In his later years he was gratified to be joined in his offices and in the Cleveland Reading Club by his son, Dr. Harry C. Garvin, a graduate of Amherst and Western Reserve Medical School.

Dr. Garvin had a 52-year career as one of Cleveland's preeminent physicians, fully immersed in all the problems of his race. He saw the city enact a municipal civil-rights law, and he was there for the riots. Only a year before his death on July 17, 1968, he was pleased to be alive to see Cleveland elect its first African American mayor, the Honorable Carl Stokes.[16]

NOTES

1. *The Crisis*, March 1912, Vol. 3 No. 5, 185.
2. http://ech.case.edu/cgi/article.pl?id=GCH (accessed October 6, 2013).
3. AMA Deceased Physicians Card, National Library of Medicine, Bethesda, MD.
4. ech.case.edu (accessed October 14, 2013).
5. Record Group 120, 92nd Division, Officers 1918, National Archives, College Park, MD.
6. Record Group 120, 92nd Division, Officers 1918, National Archives, College Park, MD.
7. John A. Garraty and Mark C. Carnes, editors, *American National Biography* (New York: Oxford University Press, 1999) 773.
8. U.S. Army Medical Department, Office of Medical History, Vol. VIII Field Operations, Chapter IV, Medical Service of the Division in Combat (Washington, D.C.: GPO, 1925) history.amedd.army.mil (accessed April 23, 2015).
9. *Ibid.*
10. www.ech.cwru.edu (accessed October 13, 2013).
11. AMA Deceased Physicians card, National Library of Medicine, Bethesda, MD.
12. Chas H. Garvin, "Index Medicus of Negro Authors," *Journal of the National Medical Association (JNMA)*, November 1935, Vol. XXVII, No. 4, 146.
13. Charles H. Garvin, "Neglected Fields for Research," *Journal of the National Medical Association (JNMA)*, October 1920, Vol. XXIII, No. 4, 179.
14. www.ech.cwru.edu (accessed October 13, 2013).
15. Rayford W. Logan and Michael R. Winston, *Dictionary of American Negro Biography* (New York: WW Norton & Co) 256.
16. W. Montague Cobb, MD, "Medical History," *Journal of the National Medical Association (JNMA)* January 1969, Vol. 1, No. 61, 85–89.

Lucius Hough GILMORE

11 January 1889–2 February 1927
Meharry Medical College, 1912

Roots and Education

Lucius H. Gilmore was the only son of Reverend John S. and Sarah J. Gilmore. His father was a minister for an African American Baptist Church in Columbia, Tennessee. Columbia is an old city (1817) in Tennessee located on the Duck River, 50 miles south of Nashville. The family lived on Eighth Street in the African American section of town.

Lucius was a graduate of Columbia High School, and in 1909 at age 20 he was accepted at the Meharry Medical College in Nashville. He graduated with his medical degree in 1912 and returned to Columbia to practice medicine.[1] On July 10, 1912, he married schoolteacher Hattie Louise Sargent. They lived at 212 East Eighth Street in downtown Columbia. Her parents were Jerry (a blacksmith) and Paralee Sargent.

Military Service

In 1917, when the America entered the First World War, he volunteered for the U.S. Army Medical Reserve Corps and was awarded a commission as a first lieutenant. In August 1917, he was ordered to Fort Des Moines, Iowa, for three months of training in military medicine at the Medical Officers Training Camp (MOTC). On November 3, 1917, he was assigned to the 365th Infantry Regiment of the 92nd Division at Camp Grant in Rockford, Illinois.

From there he was sent to France in June 1918 where he served with the 92nd Division until war's end. Five of his fellow MOTC graduates were also assigned to his same medical detachment: Captain Frederick A. Stokes, and first lieutenants Leonard Stovall, Thomas L. Zuber, Arthur J. Booker, and Dorsey B. Granberry.[2] The 365th Infantry fought particularly hard and suffered many casualties in one of the final battles of the war near Metz in eastern France.

Lieutenant Gilmore won a meritorious citation for bravery while on the front.[3] Physicians working in medical detachments with the infantry, such as his, were close to the action. They were often in company and battalion first aid stations treating casualties before sending them on the field hospitals located further behind the lines. They were often subjected to the same artillery and gas attacks as their troops.

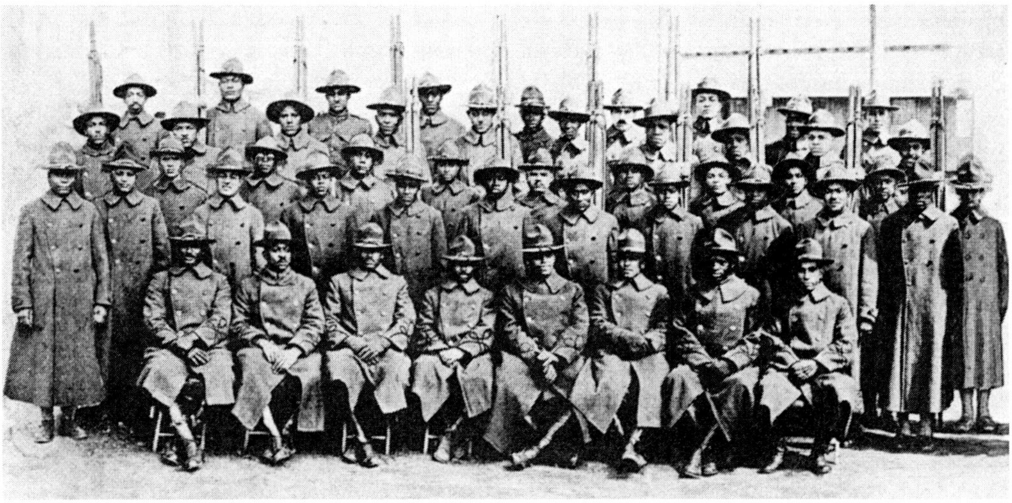

The 365th Infantry medical detachment (National Archives).

Career

Dr. Gilmore returned to Columbia after the war and resumed his practice. Interestingly, in the 1920 U.S. Census records, he was also the Census enumerator for his area. At that time, he and his wife had his 74-year-old father and his mother-in-law living with them. Sadly, Dr. Gilmore's wife Hattie suffered from pulmonary tuberculosis in 1923, and he attended her until she died a year later on April 5, 1924. She was only 34 years old, and he was the signatory on her death certificate. They had no children, and she was buried in Rose Mount Cemetery in Columbia.

Dr. Gilmore continued his general medical practice in Columbia until January 1927, when he passed away from heart disease on February 2, 1927, at the age of 38.

Although they both died prematurely, the doctor and the schoolteacher had to have been important caregivers and role models for the succeeding generation of African Americans in the town of Columbia.

NOTES

1. Report received from Meharry Medical College Archives, July 17, 2012.
2. "Returns of Medical Officers Serving in the 92d Division, for August, September and November, 1918," Record Group 120–92d Division, 317th Sanitary Train, National Archives, College Park, MD.
3. *Meharry Annual, Military Review, 1919*, p. 66, Harold D. West Collection, Meharry Medical College Archives, Nashville Tennessee.

Clarence Morgan GLOSTER

16 December 1890–25 June 1942
Meharry Medical College, 1905

Roots and Education

Gloster was born in Brownsville, Tennessee, to educators John R. and Dora Gloster. Brownsville is a small city and county seat—60 miles from Memphis, halfway to Jackson. His father taught in Brownsville and later became assistant principal at the Howe Institute in Memphis. One of his students was the renowned Miles Vandahurst Lynk, to whom he taught Latin, physics, geometry, algebra and biology. Lynk went on to become a physician and founder of the University of West Tennessee Medical College. It graduated 216 physicians before it was forced to close for financial reasons in 1923. Gloster's mother was a teacher in Brownsville, and later in Memphis. Clarence had three siblings—Claudius, Alice and the youngest, Hugh who was born much later (in 1911).

According to the 1900 U.S. Census, grandmother Alice Morris also lived with the family at their house at 439 Park Avenue in Brownsville. "His parents emphasized spiritual devotion, education, accomplishment and the social responsibility of demanding full citizenship rights."[1]

After graduating from Brownsville High School, he studied for a year at Roger Williams University in Nashville before going on to Meharry Medical College. He was awarded his medical degree in 1915. By the time he graduated, his parents and younger siblings had left Brownsville because of racial turmoil.[2] His parents and younger brother Hugh settled in Memphis. Dr. Gloster decided to return to Brownsville. His reason was likely teacher Vashti Velmer Caldwell because on August 1, 1915, he married her at her church not far from Brownsville.[3]

Military Career

Dr. Gloster registered for the draft from Brownsville, on June 5, 1917. On September 3rd, he reported to Fort Des Moines' Medical Officers Training Camp (MOTC), and after completing his basic training, was transferred to Camp Funston, Kansas. He was assigned to the 366th Ambulance Company of the 92nd Division's Sanitary Train.

According to a March 3, 1918, report by unit commander Major David B. Downing, First Lieutenant Gloster was already in charge of the infirmary of the 317th Sanitary Train. Eight of the physicians who were in training with him at Fort Des Moines were now reporting to him. He arrived in France in July 1918. Several months later, he was reassigned to the 368th Field Hospital. It was located at Griscourt on the west bank of the Moselle River, across from the main evacuation hospital at Millery. The main function of the 368th became triage. It was a sorting station. These doctors evaluated patients and sent them on to appropriate hospitals. It was a new formation in the American army, borrowed from our Allies. Triage officers were required to make quick but unhurried diagnoses and to estimate correctly the patients' needs and determine where to send them.

The task became much more difficult for the doctors as the war was nearing a close and the 92nd was engaged in the battle for Metz.

The final two days of the war (November 10 and 11) saw the division's heaviest combat and the greatest number of casualties. After the war, Lieutenant Gloster was busy sorting the wounded for the return to the United States. Doctors were also helping French and Belgian soldiers who were being repatriated. He accompanied some of the American wounded on his return to the United States in February 1919. He was discharged March 12, 1919. He continued to serve in the Army Medical Reserve Corps as a captain from March 20, 1920, until February 8, 1935, but he saw no more active duty.

Career

After the war, Dr. and Mrs. Gloster initially lived in Nashville at 1732 Firemen Street. By 1923, they had moved to Memphis where they lived with his father, mother and youngest brother Hugh at 373 South Lauderdale Street. He and the family were still on Lauderdale Street when his father died in 1933.

Unfortunately, we lose track of Dr. Gloster for the next 12 years. It is likely he was caring for patients and busy in Memphis. He reappears in 1942 at the Tuskegee Veterans Hospital where he passed away. His death certificate lists hypertension as the cause of death. He was buried in the Mobile (Alabama) National Cemetery with a Latin cross on his tombstone provided by the U.S. Army. Dr. Gloster rests there in section 6, site 1524.

Gloster's youngest brother Hugh became the best-known member of the family and gained a national reputation. He graduated from Morehouse College, Atlanta, Georgia, in 1931 and received his doctorate degree in 1943 at New York University. For 20 years he served as president of Morehouse College in Atlanta.[4]

NOTES

1. http://www.blackpast.org/aah/gloster-hugh-1911-2002 (accessed July 20, 2014).
2. *Ibid.*
3. Tennessee State Marriages, 1780–2000, ancestry.com.
4. G. James Fleming and Christian Burckel, *Who's Who in Colored America*, 1950 (Seventh Edition), 213.

Fenton Noah GOODSON

29 March 1888–1 April 1956
Meharry Medical College, 1911

Roots and Education

Fenton Goodson was born in Carrollton, Missouri, to Richard H. and Mattie Roller Goodson. Carrollton is still a small town, not far from St. Joseph. Nothing is known of his childhood.

In 1911, he graduated from Meharry Medical College in Nashville. He returned to St. Joseph and set up his medical practice. His focus was obstetrics.

In a 1917 issue of the *Journal of the National Medical Association*, Dr. Goodson wrote about "Preventive Medicine in Obstetrics." Reading the article today shows how much obstetrics has changed since early this century. He concludes with a statement that is startling to us today because it is so obvious, "since we know that more than one-half of all maternal fatalities in childbirth are from infection. We as physicians should ... make a specialty of antiseptic technique and other available methods that tend to lessen abnormal offspring and maternal fatalities."[1]

Six years after his graduation from medical school, Dr. Goodson appears to have had a busy medical practice in St. Joseph. He was a member of the First Baptist Mt. Union Church, the Knights of Pythias, the American Woodmen and the Masonic Temple.[2] He and his wife Mabel Fox Goodson bought the house at 324 East Missouri Avenue, where he would live the rest of his life.

Military Service

On July 10, 1917, at the age of 29, he owned a home, had a medical practice, a wife and a daughter Ruth, but he volunteered for service as an army physician and reported to Fort Des Moines for training on August 1.

After basic training at the Medical Officers Training Camp, Lieutenant Goodson was transferred to Camp Funston. There his difficulties began. His superior officer, Captain H. H. Walker, was an African American physician who had been with him at Fort Des Moines. On May 1, 1918, Walker wrote a poor efficiency report on him, saying he was "slow to grasp, dull of comprehension, lack of initiative, and slow of action."[3] He was honorably discharged and sent home after nine months of service. The Meharry Annual said, "Owing to the scarcity of colored physicians at his home town, he was asked to resign and return to his home to help in the threatened epidemic of Spanish Flu."

Career

Goodson returned to St. Joseph, his family and his medical practice. In 1920 Dr. Goodson was arrested in conjunction with a gruesome murder. "Murdered, beheaded and flung into Lake Contrary at St. Joseph, MO, Mrs. James R. Coleman of Iowa may have been the victim of Dr. Fenton N. Goodson, a Negro physician and surgeon of St. Joe."[4] The police thought they had enough to convict the doctor despite his refusal to speak. Mrs. Coleman had said she was going to Dr. Goodson to have an abortion. The police concluded the operation was botched, she died and Goodson beheaded her to keep her from being identified. The corpse was discovered in Lake Contrary near St. Joe by a nine-year-old girl. In the end, there was not enough evidence to convict him.

Late in 1929 Goodson was arrested again. The local newspaper reported he plead guilty to violation of the Anti-Narcotic Act. He was "bootlegging drugs" according to St. Joseph district attorney Vandeventer.[5] Goodson was sentenced to prison at the federal penitentiary in Fort Leavenworth for one year and three months.[6] His medical license was revoked because of his violation of the Federal Narcotic Act.[7] According to the 1930 U.S. Census, he was working as a nurse at the penitentiary hospital. He was certainly there on January 29, 1930, when he was unable to appear to defend himself in a $5,000 personal damage suit. It was reported that he made his deposition later from his cell at Leavenworth.[8]

After completing his sentence, Dr. Goodson was again licensed to practice medicine. He returned to St. Joseph and reestablished his practice, but it was never as prosperous as it had been before his prison term. He and Mable were still at the house on East Missouri Avenue. He also returned to active involvement in the medical societies, and he was included in a newspaper photograph in the Norfolk, Virginia, *New Journal and Guide* with four other doctors attending a medical clinic in Buffalo, New York.[9] The St. Joseph city directory continued to include his office address listing.

On November 10, 1953, his medical license was again revoked. This time he was convicted of criminal abortion.[10] Until the years after World War II the crime of abortion had a protected status because law enforcement authorities often tolerated the practice as long as the woman did not die. By the 1950s, legal authorities in some areas of the country stepped up their campaign to eliminate practitioners who provided illegal abortions.[11] Abortions were unreported income and a offered Goodson a way to supplement his income and care for his wife Mable and daughter Ruth.

Three years later, at the age of 68, Dr. Goodson died of a heart attack at his home. His obituary says he practiced medicine there for more than 40 years before retiring in 1953 due to failing health.

No mention of his time in Leavenworth or his other scrapes with the law was made in the newspaper article reporting his death. The article did mention that he was a lifelong member of the local Roy Curd American Legion Post No. 51 and the First Baptist Mount Union Church.

His survivors included his wife Mable (Mattie) and daughter Ruth. Final rites were said at the First Baptist Church. He was buried in St. Joseph's Ashland Cemetery.[12]

Dr. Goodson's problems with the law coexisted with the medical services he provided his community. His ability to resurrect and maintain his practice for more than 40 years in the face of stiff legal sanctions demonstrates his resilience and apparent contempt for authority. A charitable interpretation of his involvement with drugs and abortions would say the doctor was simply guilty of bad judgment.

NOTES

1. Goodson, *Journal of National Medical Association* (1917, April–June); 67–70.
2. John L. Thompson, *History and Views of Colored Officers Training Camp for 1917 at Fort Des Moines, Iowa* (Des Moines: The Bystander, 1917) 54.
3. Record Group 120, 92d Division, "Efficiency Report of Officers," Ambulance Company 368, May 1, 1918, National Archives, College Park, MD.
4. "Murdered and Beheaded, Her Body Discovered," *Iowa City Daily Press*, June 17, 1920, 10.
5. "St. Joseph Narcotic Case Finally Settled," Jefferson City, MO, *Post Tribune*, December 23, 1930.
6. *Ibid.*
7. AMA Deceased Physicians card, National Library of Medicine, Bethesda, MD.
8. Sherrie Kline Smith, Web Content Librarian, Missouri Valley Special Collections, Kansas City (MO) Library.
9. "Physicians Attend Buffalo Clinic," *New Journal and Guide*, October 24, 1942, B 10.
10. AMA Deceased Physicians card, National Library of Medicine, Bethesda, MD.
11. www.trustblackwomen.org/2011-05-10-03-28-12/publications-a-articles/african-americans-and-abortion-articles/31-african-american-women-and-abortion (accessed February 28, 2015).
12. "Dr. F. N. Goodson," St. Joseph, MO, *News Press*, April 2, 1956, B10.

Dorsey B. GRANBERRY

2 December 1886–26 March 1945
University of West Tennessee, 1916

Roots and Education

Dorsey Granberry was born in Mason, Tennessee, to Isaac and Elizabeth Wilson Granberry. He was one of four children (Richard, Dorsey, Alfred and Bessie) born to this farming couple. Nothing was uncovered of his early life until he enrolled in medical school.

At the age of 20, Dr. Miles V. Lynk (1871–1956) graduated from Meharry Medical College. The next year he founded the University of West Tennessee, a medical, dental and pharmacy school in Jackson, Tennessee. The school was moved to Memphis in 1907. Granberry enrolled in the school and supported himself and paid for his education by working as a druggist on Polk Street. As a result of the Flexner Report's scathing criticism of nine (five white, four black) medical schools in Tennessee, all were eventually closed and merged into the University of Tennessee College of Medicine.[1]

After receiving his medical degree in 1916, Granberry moved to Jackson and established a practice. Jackson is located 90 miles east of Memphis, almost halfway to Nashville. It became a trading town and retail center for surrounding agricultural areas, as well as a railroad town at a junction with maintenance shops for several early railroads. Its population in 1910 was about was 78,590 whites and 52,441 blacks. Although the black citizens were poor, they required medical care, and a doctor could make a living there.

Military Service

When Dr. Granberry registered for the draft, he and his wife Pearl were living at 116 High Street in Jackson. He was 30 when he reported for basic training at Fort Des Moines' Medical Officers Training Camp on Sept 18, 1917. From there he was sent to Camp Funston

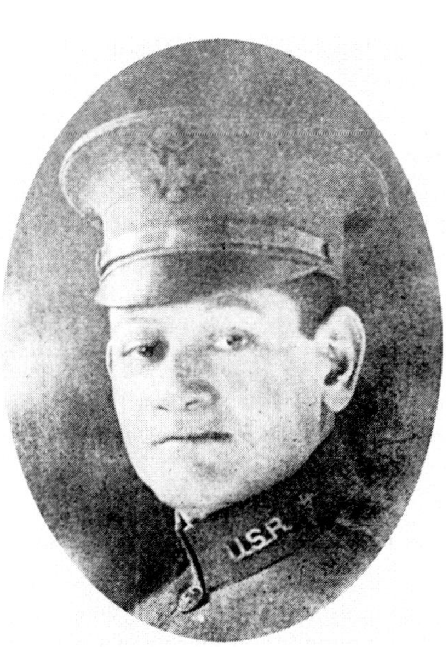

Captain Dorsey B. Granberry (courtesy General Research & Reference Division, Schomburg Center for Research in Black Culture, New York Public Library, Astor, Lenox and Tilden Foundations).

where he was assigned to its 365th Field Hospital. After arriving in France in late June 1918, he was reassigned to the 366th Ambulance Company. He was with them during the division's first major offensive in the Meuse-Argonne, the battle near Binarville (September 27–28, 1918).

Emmett J. Scott's history of the war lists some of the heroic actions of the men of the 368th Infantry during the battle of Binarville. These are a few examples of the men who were cared for by units such as Granberry's ambulance company:

> Private James went to the aid of a wounded companion under very severe machine-gun and artillery fire and brought him to cover.
>
> Private Davis voluntarily left shelter and crossed an open space fifty yards wide, swept by shell and machine-gun fire, to rescue a wounded soldier, whom they carried to a place of safety.
>
> Private Rivers, although gassed, volunteered and carried important messages through heavy barrages to the support companies. He refused first aid until his company was relieved.[2]

At the end of October, shortly before the division's big attack on Metz, Granberry joined the 365th Infantry Regiment's medical detachment, a front line unit. The 365th suffered significant casualties during the heavy fighting in the attack on November 10 and 11. He served well and honorably, and was promoted to the rank of captain by the end of the war.

Career

After the war, he returned to his Jackson practice. By 1930, he partnered with Dr. Hildreth to form the Granberry-Hildreth Clinic to serve their city's African American community.

September 21, 1931, had to have been an especially sad day for the good doctor. His friend, fellow doctor and World War I Medical Corps physician, John Q. Taylor of 692 Alston Street in Memphis, died. It was Dr. Granberry who signed the death certificate indicating his death was caused by a secondary cerebral hemorrhage. The first occurred in 1921, soon after the war.[3]

By 1933, he gathered the Jackson African American community behind his effort to take over an old hospital and renovate it to serve the African Americans of Jackson and all the surrounding country between Nashville and Memphis. This would provide needed care for the community. Dr. J. F. Lane, retired postmaster and son of the president of Lane College, and other notable leaders devoted much time to the effort.[4] They were successful. When James Worthington wrote a short history of Jackson during the 1930s for the Kansas City *Plaindealer,* he said, "The Granberry Hildreth Hospital is a real asset to Jackson."[5]

Dr. and Mrs. Granberry lived at 334 Laconte Street. They were important members of the local African American society. He was active in the local Methodist church, the Boys and Girls Clubs, and the Colored Farmers Institute. In 1941, his activities in the local Methodist Church were expanded when he was chosen lay delegate to the Tennessee Methodist Conference in McMinnville.[6]

Dr. Granberry died at the age of 56 of peritonitis from a ruptured appendix at Friendly Clinic and Hospital in Memphis. This was run by Dr. Sherman B. Hickman, one of his friends who volunteered and served in France.

He is buried in Madison County's Elmwood Cemetery. Elmwood is a large African

American cemetery adjoining Old Hickory Mall in Jackson. Many of the graves are unmarked. Granberry's just reads "Dr."[7]

NOTES

1. Patricia LaPointe McFarland and Mary Ellen Pitts, "*The Progressive Era*," Memphis Medicine: A History of Science and Service, (Legacy Publishing, 2011), 67.
2. Emmett J. Scott, *Scott's Official History of the American Negro in the World War* (Chicago: Homewood Press, 1919) 179.
3. "John Q. Taylor," Tennessee Death Records, 1908–1951.
4. "Jackson Hears Roscoe Simmons," *Spokesman*, Chicago, IL, January 14, 1933, 8.
5. "Jackson, Tenn," *The Plaindealer*, Kansas City, KS, December 13, 1935, 6.
6. *Ibid.*, October 17, 1941, 4.
7. http://www.tngenweb.org/cemeteries/index.html#!cm=1283726 (accessed July 19, 2014).

Royal William GRUBBS

15 September 1886–14 March 1937
Meharry Medical College, 1916

Roots and Education

Royal Grubbs was born in the far western tip of Kentucky in Paducah in 1886. He was the oldest of four children. He had a younger sister, who became a public school teacher, and two younger brothers. One brother became a writer and moved to Chicago. The other brother, George, became a mortician.

His grandfather, Richard Grubbs, was a slave and came to Kentucky by wagon with his wife and children. It was a hard trip and a daughter died en route. According to Grace Grubbs Newbern, the Grubbs family was very religious, and Dr. Grubbs' grandfather mortgaged his home in 1875 to help finance the building of the Clay Street (Disciples of Christ) Christian Church on 13th Street in Paducah. Richard's family, and extended family, lived on a 200-plus acre farm in Cecil, Kentucky, now part of Paducah, where family members worked together to keep it viable. Along with the usual farm animals, the families all maintained gardens. Produce and meats were sold at Paducah's famous Market House at 2nd and Broadway. After Richard's death the land was divided, and the Grubbs families moved to different places. The homestead was willed to John Grubbs, and after his death it was lost due to debt.[1]

Dr. Grubbs father, George W. Grubbs, was described as a coal and wood dealer in 1900 and the family lived in town at 915 North 8th Street. His mother Amanda was called "Annie." By 1910 his father, George, was farming and lived just across the Ohio River from Paducah in Jackson, Illinois. The family consisted of George, Amanda and three children, Royal (23), Seberlie (21), and Harry G. (18).[2] The family's religious commitment was demonstrated when they co-founded the New Bethel Methodist Church in nearby Brookport, Illinois. The neighborhood church building is still there.

After completing his undergraduate schooling at the Colored School in Paducah in June 1907,[3] Royal Grubbs went to Louisville, Kentucky, to attend Simmons University, a university established by the Baptists in 1879 to educate African American citizens. He worked to put himself through school. In 1908 he was a waiter in Paducah. Then, while he was as student in Louisville from 1910 to 1912, he worked as a houseman.[4] From Simmons University he went on to Meharry Medical College in Nashville. After earning his medical degree in April 1916,[5] he returned briefly to Louisville to work as a physician, and then in 1917 he came home to Paducah and established a practice

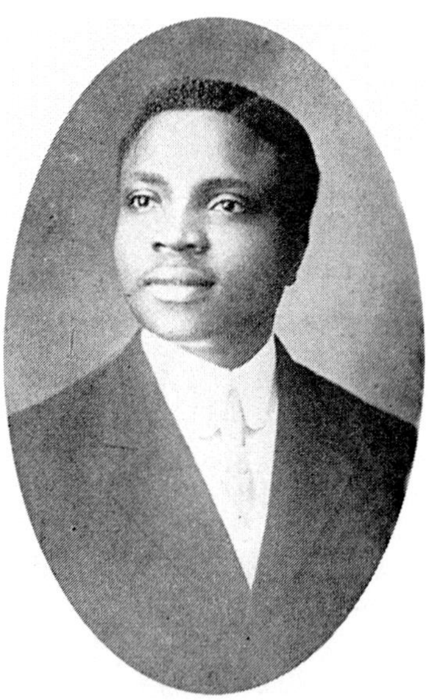

Royal W. Grubbs (courtesy Joan Dance and the Grubbs family, Paducah, Kentucky).

that he maintained there until the early 1920s.[6] He lived at 423 North 12th Street in downtown Paducah.[7] On September 3, 1917, he married Sallie B. Williams in Franklin, near Nashville where he had attended medical school.[8] The *Chicago Defender* newspaper carried a report of the wedding.[9] Ultimately they were married for 20 years.

Military Service

In response to appeals for physicians Dr. Grubbs volunteered to join the U.S. Army Medical Reserve Corps. He was commissioned a first lieutenant and sent for military training to Fort Des Moines. He was the last arrival and had scarcely arrived before the training camp closed. Because his military training lasted only 19 days (from October 24–November 11), he must have been one the least prepared of the 104 camp graduates to serve as a military doctor. Most of the other doctors received between 40 and 80 days of training.[10] Nevertheless, upon completion of his training he was ordered to the 317th Sanitary (Medical) Train, 92nd Division, at Camp Funston and then on to France.

Upon his arrival he was assigned to the 365th Field Hospital. It established a triage hospital at Raon L'Étape in the St. Dié sector when the division saw its first real combat. He served with that unit in the U.S. and France during 1917–1919, throughout the war.

The 92nd Division saw significant combat activity from September–November 1917. He undoubtedly treated numerous casualties who fell from influenza, pneumonia, gas warfare attacks, as well as victims of artillery, machine guns and knives. He also dealt with more general medical problems like broken bones and sprains, venereal disease and even administering inoculations. The training and experience he gained served him well in civilian life.

Career

Following the war Dr. Grubbs returned to Paducah in 1919 and resumed his medical practice as a general practitioner. The *Washington Bee* reported in January 1920 that he was elected finance officer of the American Legion of Kentucky, Robert Smalls Post No. 60 in Paducah.[11] This newly chartered post held its first mass meeting at the Harrison Street Baptist Church in Paducah on January 18, 1920.

The doctor and his wife lived at 1131 14th Street in Paducah in 1922 and his medical office was at 501 South 7th Street.[12] A family story passed down, and undoubtedly embellished over time, describes him as a highly spiritual, God-fearing Christian who always prayed (down on his knees) before he attended any patient, and that his patients always got well. It was said he had as many white patients as he did "colored" patients, which attested to his professional reputation.

In 1924, the doctor and his wife moved 375 miles north to Gary, Indiana. In those years, Gary was a fast growing industrial city 25 miles southeast of Chicago, Illinois. Opportunity abounded. The city was a "company town" having been created by U.S. Steel Corporation. Its population grew to about 55,000 in 1920 and more than 100,000 in 1930. There was a great need for black professionals there. After the outbreak of World War I, as European immigration ceased, African Americans from the south began migrating to Gary. In 1930 they constituted almost 18 percent of the population, and that number was growing. Dr. Grubbs and his wife pursued the opportunity. He worked and lived in the segregated African American midtown area of the city known as the Central Business District. His office was on Broadway, a main North-South Street in Gary. Their home at 2308 Connecticut was nearby, less than a mile from his office.

Throughout the 1920s the city's growth and prosperity depended on a single industry, which caused great problems during the Great Depression of the 1930s, when production at the steel mills was cut back 80 percent.[13] These turbulent economic times in Gary were difficult for the city. Dr. Grubbs was a prominent civic leader in the African American community and served as president of the board of directors of the Stewart Settlement House for six years, up until the time of his death.[14] The Stewart Settlement House was extremely important as a cultural and educational center, as well as a shelter and health facility for poor black families in Gary. It was established and supported by both the white and black communities. Dr. Grubbs was well known for treating patients there, as well as for conducting hygiene classes and training a whole cadre of women in health care. The women worked in health clinics and well baby clinics that were established in settlement houses and some church basements.[15]

Clearly, Gary had become his home and despite the hard economic times, he and Sallie stayed and helped their community. Unfortunately he was only 51 years old when he passed away on March 14, 1937, following a five-month struggle with a heart disease called cardio renal nephritis. Following services at the Trinity Methodist Episcopal church, he was buried at the Fern Oaks Cemetery in nearby Griffin, Indiana. His widow, Sallie B., remained in their home in Gary for 14 years before she passed away on May 29, 1951.[16] She is buried with him.

Dr. Grubbs was a patriot and always served his nation, his community and his people in numerous ways. In addition to maintaining a private medical practice and working with the Settlement House, he was a Trustee of the Trinity Methodist Episcopal Church, commander of the Chicago Division of the American Woodmen of the World, a member of the Indiana State Medical Association, Masonic Lodge No. 92 of Paducah, Kentucky, IOOF (the International Order of Odd Fellows), and the Negro Elks Lodge.[17] American Woodmen was a fraternal organization for Negro men emphasizing community service and family values. The IOOF was the first national fraternity consisting of men and women united together for mutual aid and providing social and practical support for each other and their communities.

Dr. Grubbs' focus on community service is reflected in his many affiliations for helping others. His prominence in his community was well deserved.

NOTES

1. Information supplied to authors in January 2013 by Grubbs cousin Joan Dance of Paducah, Kentucky.
2. 1900 & 1910 U.S. Federal Census Records.
3. "Colored Schools," *The Paducah Evening Sun*, June 1, 1907, 8.
4. *Caron's Directories of the City of Louisville,* for 1910 (p 481) and 1912 (p 537) ancestry.com.
5. "Meharry Commencement," *The Meharry News*, Vol. 14, No. 4, April 1916 http://library.mmc.edu/catalogues/MMC_news_1916_color.pdf.
6. "R. N. Grubbs, Negro Doctor of Gary, Dies, Illness of Five Months Fatal to Prominent Civic Leader," *The Gary Post-Tribune*, March 15, 1937, 6.
7. World War I Draft Registration Cards (1917–1918), ancestry.com.
8. Tennessee State Marriages, 1780–2002, ancestry.com.
9. "The Blue Grass State," *Chicago Defender*, September 15, 1917, 12.
10. Table of Medical Reserve Corps—Colored—Receiving Instruction, Medical Training Camp, Fort Des Moines, Iowa, RG-112, Records of the Army Surgeon General, National Archives, College Park, MD.
11. *Washington Bee*, January 10, 1920, 8.
12. *Caron's Paducah Directory*, 1922, 237, ancestry.com.
13. *Encyclopedia of Chicago* http://www.encyclopedia.chicagohistory.org/pages/503.html (accessed March 20, 2014).
14. "R. N. Grubbs, Negro Doctor of Gary, Dies, Illness of Five Months Fatal to Prominent Civic Leader," *The Gary Post-Tribune*, March 15, 1937, 6.
15. Dharathula (Dolly) Millender, "*Gary's Central Business Community*," Images of America (Charleston, SC: Arcadia Publishing, 2003) 18, 57, 64, 110.
16. "*Gary, Indiana City Directory, 1945*," U.S. City Directories, 1821–1989, ancestry.com.
17. "R. N. Grubbs, Negro Doctor of Gary, Dies, Illness of Five Months Fatal to Prominent Civic Leader," *The Gary Post-Tribune*, March 15, 1937, 6.

William Alfred HARRIS

2 October 1887–26 June 1938
Leonard Medical School, 1913

Roots and Education

William A. Harris was born in Madison, a small city and the county seat of Morgan County, Georgia. His father Harrison was a shoemaker, and his mother Hasaline was a washer woman. He had two older siblings, Mamie and Charlie.[1] Madison's first school for African Americans dated back to 1867 when the Freedmen's Bureau purchased land on Hill Street for a school. Local public schools have been important to the community, and by 1900, a quality public school education was available to all children. Young William attended those schools and after graduation from Madison High School, he earned his undergraduate degree from Morris Brown College in Atlanta. He was a member of the AME Church.[2]

The college was founded in 1881 by The AME Church "as an educational institution in Atlanta for the moral, spiritual, and intellectual growth of Negro boys and girls. It formally opened its doors on October 15, 1885, with 107 students and nine teachers. Morris Brown was the first educational institution in Georgia under sole African American patronage."[3]

From there Harris studied at the Leonard Medical School of Shaw University in Raleigh, North Carolina. He was awarded his medical degree in 1913. Egbert T. Scott was in his graduating class at Leonard. Arthur Browne, Andrew McKenzie, and Rufus Vass had graduated the previous year. There were only about 25 in each class and so he likely knew these men well. He would encounter them all again at Fort Des Moines in 1917.

Dr. Harris continued his medical training with a one-year internship at John A. Andrew Memorial Hospital, Tuskegee Institute, Alabama. Then he settled in Athens, the home of the University of Georgia, where he practiced medicine for three years. Athens is located 30 miles north of the family home in Madison. He was single and lived at 1487 East Broad Street with his office in the Morton Building. He helped care for his family by serving as administrator of his father's estate after his death in 1915. His father had been prominent as Chairman the local Morgan County Republican Party, having once run unsuccessfully for the Georgia legislature, and had engaged in a number of real estate transactions that left an estate large enough to support the family.[4]

Military Career

When America entered the First World War, Dr. Harris volunteered. On August 3, 1917, he received a commission as a first lieutenant in the Army Medical Reserve Corps. He reported for basic training at the Medical Officers Training Camp at Fort Des Moines, Iowa, on August 17. On November 3, he was sent to Camp Meade, Maryland, where he was assigned to the medical detachment of the 368th Infantry Regiment.

In June 1918, the 92nd Division and Lieutenant Harris were moved to Hoboken, New Jersey, and departed for France. He served in the medical detachment of the 2nd Battalion of the 368th Infantry throughout the war. Several classmates from Leonard and Fort Des Moines served with him in the 368th. James M. Ponder was with the 1st Battalion, T. E. Jones with the 3rd Battalion. James A. Whittico was also assigned with the regiment.

In mid–September Pershing's battle plan for the first major battle of the Argonne was discovered to have a flaw. There was a gap on the left flank between the American 77th Division and the French 4th Army. The 368th was moved from the relative quiet of the St. Dié trenches to join a dismounted French cavalry regiment in the Groupement Durand. The Americans arrived exhausted and hungry. There had been no food for two days. No good maps were available so some of the officers got lost. What wire cutters there were had great difficulty cutting the wire with its one-and-one-half inch barbs spaced less than an inch apart.[5]

The Germans had been in the area so long that they had dug tunnels between the trenches and were able to attack from the tunnels at night. Once this was detected, some of the 368th equipped with grenades began seeking out the tunnels and tossing grenades inside before blocking the entrances.

Unfortunately "The Groupement Durand failed. And for at least thirty years to come, it would be pointed to as proof of the inadequacy of black solders and officers and would prevent their rise in the army."[6]

Whatever the views of the white leadership, Lieutenant Harris and the other members of the 368th Medical Detachment were busy. When the 368th was finally relieved on September 30, casualties of those first five days brought those four doctors and their teams of medics more than 250 soldiers. Forty-two were killed and 16 died of their wounds, and more than 200 were wounded.[7]

Two months later the 368th was held in reserve during the final battle at Metz on November 10, 1918. The war ended the next day. Physicians and medics accompanied the wounded as they returned from France on February 14, 1919. Dr. Harris was kept in service helping care for the wounded at Camp Upton, New York, until March 7 when he was discharged.

Career

Soon after his return to civilian life, he left Georgia and married Mabel N. Thompson of Baltimore, Maryland. By 1920 the couple had moved into her parents' (Rufus and Nellie Thompson) home at 1204 Division Street in Baltimore.[8] He opened his office at 703 Dolphin Street.

Three years later, Dr. Harris relocated his office to 1200 Pennsylvania Avenue, and the couple moved to 1132 Etting Street.[9] Pennsylvania Avenue was the city's central cultural and commercial area for African Americans. It was home to professionals such as doctors and lawyers, retailers who served a middle-class and upscale clientele, jazz clubs, dance halls, theaters, and other public and private institutions for the black community.[10]

This is the area now known as Old West Baltimore Historic District. The Henry Highland Garnet School on Division Street is still there. U.S. Supreme Court justice Thurgood Marshall attended that school. Within the district of grand mansions and alley houses are churches, public buildings, and civic monuments related to Baltimore's premier historic African-American community.

Dr. Harris remained in his adopted Baltimore community and practiced medicine from his office on Pennsylvania Avenue for the next 16 years.

In 1926 he was named to a committee formed to help with the expansion of the Elks organization in Baltimore.[11] In 1927 he was credited with caring for a seriously injured woman involved in a car crash.[12] In 1932 he attended a meeting of Shaw University alumni in Baltimore when the president of the university paid a visit to the city.[13]

When he died in 1938 at the age of 51, he was buried in the Officer Section of Baltimore's Loudon Park National Cemetery. That cemetery was one of the 14 original National Cemeteries established under the National Cemetery Act on July 17, 1862.[14] He was survived by his wife, Mabel, and two boys, William A. Harris (19) and Willie H. Harris (14). Mabel was working as a clerk at the U.S. Census Bureau. She, the boys and her parents lived together at her parents' home on Division Street.[15]

Notes

1. 1900 U.S. Census.
2. John L. Thompson, *History and Views of Colored Officers Training Camp* (Des Moines, Iowa: The Bystander, 1917), 57.
3. http://en.wikipedia.org/wiki/Morris_Brown_College#Establishment (accessed June 3, 2014).
4. Marshall Williams, Archivist, Morgan County Archives, *Ordinary Minutes Book for 1916,* 226.
5. Arthur E. Barbeau and Florette Henri, *The Unknown Soldiers African-American Troops in World War I* (Philadelphia: Temple University Press, 1974), 159.
6. Barbeau and Henri, *The Unknown Soldiers*, 149–150.
7. Ibid., 151.
8. 1920 U.S. Census.
9. James N. Simms, Compiler and Publisher, *Simms' Blue Book* (Chicago: Simms Publishing, 1923) 159.
10. http://en.wikipedia.org/wiki/Upton,_Baltimore (accessed May 24, 2015).
11. "Elks Here Plan Big Expansion Program," *Afro-American*, October 2, 1926, 7.
12. "Man Hurt in Crash," *Afro-American,* May 21, 1927, 12.
13. "Visiting Alumni in D.C., N.Y., Boston and Philly," *Afro-American*, February 13, 1932, 2.
14. http://en.wikipedia.org/wiki/Loudon_Park_National_Cemetery (accessed May 26, 2015).
15. 1940 U.S. Census.

Sherman Booker HICKMAN

22 September 1888–3 June 1953
Meharry Medical College, 1911

Roots and Education

Sherman Hickman was the youngest of three boys born to William and Martha Hickman. The 1895 Kansas Census shows his family lived on the eastern Kansas border in Fort Scott, 90 miles due south of Kansas City, Missouri. Five years later, he, his mother and older brother Jason Otis were living with Jasper N. Kemp at 819 East Washington Street in Springfield, Illinois. Kemp operated a restaurant there and Martha worked as a cook. She and the boys lived with her employer and the boys attended local public school. Sherman went to Springfield High School. From there they moved to Little Rock, Arkansas. Sherman's older brother Jason left to attend Meharry Medical College in Nashville. After Jason graduated in 1904, he returned to Little Rock to practice medicine. Sherman and his mother lived with him at 1203 Broadway. Young Sherman followed in his older brother's footsteps. Sherman worked his way through school. In 1907 and 1908, he earned money as a messenger and bellboy at the Hotel Marion in Little Rock.

He left for Meharry Medical College in

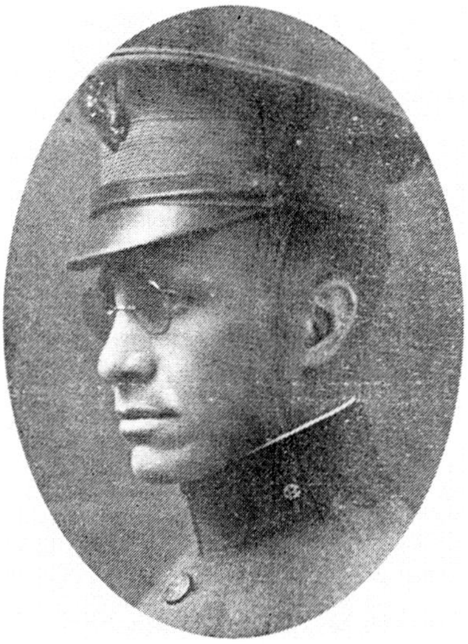

Captain Sherman B. Hickman (courtesy General Research & Reference Division, Schomburg Center for Research in Black Culture, New York Public Library, Astor, Lenox and Tilden Foundations).

1909. Two years later, he graduated with his M.D. in 1911. He returned to Little Rock and in 1912, established his medical practice at 515½ East Washington Avenue.[1] In 1913, he joined his brother in his medical office at 703½ Main Street.[2] In 1915, Sherman managed to secure an appointment as physician for the Arkansas School for the Deaf.[3] The school was an integral part of the state vocational education system and admitted students between ages six and 21. By law deaf children were allowed to attend the state residential school for up to 13 years. The school housed more than 100 students at that time.

Dr. Sherman soon found another opportunity in Memphis, Tennessee, about 140 miles east of Little Rock. Memphis had a large African American community. Its active social scene and music may have also attracted him. He moved there and remained for the rest his life. In 1917, his medical office was located downtown at 149 Beale Avenue and his residence at 672 Alston Avenue.[4] As the United States prepared to enter the First World War, he registered for the draft that June. His draft card revealed he was 29 years old, self employed as a physician and surgeon and married to a woman named Myrtle, whose race was described as Ethiopian. Interestingly, under prior military experience he wrote he had been a Sergeant and Trumpeter in the Illinois National Guard for three years.[5] His interest in music was an important feature of Hickman's life.

Military Service

Dr. Hickman volunteered and received a commission as a first lieutenant in the army's Medical Reserve Corps. He was called to active duty and sent to the Medical Officers Training Camp (MOTC) at Fort Des Moines on August 25, 1917. The MOTC commanding officer, Lieutenant Colonel Bingham, identified Lieutenant Hickman as one of four officers in camp who had the ability to command an ambulance company. Further, he recommended the four officers for promotion to captain on account of "exceptional ability and qualifications, their ability to command men and loyalty to their superiors."

After successfully completing 71 days of training there, Hickman was sent to Camp Funston at Fort Riley, Kansas, and assigned to the 317th Sanitary (Medical) Train of the 92nd Division. At Camp Funston Lieutenant Hickman was promoted to captain and assigned as commander of the 365th Ambulance Company. The unit had a complement of five medical officers and 100–120 enlisted men.

After arriving in France at the end of June 1918, his ambulance company was first sent to the 92nd Division training area at Bourbonne-les-Bains. In late August, the division entered into its first combat in the St. Dié sector of the Vosges mountains. His company established dressing stations at Sells and Virge Clarice, with its headquarters at Raon L'Étape. In late September, his unit was reassigned to Ste. Menehould in the Meuse-Argonne sector where the division was sent to support a major offensive.

By October, the division moved to the Marbache sector in preparation for an attack on the German stronghold at Metz. There his company established a dressing station near the front at Atton, and was responsible for furnishing ambulance service from the front line, via Pont-à-Mousson—Atton—Loisy—Millery (where the triage hospital was located). There were three motor trucks assigned to move each dressing station forward for the attack. They were involved in serious full-scale combat operations when the American Second Army launched its attack in early November. It ended on November 11 with the armistice.[6]

Fellow MOTC graduates who served under his command at various times include Lieutenant Elisha Jones, Lieutenant Joseph C. Bradfield, Lieutenant Everett R. Bailey, Lieutenant John D. Carr (August 27, 1918, report—work not satisfactory, lazy and inefficient in every way), Lieutenant Thomas E. Miller, Jr., Orlando W. Hodge (who replaced Lieutenant William W. Wallace August 1, 1918), Lieutenant Horace S. Brannon, Lieutenant James L. Martin, and Lieutenant Vanderbilt Brown (reassigned to 366th Ambulance Company in December 1918).[7] The record indicates that Captain Hickman performed his 18 months of military service in an exemplary manner. He returned to the U.S. with the 92nd Division in February 1919, and after nearly two months caring for the wounded, was discharged in April.

Career

Hickman returned home to his wife Myrtle and resumed his medical practice in Memphis. Annual city directories show he maintained his office at 149½ Beale Street for ten more years. Then in 1930 he relocated his office to 327½ Beale Street where it remained for another ten years. When he and his wife separated in 1927, his residence changed to his office address.

He maintained a connection to the military through his involvement with veterans in the American Legion. Memphis was the home of the world's largest African American Legion Post, the Austress Russell Post No. 27. Hickman directed its Drum and Bugle Corps. In early September 1931, he went to Nashville for the Tennessee State American Legion Convention where members of his Post worked to draw attention to the poor conditions for African American veterans at the Tennessee Veterans Hospital located in Memphis. The next month, Hickman was installed as Post Commander.

In 1933, Dr. Hickman married Anna Byrd, a much younger woman. She became queen of the annual Cotton Maker's Jubilee in Memphis in May of 1937. The Cotton Maker's Jubilee was started in 1935 and was a major social event for the African American community in Memphis for close to 50 years. Dr. Hickman was one of five men who formed the non-profit organization that planned and supported the event. In 1938, more than 25,000 people watched the parade, which included 20 floats and a marching band with Dr. Hickman playing trumpet.[8] There were actually three parades, a coronation parade, and children's parade and the grand jubilee parade.

By 1939, he was in charge of all the music for the annual jubilee.[9] In 1943, he was still involved in the planning of the Jubilee and was a member of its board of directors.[10] By 1952, the *Memphis World* newspaper article headlined "Cotton Makers Jubilee Takes Spotlight Here. South's Biggest Show to Attract Over 600,000."[11]

Dr. Hickman and John Arnold, Jr., started the Friendly Clinic in the late 1930s. Its focus was syphilis and tuberculosis treatment. The clinic was run on a non-profit basis and about one third of the work was charity. According to Arnold, "A patient at the Clinic pays only $1 dollar for an examination, which includes three tests for syphilis, tests for other diseases, tuberculosis, and for defects of the heart, lungs, skin, teeth, eyes, ears, nose, and throat. With the examination the patient receives a health card that was renewed twice a year. This card either gives him a clean bill of health or lists his physical defects and whatever treatment is underway. Cooperation from white and African American organizations as well as from prominent Memphis physicians who serve as consultant staff, have been most satisfactory."[12] By 1940, he had become the medical director for the Friendly Clinic. The clinic treated 58,000 people in one year.

Hickman was also named a medical director for the Tri-State (Tennessee, Arkansas, and Mississippi) Amateur Boxing Association.[13]

In mid–1941, Dr. Hickman organized a Traffic Safety Parade. He served as chairman of the parade committee. Hickman declared, "This is purely a civic campaign designed as an effective way for colored citizens to cooperate with the Memphis Police Department and Sherriff's office in their efforts to curb traffic fatalities and accidents."[14] He was also described as a prominent Memphis physician and Drum and Bugle Corps organizer for the two high schools, the Booker T. Washington and Manassas.

In 1944, during the Second World War, he was one of 25 influential members of the African American community who were on the Executive Committee for the Fifth War Loan Drive. Led by an African American political activist and Beale Street music promoter, Lieutenant George W. Lee, a bond rally was held for the Negro Division of the Memphis-Shelby County Finance Committee.[15]

Hickman's prominence in the community continued. By 1950, he was a member of the prestigious Omega Psi Phi fraternity, and participated in an event honoring its graduates that drew 1,300 people.[16]

On June 3, 1953, after suffering from renal hypertension for six months, Dr. Hickman succumbed to a heart attack. He was nearly 65 years old. His wife, Annie Byrd Hickman, and a niece, Grendetta Hickman Scott of Little Rock, survived him. He was buried at the Memphis National Cemetery.[17]

His obituary ran on the front page of the *Memphis World*. It included a large photograph of Dr. and Mrs. Hickman standing together in front of his office at 514 Beale Street, the home of the Friendly Clinic. It said he was considered "one of the best-prepared medics there and was well liked by all who knew him." He was a staunch supporter of the American Legion, an Elk and a devout Catholic and member of St. Augustine Church.[18]

Dr. Hickman's many civic activities, especially his musical endeavors, were secondary to the significant contributions he made to the health of the Memphis African American community he served for more than 35 years.

NOTES

1. *Little Rock City Directory 1912*, 709, ancestry.com.
2. *Little Rock City Directory 1913*, 259, ancestry.com.
3. "Medical News, Arkansas," *Journal of the American Medical Association (JAMA)*, October 23, 1915, Vol. 65, No. 17.
4. *Memphis City Directory 1917*, 581, ancestry.com.
5. World War I Draft Registration Card, ancestry.com.
6. RG-120, Records of the American Expeditionary Forces (World War I), 92nd Division, Office of the Surgeon General, U.S. Army, Medical History of the 92nd Division, National Archives, College Park, MD, 10.
7. RG-120, Records of the American Expeditionary Forces (World War I), 92nd Division, 317th Sanitary Train Records; Rosters of Officers Aug, September & Nov, 1918; Weekly Report, 14 December 1918; Special Orders 6, 29, F.H. 366, Gas cases received and treated 14 to 31 October 1918; Supplemental list of officers for reassignment, 27 August 1918.
8. Dr. Beverly G. Bond and Dr. Janann Sherman, "*Beale Street*" (Mount Pleasant, SC:Arcadia Publishing Co., 2006), 61.
9. "Memphis, Down in Dixie, the Cotton Makers Jubilee," *Pittsburgh Courier*, March 23, 1939, 23.
10. "Memphis Planning for Cotton Makers Jubilee," *Pittsburgh Courier*, March 6, 1943, 17.
11. "Cotton Makers Jubilee Takes Spotlight Here," *Memphis World*, May 13, 1952, Vol. 20, Edition 92.
12. "Beale Street Clinic 58,000 in One Year," *The Plaindealer*, August 16, 1940, Vol. 42, Issue 33, 5.
13. *The Sphinx* [Alpha Phi Alpha Fraternity], Winter December 1940, Vol. 26, No. 4.
14. "Traffic Safety Parade a Success," *The Plaindealer*, August 1, 1941, Vol. 43, Issue No. 32, 4.
15. "Memphis All Set for Big Bond Drive," *The Plaindealer*, June 16, 1944, Vol. 46, Issue No. 23, 4.
16. "Bluff City Society, Omegas Give First Annual Showboat," October 6, 1950, *Memphis World*, Vol. 19, Edition 31, www.crossroadstofreedom.org.
17. "Report of Interment," Memphis National Cemetery, Hickman, Sherman Booker, The Quartermaster General, Washington, D.C., September 1, 1953, ancestry.com.
18. "Heart Attack Proves Fatal to Dr. Hickman," *Memphis World*, June 5, 1952, Front Page, www.crossroadstofreedom.org (accessed January 3, 2015).

Louis Archibald HILTON

3 September 1888–19 July 1961
Howard Medical College, 1910

Roots and Education

Louis Hilton was born in Newark, New Jersey, to Ralph and Lucretia Hilton. His older brother was Arthur R. Hilton. His father worked as a letter carrier. In 1900 the family resided at 312 Halsey Street. After public school, Louis went on to study at the Howard University College of Medicine in Washington, D.C. At age 22 he received his medical degree in 1910.

After graduation, he moved to Princeton in southern West Virginia to begin to practice his craft. Princeton was a small but growing rail hub between Roanoke, Virginia, and the west. Soon he moved 30 miles further west into McDowell County, following the highway and rail line to Kimball, West Virginia, near Welch, the county seat.

This was coal country and the industry was growing rapidly as was the population of African American miners. The towns and mines located along the deep valleys were linked by dirt roads and railroads. As the Norfolk and Western Railroad expanded into this region, pushing westward, it spurred economic growth. As these coalfields grew, they were linked by rail to the great booming steel industry in Pennsylvania, Ohio, and Indiana. At this time the population of Kimball was 1,603 people, many of whom were African American miners and laborers. There were separate schools for the white and black communities.

Hilton worked and received training at Harrison Memorial Hospital, a private hospital opened in 1908 to serve the African American community. The hospital was located on the main street in a sturdy two-story stone building. Dr. Roscoe C. Harrison, who owned and operated the hospital, "was considered the dean of black physicians and surgeons in the area."[1]

Dr. Hilton became a member of the West Virginia Medical Society, and as early as 1912 he led a discussion on "Life and Death" at their annual meeting in Huntington, West Virginia.[2]

By 1912, Hilton had opened a private practice in his home at Wilcoe. In 1915, he and Ann Gray Moorehead of Zanesville, Ohio, were married in nearby Gary, West Virginia. U.S. Steel Corporation built a hospital in Gary in 1908 that served all the regional mining operations of its subsidiary, United States Coal & Coke (USC&C).[3]

Hilton lived and worked in McDowell County for seven years. He cared for coal miners, railroaders, loggers, their families, and others who lived in the mountains and worked to support those industries. While most of his patients would have been African American, he would have certainly treated some white patients as well.

Military Service

Howard University encouraged graduates to serve their country, and Hilton responded quickly. He closed his practice and was commissioned a first lieutenant in the Medical Reserve Corps. On August 2, 1917, he was among the earliest arrivals at the Medical Officers Training Camp (MOTC) at Fort Des Moines, Iowa. He gave 140 Somerset Street in Newark as his address at that time.[4] He completed his training three months later and was assigned to medical duty at Camp Dix, New Jersey, with the 349th Field Artillery of the 92nd Division. The camp was located about 60 miles south of his family home in Newark. His active service in the army ended after roughly six months when he was discharged to return to West Virginia in early 1918. It is likely he was needed there to care for the miners who were supporting the war effort by supplying coal to the steel industry and to the U.S. Navy for its ships. He was proud of his military service and later became an active member and supporter of the American Legion and the Veterans of Foreign Wars.

Career

Soon after the war, Hilton and his wife decided to return to New Jersey. By 1920 he had established a private practice in downtown Newark. Initially, their residence was at 137 Somerset Street. A few years later, he and Anna settled a mile away at 95 Mercer Street.

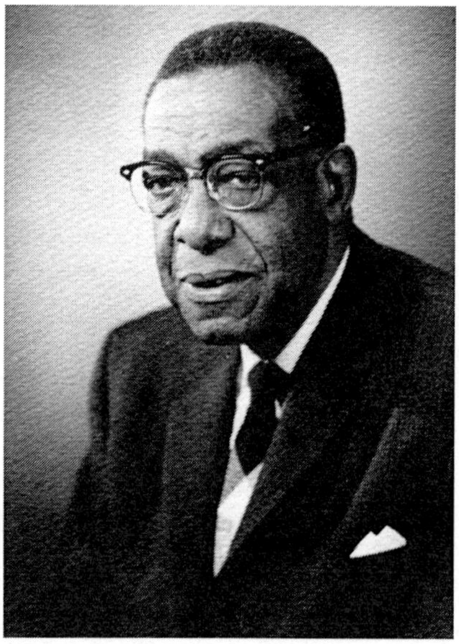

Dr. Louis A. Hilton portrait, 1960, Newark, New Jersey (courtesy Newark Public Library).

Newark's black population had grown to 25,000 by the mid–1920s. Professor Clement A. Price, a Rutgers University historian, wrote, "From 1910–1930, the early years of significant black migration to Newark, contemporary observers claimed that the city's racial climate was congenial.... [this] was not meant to suggest that Newark blacks enjoyed markedly better living conditions than blacks in New York, Chicago or East St. Louis. ... however, favorable race relations in Newark were shaped by the city's long history of benign labor relations, a booster spirit to which black leaders subscribed, a relatively flexible pattern of black settlement before World War 1, and an established dialogue between influential whites and a few black ministers, businessmen and professionals."[5]

Things changed with the Great Depression of the 1930s, and it took until the mid–1940s for African American physicians to finally be allowed to practice at the Newark City Hospital. They were forced to use smaller private facilities such as Community Hospital, which was opened in 1927 by the renowned Dr. John A. Kenney. It was administered by African American doctors. Hilton almost certainly saw patients at Community Hospital.

He remained professionally active and civically engaged in Newark for 41 years. Hilton's numerous activities and ventures were chronicled in various journals and newspapers beginning as early as 1912.

In July 1924, the *Pittsburgh Courier* reported that Dr. Hilton helped disarm and hold a jealous Newark woman who had just shot and killed her husband.[6] In March 1927, the *New York Amsterdam News* reported that Dr. Hilton was one of the distinguished members of the "newly formed" Twenty Club of North Jersey.[7]

In April 1932, Dr. Hilton as Secretary of the National Negro Business Progress Association gave a stirring talk about "the association's plan to start at once in the manufacture of shirts and handkerchiefs."[8] He was also one of eight directors and was instrumental in bringing its annual convention to Newark.[9] In 1933, this organization was reportedly behind a movement to establish a cooperative department store in Harlem to employ mostly African Americans.[10]

In November 1939 the *New York Amsterdam News* reported that Dr. Hilton was among those at a testimonial banquet in Newark who presented a gift to Dr. John A. Kenney, founder of the city's Community Hospital.[11]

In March 1940, the *Afro-American* reported that Hilton was one of the leaders of a "revolt movement" in the New Jersey Democratic Party.[12] Hilton was also a member of the 1942 Newark American Legion Post committee that created a historical pageant "Salute to Negro Troops" that dramatized the Negro's contribution to the defense of America from the Revolutionary War to the present.[13]

In January 1943, a *New York Amsterdam News* article headlined "Doctor Wins $200 Verdict in Color Bar." It gave the details of a discrimination case that Hilton had brought because a restaurant in his neighborhood he had frequented for years refused him service. The owner, Isadora Kreigel, was reprimanded by the judge for "practicing the thing that Hitler has been preaching."[14]

Hilton was appointed a New Jersey state boxing physician in 1944.[15] His job was to determine the physical fitness of all boxers before they were allowed to fight in the state. The *Atlanta Daily World*'s coverage of the appointment described the doctor as a "prominent physician and fraternal leader." He was also a member of the State Fair Employment Practices Committee (FEPC), the Committee on Human Resources, the North Jersey Medical Society and the New Jersey Medical Association.

In November 1947, the *Philadelphia Tribune* reported that Dr. Hilton was one of the speakers who gathered to honor a Negro assistant attorney general who, at the state's first constitutional convention in 103 years, inserted in the new State Constitution's "Bill of Rights" the most liberal clauses of any state in the union.[16] The law was passed and took effect January 1, 1948.

In May 1949, the *New York Age* said that Hilton was appointed as a city physician by Newark's public works director, Meyer Ellenstein.[17] Then in May 1951, a feature column entitled "Broadway Patrol" in the same newspaper reported, "One of the best-liked men on the

New Jersey State Athletic Commission is Dr. Louis A. Hilton, the Negro doctor who examines the wrestlers in Newark at the Laurel Gardens."[18]

The *New York Times* reported in October 1951 that New Jersey State Boxing Commission physician Dr. Lewis [*sic*] Hilton had ended a fight at Laurel Garden with a ruling that an injury to a fighter was too serious for the fight to continue.[19]

In 1957 the Old Time Athlete Association of New Jersey, where he was a longtime member, presented him with an award for his outstanding services in civic affairs.

In 1960, he received the golden merit award from the Medical Society of New Jersey for having practiced medicine for 50 years. He received a similar award from his alma mater, Howard University.[20]

Dr. Hilton fell ill in 1961 at 72 and was hospitalized in early July at Presbyterian Hospital, where he passed away on July 19 with kidney failure. Obituaries appeared in several newspapers including the *Newark Evening Star*, "Dr. Hilton Dies at 72," and the *New Journal and Guide*, "Dr. L. Hilton, Veteran Medic, Dies in Jersey." He was survived by his wife.

His service to his community went well beyond caring for the sick. He was a prominent member of the New Jersey and Newark medical community, but he was also deeply involved in state and local politics and active in many fraternal organizations, including the Masons and American Legion. He always worked effectively and diligently to reduce racism and ensure that opportunities for the African American community would be protected and expanded.

NOTES

1. Alex P. Shust, "*Billion Dollar Coalfield," West Virginia's McDowell County and the Industrialization of America* (Harwood, MD: Two Mule Publishing, 2010), 210.
2. "West Virginia News," *Journal of the National Medical Association (JNMA)*, Vol. 4, No. 3, July–September 1912, 278.
3. Alex P. Shust, "*Billion Dollar Coalfield," West Virginia's McDowell County and the Industrialization of America* (Harwood, MD: Two Mule Publishing, 2010), 262–264.
4. John L. Thompson, *History and Views of Colored Officers Training Camp for 1917 at Fort Des Moines, Iowa* (Des Moines: The Bystander, 1917), 61.
5. Clement A. Price, "*The Struggle to Desegregate Newark: Black Middle Class Militancy in New Jersey, 1932–1947*," New Jersey History, New Jersey Historical Society, Fall-Winter 1981, 216.
6. "Jealousy and 'Other Woman' Cause Killing," *Pittsburgh Courier*, July 5, 1924, 1.
7. "N.J. Twenty Club Gives Pre-Lenten Reception," *New York Amsterdam News*, March 2, 1927, 7.
8. "Natl Business Asso. to Make Shirts," *Afro-American*, April 30, 1932, 23.
9. "Simmons, Jackson to Talk at Meet in Newark, N.J.," *Atlanta Daily World*, August 20, 1932, 1.
10. "Movement to Open Co-Operative Dept. Store in Harlem," *New York Age*, August 26, 1933, 1.
11. "Leaders Laud Dr. J. Kenney," *New York Amsterdam News*, November 4, 1939, 9.
12. "Hartgrove Not Alarmed Over Leadership War," *Afro-American,* March 23 1940, 23.
13. "Set to Honor Race Soldiers of U.S. Wars," *Chicago Defender*, May 2, 1942, 4.
14. "Doctor Wins $200 Verdict in Color Bar," *New York Amsterdam Star-News,* January 23, 1943, 23.
15. "Negro Physician Gets Boxing Post," *Atlanta Daily World*, June 7, 1944, p. 5.
16. "Randolph Lauded by Fellow Citizens," *Philadelphia Tribune*, November 11, 1947, 14.
17. "Newark," *The New York Age*, May 7, 1949, 10.
18. "Broadway Patrol, by Ben Feingold," *The New York Age*, May 19, 1951, 10.
19. "Saxton Victor Over La Board," *New York Times*, October 10, 1951, 27.
20. "Obituary: Dr. Hilton Dies at 72," *Newark Evening News*, July 23, 1961.

DeHaven HINKSON

5 December 1891–1 November 1975
Medico-Chirurgical College, 1915

Roots and Education

Hinkson was born in West Philadelphia, the first of six children born to DeHaven Hinkson, Sr., and Mary Louisa (Luter) Hinkson. His father drove horse moving vans for a living. He spoke of his childhood, "I distinguished myself neither at school nor at home.... If I didn't get licked every day, the world was coming to an end. And I had those lickings coming, too!"[1] At the age of nine, he had typhoid fever. His doctor was a "fine old colored doctor, complete with goatee, wisdom and bedside manner." That image stayed with him and inspired him to become a doctor.[2]

After graduation from Philadelphia's Central High School in 1911, he went directly to the Graduate School of Medicine at the University of Pennsylvania. He earned his college expenses during the summer as a bellman at a hotel in Cape May, New Jersey. In 1915, he interned at Philadelphia's Mercy Hospital. While there, he joined the Alpha Phi Alpha fraternity, and he met his future wife Cordelia S. Chew.

After passing the Pennsylvania State Board in 1916, Dr. Hinkson set up practice in the nearby steel-mill town of Coatesville.[3] He was there when he registered for the draft in 1917. As Dr. Hinkson tells it: "My draft number had come up third from the top." He really didn't think he would get called when he applied for a commission in the Army Medical Corps. He didn't think African Americans would be asked to serve.[4]

Military Service

Hinkson was indeed called up. He reported for basic training at Fort Des Moines' Medical Officers Training Camp (MOTC) on Sept 18, 1917. Fourteen other physician members of his Alpha Phi Alpha fraternity were there. A picture of the group hung in his medical office long after the war.

From Des Moines, First Lieutenant Hinkson was assigned to the 365th Field Hospital of the 92nd Division at Camp Funston, Kansas, and then sent to France. He was especially proud of the report Colonel C. R. Reynolds, Medical Corps, wrote praising the work of the 92nd Division's work at the field hospital at Millery, France, where Hinkson was stationed. Although Hinkson was recommended for captain while serving at the 365th Field Hospital, he was discharged before the promotion came through.

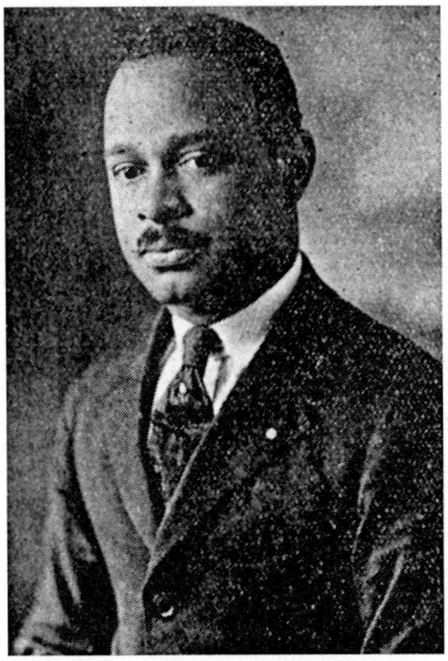

Dr. DeHaven Hinkson (national pictorial, members of the National Medical Association, 1925, courtesy Kansas City Public Library).

Hinkson was discharged in March 1919, and received notification of his promotion to captain in May. He continued in the reserves and rose to the rank of major before the Second World War. Four times, he was commander of the Philadelphia "Colored" American Legion Post.[5]

As late as 1926, Dr. Hinkson was still urging the American Battle Monuments Commission to recognize the efforts of the 93rd Division during the First World War. It was his belief that such a monument would offset the critics of the black soldiers.[6] He appealed to the NAACP to help him with the monument, but was told the commission had a firm policy against individual regiment monuments.[7] Finally, Senator Reed, chairman of the commission, replied. He declined to pursue the monument. Further he said, "The idea that we are in any way discriminating against the 93rd Division because of its color is absurd and unfair."[8] The idea was dead.

Career

Dr. Hinkson returned to Philadelphia, bought a house at 329 North 40th Street and set up his practice. He also worked at Douglass Hospital with Dr. Felix Antoine in the gynecology department. In 1922 he married Cordelia. They had two daughters, Cordelia (called Betty) and Mary.

In 1932, he received a Barnes Foundation fellowship to study gynecology and endocrinology in Paris and Vienna. His wife "Dede" and the daughters accompanied him. The next year, he returned to his practice in Philadelphia and, after a few years, he and Dr. Douglass Stubbs were the first African Americans to be appointed to the staff of Philadelphia General Hospital.

In 1934, he tried his hand at politics and ran for Congress. He was defeated in a bitter fight. He was a lifelong Republican and served as an elector in the 1940 convention.[9]

Return to Military Service—World War II

In 1941, Major Hinkson was still in the reserves and 49 years old when he received orders for active duty. He reported to Tuskegee Army Flying School to head the station hospital, a 25-bed facility with one operating room. He and four other physicians were to "guard" the health of the pilots of the 99th Pursuit Squadron.[10] During the year under his leadership, the facility saw the addition of an x-ray room, laboratories, examining rooms, and a pharmacy that were furnished throughout with modern equipment.[11] It also saw the arrival of five African American nurses, all army officers.[12]

In 1942, he was ordered to Fort Huachuca, Arizona, where the station hospital was being expanded to 1,000 beds and trainees were coming in. They would become the African American medical, dental and nursing officers in World War II. Major Hinkson became second in command at the hospital behind Lieutenant Colonel Midion O. Bousfield.

In 1944, Major Hinkson was promoted to the rank of lieutenant colonel at Ft. Huachuca's Station Hospital No. 1.[13] By June 1945, Dr. Hinkson was separated from service in Fort Dix, New Jersey, with the rank of lieutenant colonel. As late as 1972, Dr. Hinkson wrote articles for the *Journal of the National Medical Association* about African American military service in both world wars.[14]

Career

After the Second World War, Dr. and Mrs. Hinkson returned to Philadelphia. He worked in the gynecology departments of both Mercy and Douglass hospitals until their merger in 1948. Soon afterward the combined hospital built a new and fully modern facility. Through much of its existence, this institution was largely funded by the community it served. Desegregation of the city's hospitals meant Mercy-Douglass was no longer needed by the African American community. It closed in 1973.[15]

In the 1940s, the NAACP asked Dr. Hinkson and a few other Philadelphia physicians to approach the Mayor about the appointment of "capable" African American interns at Philadelphia General Hospital, a public hospital. The group was successful with, according to Dr. Hinkson, "no picketing, just frank confrontation."[16]

In 1953, Dr. Hinkson was elected president of the Urban League of Philadelphia. That was not unexpected as the good doctor had been a longtime member of its predecessor, the Armstrong Association. The *Philadelphia Tribune* noted that he was a member of the American Medical Association, the Medical Society of Pennsylvania, and the Obstetrical Society of Philadelphia. He was also on the staff of Philadelphia General and Mercy-Douglass hospitals.[17]

In 1956, Dr. Hinkson received the American Legion's Distinguished Service Award "in recognition of his more than 50 years of service to mankind." The article in the *Philadelphia Tribune* noted previous recipients included Dr. Jonas Salk.[18]

In Dr. Lorenzo Walker's extraordinary 1974 article in the NMA journal about Dr. Hinkson, he included a quote from Hinkson himself: "I am an optimist. I have lived over such a span of years to make me an optimist. I have seen so many improvements and so much progress come to the race in so many aspects."

Dr. Walker closed his article with "As we salute this great man, let us also try to emulate his greatness through study, through work, through healing, and through genuine consideration for our fellow man."[19] Hinkson died the following year. How extraordinary that he was able to hear this tribute before his death.

NOTES

1. "Meet the Hinksons," *Ladies Home Journal*, August 1942.
2. M. Lorenzo Walker, MD, "Dehaven Hinkson, M.D.," *Journal of the National Medical Association (JNMA)*, July 1974, 339.
3. *Ibid.*
4. *Ibid.*
5. *Ibid.*, 340–341.
6. "Bringing Pressure to Bear," *Pittsburgh Courier*, June 5, 1926, 11.
7. "The Letter to the NAACP," *Pittsburgh Courier*, June 5, 1926, 11.
8. "Senator Reed Makes Reply," *Pittsburgh Courier*, June 5, 1926, 11.
9. "Wilkie Approves List of State's G.O.P. Electors," *The Evening News*, July 30, 1940, 1.
10. "99th Pursuit Squadron Gets Medical Corps," *Chicago Defender*, September 20, 1941, 6.
11. "Air Corps Medical Unit Almost Ready," *New Journal and Guide*, March 14, 1942, 2.
12. "Virginia Army Nurses Report at the Air Base," *New Journal and Guide*, April 18, 1942, B11.
13. "Huachuca's Four Staff Officers Recently Promoted to Colonelcy," *The New York Age*, March 25, 1944, 3.

14. "The Role of the Negro Physician in the Military Services from World War I Through World War II," DeHaven Hinkson, MD, *Journal of the National Medical Association (JNMA)*, January 1972, 75.
15. http://jeffline.jefferson.edu/SML/archives/exhibits/diverse/mercy.html (accessed August 13, 2014).
16. M. L. Walker, "Dehaven Hinkson, M.D.," *Journal of the National Medical Association (JNMA)*, July 1974, 342.
17. "Dr. Hinkson Heads Urban League," *Philadelphia Tribune*, February 17, 1953, 9.
18. "The Highest Award," *Philadelphia Tribune*, August 5, 1969, 4.
19. M. L. Walker, "Dehaven Hinkson, M.D.," *Journal of the National Medical Association (JNMA)*, July 1974, 342.

Orlando Waldo HODGE

8 July 1886–6 August 1938
University of West Tennessee, 1910

Roots and Education

Orlando Hodge was born in Montgomery, West Virginia. The city is located near the center of the state about 30 miles southeast of the capital Charleston, on the Kanawha River among the picturesque mountains of Appalachia. His parents were Thomas and Lucy Davis Hodge. His father died when Orlando was young. He was educated in the Montgomery elementary schools and later took his college course at West Virginia State College.

Hodge had quite a varied higher education experience. He studied at Howard University in Washington, D.C., for three years and then studied for a year at Meharry Medical College in Nashville. He actually received his medical degree from the University of West Tennessee in Memphis in 1910. During his time in Memphis, he met and married Marie Colleen Moore. The couple had two sons before she died in 1913. The next year he left Memphis for graduate work in medicine at Chicago University in 1914–15. His early medical practices were in Montgomery, West Virginia, and Johnson City, Tennessee.

Dr. Hodge and his sons returned to Memphis, and he established what would become a lucrative practice.[1] In early 1917, Hodge was introduced in Memphis at the inaugural reception of the Young Men's Business Club, attended by 52 people.[2] In April, he was one of several speakers at a Howe Institute Sophomore Class public banquet in Memphis.[3]

Military Service

In 1917, as America entered World War I, Dr. Hodge volunteered to serve as an army physician. He was commissioned first lieutenant in the Army's Medical Reserve Corps and reported to Fort Des Moines, Iowa. The camp was already occupied by line officers so the medical officers got whatever facilities were left. Some officers got quarters in the band barracks while others were housed in old stables. An old nearby National Guard building was razed so the lumber could be used as flooring in the stable. It lacked heat and light and became most uncomfortable once the weather turned cold.[4] He trained there for 79 days[5] and was then assigned to the medical detachment of the 317th Engineers Battalion at Camp Sherman, Ohio. After arriving in France in June 1918, he was attached to the 92nd Division Sanitary (Medical) Train and subsequently assigned to its 365th Ambulance Company in August 1918. In November 1918 he was reassigned to the division's 325th Field Signal Battalion and put in charge of its medical detachment.

Throughout the war some members of the Medical Corps were moved around as needed. It meant they had to be prepared to deal with a variety of medical needs. With the Engineer Battalion in Ohio he experienced the sudden influx of men from all over the United States. He needed to discover, treat, and quarantine troops if necessary, to avoid spreading diseases such as meningitis, tuberculosis, influenza, pneumonia, and venereal diseases. In France, with the 317th Sanitary Train headquarters, he was called upon to respond to all aspects of the division's health needs. When he joined the ambulance company, his medical job expanded to include treating and transporting ill and wounded from front line dressing stations to field hospitals, in addition to maintaining the health of his unit. Finally, as commanding officer of the medical detachment of the 325th Field Signal Battalion he gained command and leadership responsibility.

After the armistice on November 11, Lieutenant Hodge returned home with the 92nd Division in February 1919. He was discharged in May after serving his country for nearly two years.

Career

Initially, Hodge returned to his mother's home in Montgomery, West Virginia. His sons had stayed with their grandmother while he served in the army. He rested and visited there for three months and spent time with his sons before returning with them to Memphis. He resumed his medical career and became socially and professionally involved in the city.

Several years later in 1923, he had a run-in with the law over whether he had sold a narcotic unlawfully.[6] A jury found him guilty of making two illegal sales of heroin to a man who was in fact a narcotics inspector posing as an addict. He admitted furnishing heroin on two occasions to the man but maintained he was dispensing it in good faith to relieve severe rheumatic pain.[7] Such incidents do not appear to have been that uncommon for the medical community under the Harrison Narcotics Act of 1914. The case does not appear to have affected his ability to practice medicine.

Hodge, an only child, always remained very close to his mother and as she aged he visited her in West Virginia regularly. It was a long drive from Memphis, 700 miles, and it took almost two days to get there. The press in the early half of the 1900s carried numerous brief social items about him. For example, in December 1913, his mother took his son O. W. Hodge, Jr., on a trip to Chicago "to visit grandma."[8] Then, in 1934, Hodge and one of his sons paid his mother a visit in Montgomery, West Virginia.[9] In 1936, his mother returned from an extended visit with him in Memphis, during which the family traveled to Dallas for an Exposition and to Hot Springs, Arkansas.[10] The most dramatic tale was about a mid-winter trip he made in February 1938. He drove from his home at 1306 South Parkway East in Memphis without stopping, because his mother's health at 77 was failing dramatically.

After he arrived she fell during the night when getting out of bed, and he detected her heart rate slowing, and then it stopped altogether. It appeared she was dead. He was able to restore her heartbeat by injecting her heart directly with adrenaline hydrochloride, a drug used in emergency situations for people whose hearts have suddenly stopped.

Fortunately, he was with her and had the right drug and equipment on hand to bring her back to life. When he returned to Memphis Hodge seemed to be in the best of health. Then in late July and early August he suffered with a throat infection for two weeks that developed into pneumonia. He was receiving treatment in the Collins Chapel Hospital, a regional black hospital with 75 beds, with his mother at his side when he passed away. Ironically, his elderly mother outlived her son.

Hodge was well regarded in Memphis as a heart specialist, as well as nose and eye infection specialist. The *Atlanta Daily World* commented that he was well known in civic and fraternal circles in Memphis as well. He was a Mason, a member of the Knights of Pythias and an officer of the Bluff City Lodge 96 of the Elks of the World. In 1937, he was even one of three candidates for "King" of the big annual Cotton Carnival.[11]

Besides his mother, Mrs. Lucy Davis Hodge, two sons, Orlando Jr., and Arthur Hodge of Chicago, and a granddaughter, Jeanette Marie Hodge, survived him.[12] His body was returned to Montgomery, West Virginia, for burial. The U.S. Army supplied an upright headstone to mark his grave.

NOTES

1. "Death Takes Dr. O. W. Hodge," *Atlanta Daily World*, August 10, 1938, 2.
2. "Down in Tennessee by Fred H. Lester," *Chicago Defender*, March 24, 1917, 5.
3. "Tennessee by Fred H. Lester," *Chicago Defender*, April 21, 1917, 6.
4. The Medical Department of the U.S. Army in the World War, Vol. VII, Training (Washington, D.C.: GPO, 1927) 267.
5. Table of Medical Reserve Corps—Colored—Receiving Instruction, Medical Training Camp, Fort Des Moines, Iowa, RG-112, Records of the Army Surgeon General, National Archives, College Park, MD.
6. "Tennessee: Memphis, Tenn.," *Chicago Defender*, December 15, 1923, A5.
7. *Ibid.*
8. "Chicago and Its Suburbs: Local Department," *Chicago Defender*, 1930, 5.
9. "West Virginia, Montgomery, W. Va.," *Chicago Defender*, October 13, 1934. 23.
10. "West Virginia, Montgomery, W. Va.," *Chicago Defender*, October 17, 1936, 22.
11. "Tennessee State: Meanderings Around Memphis Tennessee," *Chicago Defender*, May 1, 1937, 22.

12. "Death Takes Dr. O. W. Hodge," *Atlanta Daily World*, August 10, 1938, 2.

William James HOWARD, Jr.

25 December 1881–6 July 1945
University of Illinois, 1908

Roots and Education

Reverend William J. Howard and Alverta had a large family with eight children. He was a prominent, esteemed clergyman and pastor of the very successful Mount Zion Baptist Church in Washington, D.C. In 1916, he observed the 30th anniversary of his pastorate there.[1] His tenure extended even longer, well into the 1920s. Rev. Howard was deeply committed to the community and as early as 1905 he served on the board of directors of the Manassas Industrial School, a school that "opened its doors to colored youths of both sexes on September 4, 1894, when Frederick Douglass delivered its dedication address."[2] The school was honored at the White House in 1905 by President Theodore Roosevelt when he received some of its pupils.[3] The Rev. Howard was well known in the Washington, D.C., Baptist community, and in 1920 he was one of three church leaders appointed as supervisors by the District Supreme Court to monitor an election at the Mt. Nebo Baptist Church.[4]

The Reverend Howard's third child, and first-born son, William J. Howard, Jr., made his appearance on Christmas Day in 1881. He was born in the District of Columbia, where he was educated and later made his home. He attended D.C. public schools before being admitted to one of the nation's top preparatory schools, Phillips Exeter Academy, in Exeter, New Hampshire. He arrived at Exeter on September 25, 1900, at age 19, and studied at the school for two academic years. "Willie" as he was known, served as class president, class agent, class correspondent and long-range giving chairman and maintained close ties to Exeter Academy for many years. The 1902 yearbook shows he was a member of their renowned Golden Branch Debating Society, the Class Drill Squad and the football team.[5]

From Exeter he went to Harvard, before earning his medical degree in 1908 from the University of Illinois School of Medicine in Chicago. He returned home to Washington, D.C., to practice medicine. In 1909, he moved back into his family's large home, not far from the U.S. Capitol at 100 Massachusetts Avenue, NW. That year he received his medical license to practice in the District of Columbia. He opened a practice nearby at 232 F Street, SW.[6] By 1913, he had relocated his practice into part of the family home on Massachusetts Avenue, where it remained for at least 30 years.

On New Year's Eve, December 31, 1915, Dr. Howard married a local Washington, D.C., woman named Dorothy Mae Waring at a small ceremony at the home of a friend in Baltimore. His father, the Reverend Howard, came from D.C. to officiate. Dorothy was also very well educated and had been a student at the high school where her father was principal. She was a graduate of the M Street High School and Miner Normal Institute (teachers college) in Washington, as well as Columbia University where she studied early childhood education.[7] The couple moved into the large family home on Massachusetts Avenue. In 1916, Dr. Howard addressed a Colored Undertakers Association meeting on the subject of "Anatomy." It seems quite logical for him to use such an opportunity to promote himself as a medical professional and perhaps expand his business.[8]

Military Service

When the United States entered the First World War, Dr. Howard volunteered as a medical officer and received a commission as a first lieutenant in the Army Medical Reserve Corps. He was familiar with the military because during his early high school years in D.C. he had participated in a military cadet program.[9] In the summer of 1917, he was sent to Fort Des Moines, Iowa, for training for two months before his assignment with the 92nd Division at Camp Meade, Maryland. He was assigned to the Medical Detachment for the 351st Field Artillery Regiment, and served as a medical officer with the 1st Battalion of that unit in France.

The 351st trained for weeks at Camp La Courtine in central France, one of the largest artillery camps. The soldiers fired their cannons, went on long hikes with gas masks, visited gas proof dugouts, and went into gas houses where they were led into a room filled with gas where they were made to remove and put back on their masks. In early October the deadly Spanish influenza raced through the camp, keeping the medical personnel very busy until the epidemic was checked.

At the end of October 1918, his unit moved to the front where it experienced heavy combat during the final weeks of the war. The unit took part in the 92nd Division attacks on Metz that were launched near Pont-à-Mousson in eastern France.[10] The division suffered more than 1,600 casualties before the war ended. He undoubtedly saw and learned quite a lot about traumatic injury and many different kinds of wounds during his year and a half of service. Serious injuries from artillery shrapnel, gas attacks, and machine guns were commonplace. He cared for many sick and injured soldiers and served his country honorably.

Early in 1919, following his return from France and discharge from the army, he returned to the District of Columbia and to his wife Dorothy, who was working as a government clerk at the War Department.

Career

During the 1920s, Dr. Howard continued to practice medicine in downtown D.C. He must have been quite successful because by 1927 he had bought a large, impressive three-story brick home at 1728 S Street, NW, for his wife and their only daughter, Carolyn Alverda Howard. She was born January 23, 1927, at Carson's Hospital in D.C.

During the 1930s, he worked as a house physician at Freedmen's Hospital in D.C. and taught at Howard University as a clinical assistant. He maintained his medical practice in dermatology at 100 Massachusetts Avenue, and his residence was still on S Street near Dupont Circle through the 1930s and early 1940s.[11]

His wife, Dorothy, a highly intelligent and energetic person, opened a nursery school for children there in 1929 called "Garden of Children." According to her *Washington Post* obituary on September 1, 1988, it was the second nursery school chartered by the District and the first established for black children. It operated more than 30 years, until 1961, when it was closed. The first class had fewer than a dozen students and included her daughter. Later it averaged 30–40 pupils each year, with four teachers. Besides Mrs. Howard, the faculty included her daughter, Mrs. French, and Miss Nanette Binford, all of whom held teaching degrees. Her pupils included the children of diplomats, university presidents, and at least one Nobel laureate, and a former U.N. ambassador, Ralph Bunche.

As World War II ended, Dr. Howard passed away at age 63 following a prostatectomy at Freedmen's Hospital in Washington, D.C. He was buried at Arlington National Cemetery among fellow medical officers and veterans of World War I. His wife, Dorothy Waring Howard, survived another 43 years before joining him at Arlington. They are buried side-by-side on a gentle hillside in Section 8, Site 5482.

Their daughter Carolyn Alverda Howard received an excellent education at a number of quality Washington area schools and attended Mt. Holyoke College in Massachusetts. Six months after the death of her father, she married Dr. David Marshall French of Ohio in December 1945. They lived full and active professional lives, raised a family and in 1995 celebrated their 50th wedding anniversary. Carolyn passed away in 2009 and her husband David followed suit in 2011 in Barboursville, Virginia.

A *New York Times* obituary dated April 5, 2011, said Dr. David M. French, 86, a surgeon, helped found an organization of doctors that provided medical care to marchers during the civil rights era and who later organized health care programs in 20 African nations.

Dr. French was an organizer of the Medical Committee for Human Rights and in March 1965 led more that 120 of its members in the third, and finally successful, attempt by voting-rights advocates to march from Selma, Alabama, to Montgomery, the state capital.[12] The legacy of community service by members of this extended Howard family continued.

NOTES

1. "His 30th Anniversary," *Washington Bee*, July 15, 1916, 1.

2. "To Help the Negro," *The Evening Star*, December 20, 1905, 1.
3. *Ibid.*
4. "Pastor Voted Out," *Washington Bee*, October 23, 1920, 1.
5. Alumni Records for Phillips Exeter Academy, Class of 1902, Exeter, New Hampshire.
6. U.S. City Directories 1821–1989 (Beta), 1910, Washington City, ancestry.com.
7. "Miss Waring Marries in Baltimore," *Washington Bee*, January 15, 1916, 6.
8. "The Week in Society," *Washington Bee*, May 6, 1916, 5.
9. "High School Cadets Military Science. Our High School Cadets—What They Have Accomplished," *Washington Bee*, June 8, 1918, 1.
10. "With the 351st in France, a Diary Compiled by Sergeant William O. Ross and Corporal Duke L. Slaughter," Published by the Afro-American Company, Baltimore, Maryland, Pennsylvania State Archives, Harrisburg, PA.
11. *U.S. City Directories 1821–1989 (Beta), 1921, 1922, 1927, 1929, 1933, 1939 Washington City*, ancestry.com.
12. "Obituary: Dr. D.M. French Dies at 86; Treated '60s Marchers," *New York Times*, April 5, 2011, http://www.nytimes.com/2011/04/06/us/06french.html.

Raymond Nathaniel JACKSON

7 September 1883–11 May 1936
Meharry Medical College, 1905

Roots and Education

Jackson was born in Union Springs, Alabama, the son of the Reverend Alfred and Georgia Jackson. His family moved to Brunswick, Georgia, where his father was a preacher and his mother a seamstress. Brunswick is a small coastal city in the low country of southeastern Georgia. His father's affiliation with the Baptist Church likely enabled him to do his college preparatory work at Claflin in Orangeburg, South Carolina, before going on to the University of North Carolina where he graduated in 1901. He then graduated from Meharry Medical College in 1905, returned to Brunswick and opened his medical practice.

While still in his 20s, he met and married Arneta. The two of them lived at 528 Stonewall Street and took his parents in with them. Even at this young age, Dr. Jackson took a leading role in the African American community. In 1910, the *Savannah Tribune* reported on a "great gathering of doctors" when the National Medical Association (NMA) held its meeting. Dr. Jackson led the discussion of one session where he presented a paper on meningitis and scarlet fever.[1] He was also a member of the Methodist Episcopal Church, the Odd Fellows, and the Knights of Pythias.[2] When the Knights of Pythias met in Savannah, Dr. Jackson was in charge of housing the current and past officers.[3]

Military Career

By the time Jackson registered for the draft in June 1917, he and Arneta and their five-year-old daughter Irma were living at 1506 Albany Street in Brunswick. He was 34 when he volunteered on June 14, 1917. He reported for duty at Fort Des Moines Medical Officers Training Camp (MOTC) on August 25 and received training there for 71 days. During his training, Arneta and Irma came to Kansas for a visit.

First Lieutenant Jackson became one of the camp instructors and was among the 12 officers singled out by the camp commandant Lieutenant Colonel Bingham, MC, in his final report of the camp, for "his exceptional ability and qualifications, [his] ability to command men and loyalty to superiors." He was recommended for promotion to captain. This meant his army pay was raised to $200 a month when his promotion came through in December 1917.[4]

Following his training at Fort Des Moines, Jackson was assigned to the 368th Infantry Regiment Medical Detachment at Camp Meade, Maryland. He spent the winter of 1917–18 there. In April 1918, following a review by a board of officers, he was honorably discharged from active duty and returned home at the end of April. The record is unclear as to the reasons for his release but it could have been for a variety of reasons including his health, his performance, or even his request for a compassionate release, perhaps to care for family.

Career

In April 1918, Dr. Jackson returned to his practice in Brunswick and worked the rest of his life in his hometown. He was among the leaders of the Brunswick African American community. In 1922, for example, he was on the podium at the opening of a new school for black children. He made some "well chosen remarks about 'race progress'" and introduced A. V. Wood, the president of the board of education.[5] The same newspaper column mentioned his hunting party, which took place the next day. Hunting seems to have been a favorite activity of the good doctor. Several other social columns mention his hunting with good friend, Joe Williams.[6]

In 1928 he was elected first vice-president of Claflin University's alumni board of trustees. Throughout his career, Dr. Jackson was often called upon to introduce speakers and act as master of ceremony.[7] He was also often in Savannah for social events.

During the 1930s the leading causes of death were heart disease, cancer, pneumonia and infectious diseases including influenza, tuberculosis and syphilis. One of the biggest health concerns during the 1930s was how the patient would pay for any medical needs.[8] No doubt Dr. Jackson saw some patients on a charity basis and raised the prices for those who could afford to pay. Of all professions, physicians fared better than any other group during the Great Depression, but most saw their incomes reduced to half what they made in the 1920s.

According to the American Medical Association, Dr. Jackson died at the age of 52 of heart and kidney disease.[9] His wife Arneta saw to it that their daughter Irma was educated.

Irma graduated from Fisk University and Atlanta University. She lived in Chicago, Illinois, where she was a social worker. In 1942, Irma applied for entrance into the Women's Auxiliary Army Corps. She was accepted and did her basic training at Fort Des Moines where her father had completed his years before. She was posted in Washington, D.C., Fort Huachuca, Arizona, and Fort Lewis, Washington. After her stint in the army, she married and spent the rest of her life in Detroit, Michigan, where she was active in her community.[10]

NOTES

1. "Great Gathering of Doctors," *The Savannah Tribune*, May 14, 1910, 1.
2. John L. Thompson, *History and Views of Colored Officers Training Camp for 1917 at Fort Des Moines, Iowa* (Des Moines: The Bystander, 1917) 64.
3. *Ibid.*, June 21, 1913, 4.
4. "U.S. Army Finance Records—Jackson, Raymond N., Capt., M.R.C.," National Archives, National Personnel Records Center, St. Louis, MO.
5. "Out of Town News," *The Savannah Tribune*, December 7, 1922, 4.
6. *Ibid.*, *Savannah Tribune*, November 2, 1922, 2.
7. *Ibid.*, *Savannah Tribune*, February 15, 1919, 1.
8. http://ic.galegroup.com/ic/suic (accessed October 18, 2014).
9. AMA Deceased Physicians card, National Library of Medicine, Bethesda, MD.
10. www.blackpast.orgh/aah/wertz-irma-jackson-cayton-1911-2007 (accessed August 22, 2014).

Walter Jardon JACKSON

5 September 1888–11 September 1937
Howard Medical College, 1913

Roots and Education

Walter Jackson was born in Augusta, Georgia, to Joseph C. and Alice L. Jackson. His father was the foreman of a brick works company there.[1] Nothing more is known of his early life.

Jackson graduated from Howard University College of Medicine in 1913 and settled in Baltimore, Maryland. In 1914, Dr. Jackson made news when he challenged a man leaving the home of a woman who had died from whatever "strange mixture" she had been given by this faith healer. Dr. Jackson asked the man if he had a license to practice medicine. The reply was "No, but I have been intending to get one of those things—how much do they cost, anyhow?" The man was arrested.[2]

Military Service

First Lieutenant Jackson reported for duty at Fort Des Moines' Medical Officers Training Camp (MOTC) on September 1, 1917. Training was focused on fieldwork and administration. Some time was spent on medical matters, especially on diseases like tuberculosis, cardiovascular conditions and orthopedics. Special evening classes focused on army paperwork—how to complete all the regular reports. Time was also spent on drilling, marching in the cold fall Iowa air.

After 64 days of basic training, Jackson was transferred to Camp Upton, New York, and assigned to the medical detachment of the 367th Infantry Regiment. While there he had time to "visit with Miss Helen C. Edwards during the holidays" and get a mention in the society column of the *Washington Bee*.[3] He went to France with this combat unit on June 10, 1918. Its offensive engagements included the Meuse-Argonne, and its defensive roles were at

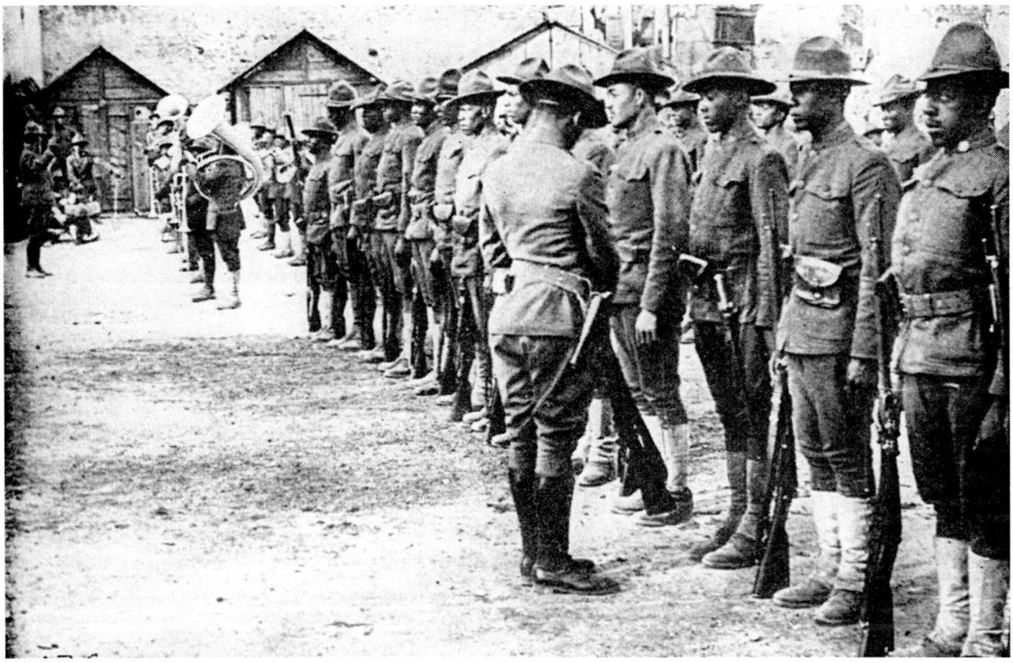

The 92nd Division in eastern France (National Archives).

St. Dié and Marbache. The 367th Infantry, known as the "Buffaloes," was made up largely of New Yorkers. It was hailed in New York City with a giant parade upon its return home on February 17, 1919. Jackson was honorably discharged in April.

Career

After World War I, Dr. Jackson resumed his medical practice in Baltimore. He married Alma Roberts. The couple had two children—Doris and Justin. In 1922 he was named a member of a new "Colored" unit of the Baltimore Public Health Department. Among other duties, he and Dr. Ralph Young operated a venereal clinic two nights a week at Provident Hospital.[4] Friends reported that "Doc" was quite a baseball fan.[5] He and Alma were also members of the elite in the city's African American society. They were among those at a party given by Dr. Joseph Thomas in Baltimore where his garden was transformed into a Japanese tea garden. Drs. Curtis and Jones from Washington, D.C., who had served with Jackson in France, were among the guests of honor.[6]

In 1932, Dr. W. H. Montague opened a renovated sanatorium for African Americans. It had 50 beds and was located at 1930 Madison Avenue in Baltimore. It was specifically established for the treatment of eye, ear, nose and throat ailments but included a number of other specialties. Dr. Jackson was put in charge of genitourinary diseases, those related to the genital and urinary organs.[7] He also continued to work with Baltimore's Public Health Department.

Dr. Jackson died suddenly at age 49 of myocarditis, an inflammatory disease of the heart muscle. His military funeral included salutes from many uniformed members of the National Guard's First Separate Company of Maryland. It was held at St. Mary's P.E. Church.[8] He is buried in the Officers Section of Loudon Park National Cemetery in Baltimore.

NOTES

1. 1910 U.S. Federal Census.
2. "Healer Jailed When Female Patient Dies," *Baltimore Afro-American*, November 10, 1914, 9.
3. "The Week in Society," *Washington Bee*, January 5, 1918, 5.
4. "Will Serve Health Department," *Baltimore Afro-American*, February 24, 1922, 12.
5. "Letter to the Editor," *Chicago Defender*, January 28, 1924, 8.
6. "Sparrows Pt. Physician Give Garden Party," *Baltimore Afro-American*, August 13, 1927, 13.

7. "New Hospital to Open Here," *Baltimore Afro-American*, July 9, 1932, 11.
8. "Photonews," *Baltimore Afro-American*, September 24, 1937, 17.

Clarence Sumner JANIFER

18 March 1886–13 November 1950
New York Homeopathic Medical College, 1915

Roots and Education

Clarence and his brother George were born in Virginia. When they were quite young, their mother died. Their father George Sr., moved the family to Newark where he got work as a school janitor. The boys' uncle Joe and housekeeper Maria Corsby (also a janitor) lived with them in the upper unit of a house at 190 Ridge Street.

In 1906, Janifer graduated with honors from Newark High School. He went on to college at Syracuse University in New York. In 1915, he graduated from the Homeopathic Medical College and Flower Hospital in New York City. After his internship at Mercy Hospital in Philadelphia, Dr. Janifer passed the New Jersey board on his first attempt and returned to Newark.[1] He then passed his examination for city clinic physician with a 99.09 percent during his first year of practice[2] as a pediatrician. In 1916, he joined the National Medical Association (NMA), and he became the first African American member of the Medical Society of New Jersey. He was single and living at 3172 Parker Street in Newark and was a member of the Alpha Phi Alpha fraternity, the Odd Fellows and the Methodist Episcopal Church. He was also a member of the Newark City Dispensary Staff.[3]

Military Service

In the summer of 1917, Janifer volunteered for service in the army's Medical Reserve Corps. In August he reported to Fort Des Moines for basic training at the Medical Officers Training Camp. Following his training, in November, he was assigned to the Third Battalion, 372nd Infantry Regiment Medical Corps of the 93rd Division. The 93rd Division had been organized in December 1917 from many National Guard units, including the famous 15th New York, called the Harlem Hell Fighters. The 372nd was designated one of the division's four regiments. Formed at Camp Stuart at Newport News, Virginia, in January 1918, it sailed for France from Newport News on March 30, 1918.[4]

The division had never been completely organized, and it was one of the first American units to arrive in France. The French had been lobbying hard to have the new American troops turned over to them to build up their beleaguered battalions. General Pershing was not ready to deal with African American troops on the ground so turned them over to the French. The soldiers traded U.S. weapons and insignia for those of the French and fought with its forces. They became known as the "Blue Helmets." The 93rd was a spark from America that the French soldiers needed to continue this long and bloody war.

Trench foot in France was common. It was often caused by men standing in trench water for so long a period that any infection caused the flesh of the foot to decay and die. Leg wounds, often caused by explosive artillery shells, were common. Legs were often amputated.[5] Janifer learned how to deal with these and a host of other traumatic wounds.

The heroism of these American troops became legend. Lieutenant Janifer was among them. On December 23, 1918, he was awarded the Croix de Guerre for courage under fire. His citation from Captain Preston F. Walsh states, "Fearless to danger, [Janifer] established his First Aid Post on the battlefield in Front of Bussy Farm [on] September 28, 1918, following the Battalion in the open fields, giving help and relief to the wounded and dying at first hand."[6]

As the war ended, Janifer, as well as the other African American doctors in the 372nd, was reassigned to the 92nd Division. There he rejoined many of the physicians with whom he had trained at Fort Des Moines.

Career

Janifer returned to Newark and practiced medicine there for the next 35 years. Clement Price's article on Newark's desegregation tells of the black migration to Newark between

1920 and 1940. The black population more than doubled. Much of the city government and its services (including the hospitals) remained segregated. "Racial discrimination in employment and housing forced all but a few of them into the central city, primarily the notorious old Third Ward in the Hill District" currently known as the Central Ward.[7] This was one of the worst slums in the country. Much of it was destroyed during the racial unrest of the 1960s.

It was in this area of the poorest that Janifer spent 35 years assisting the Newark Health Department. Most of his early years were in part-time positions, but after a time he was put in charge of the city's Well Baby Clinic for African Americans.

Since Newark City Hospital was segregated, he continued his work with Philadelphia's Mercy Hospital. By the mid 1920s he was a member of its surgical team. There he worked with some of the same officers who had served in the First World War, including Frank E. Boston and Egbert T. Scott. On the other hand, Janifer was occasionally the only African American included in medical events. In 1922, for example, he attended the New Jersey State Medical Society annual meeting in Springlake Beach.[8]

Dr. Janifer and his wife Una Marie had one son, Clarence Jr., in the early 1920s. Una was born in Auburn, New York, and was a graduate of Syracuse University. She had taught school in Texas and Virginia and at the Tuskegee Institute in Alabama before coming to New Jersey.[9] The couple lived at 208 Parker Street while he practiced medicine and continued his education earning a master's degree in public health.

One of the highlights of the Janifers' social life had to be the annual pre–Lenten promenade and party of the Twenty Club. It was described as "one of the most pretentious and exclusive affairs ever given in New Jersey." The 1927 event at the Knights of Columbus clubhouse included dances by the Ziegfeld Follies, dance selections, a "midnight buffet and a promenade at 2 a.m. in a riot of mirth, laughter, confetti and vari-colored bombing streamers."[10]

Professionally, Janifer shared the information he gathered from his position with the city's Well Baby Clinics with other African American doctors through NMA's journal. In 1929, he wrote about the symptoms of syphilis in infants.[11] The next year, he wrote on "Negro Infant Mortality Rates." In succeeding years he published articles on related subjects, always promoting the success of his well-baby clinics. He offered ways to combat the high mortality of African American children by educating mothers and care givers to the importance of child hygiene and nutrition.

The most bizarre delivery of Dr. Janifer's career was a two-headed baby boy born in 1934. Dr. Janifer reported the baby had "two perfectly formed heads on two necks. Eyes, nose and ears were all well formed, too. The infant was dead at birth. The parents had the body displayed for three days at the undertaker. More than 40,000 people came to see it before the police ordered the exhibition stopped."[12]

When the John A. Andrew Clinical Society scheduled its 1942 annual meeting at the Tuskegee Institute Hospital, 153 physicians attended, and Dr. Janifer delivered one of the papers.

It was not until 1946 that Dr. Janifer was asked to join the Newark City Hospital as a member of the pediatrics department. He was only the second African American to be invited to do so. The first (also in 1946) was a woman, Dr. E. Mae McCarrol. Two years later, he was among 42 distinguished citizens named to the *New Jersey Herald Times*' Hall of Fame in 1948.[13]

He died two years later at the age of 64 of carcinoma of the prostate. Una survived her husband by 13 years. She continued as an activist. Among the accolades she received were the Brotherhood Award from the Newark Human Rights Commission and a citation from the Council Against Intolerance in America.

NOTES

1. *The New York Age*, April 19, 1919, 7.
2. "France Honors Newark Doctor," *New York Amsterdam News*, March 16, 1927, 17.
3. John L. Thompson, *History and Views of Colored Officers Training Camp for 1917 at Fort Des Moines, Iowa* (Des Moines: *The Bystander*, 1917) 65.

4. Frank E. Roberts, *The American Foreign Legion* (Annapolis, MD: Naval Institute Press, 2004) 36–41.
5. "Sossatimothy, the Impact of Medical Treatment in WWI," www.worldhistoryiiwwi.wordpress.com (accessed October 24, 2014).
6. Emmett J. Scott, *Scott's Official History of the American Negro in the World War* (Homewood Press: 1919), 188.
7. "The Struggle to Desegregate Newark: Black Middle Class Militancy in New Jersey, 1932–1947," *New Jersey History*, New Jersey Historical Society, Vol. XCIX, 209.
8. *Ibid.*
9. "Newark Biography, October 29, 1963," New Jersey Reference Newark Library.
10. "Twenty Club of North Jersey Gives Pre-Lenten Promenade at Orange," *The New York Age*, March 5, 1927.
11. "Some Objective Symptoms of Syphilis in Infants," *Journal of the National Medical Association*, Vol. XXI, No. 4, 1929, 156–157.
12. "2 Headed Baby Born in Newark, NJ; Body May Be Exhibited," *The New York Age*, September 8, 1934, 1.
13. "N.J. Herald Elects 42 Distinguished Citizens to Hall of Fame," *New Journal and Guide*, November 13, 1948, 17.

Douglas Beverly JOHNSON

27 February 1888–5 November 1925
University of Vermont, 1914

Roots and Education

Douglas Johnson was born in Petersburg, Virginia, to Professor Walter P. and Mariah Beverly Johnson. His father was on the faculty at the Virginia Normal and Collegiate Institute (now Virginia State University) for more than 30 years, beginning in 1887. It is a historically black land-grant school near Petersburg. Douglas was born the year after his father became a professor of applied mathematics. He graduated from Virginia Normal and went on to Virginia Union University in Richmond, Virginia. He continued his graduate education at Howard University in Washington, D.C., and then earned his medical degree from the Medical College of the University of Vermont in Burlington in 1914.[1]

Dr. Johnson returned to Petersburg to practice medicine. In 1915, he sat for the Virginia State Medical Board exam and passed it with the highest average among 75 contestants. In October 1916, he joined with other Petersburg notable African American residents to found the William A. Crowder Memorial Hospital in Petersburg. It was formally opened in October 1916 and chartered by the State in February 1917. He lived at 39 Oak Street in Petersburg when he registered for the World War I draft in June 1917, and he gave his home address in August as 514 Byrne Street. He also was a member of the Episcopal Church.[2]

Military Service

Dr. Johnson volunteered to serve in the U.S. Army and received his commission as a first lieutenant in the Medical Reserve Corps. Lieutenant Johnson was called into active duty and reported for training at the Medical Officers Training Camp (MOTC) in Fort Des Moines on August 6, 1917. He was one of the early arrivals at camp and completed 90 days of training. On November 3, 1917, Lieutenant Johnson was assigned to the 92nd Division and was ordered to Camp Upton on Long Island near New York City. There he had to deal with health problems associated with a large influx of men, things like meningitis, tuberculosis, influenza, pneumonia and venereal diseases.

Johnson was appointed surgeon for the 351st Machine Gun Battalion, which consisted of three machine gun companies. The 367th Infantry Regiment, which his unit supported in combat, was also formed there. He led the 351st Machine Gun Battalion's medical detachment throughout the war and was assisted by a dental surgeon.

In June 1918, he sailed to France with the 351st. Once in France, his medical responsibilities expanded. As Battalion Surgeon, he gained command and leadership experience while treating the ill, injured and wounded. Machine gun companies were assigned to support the infantry. The machine gun had proved a fearsome defensive weapon in fixed strong points covering potential enemy attack routes.

Combat injuries in the 351st Machine Gun Battalion were limited while it was assigned in defensive trench areas of St. Dié in the Vosges Mountains, but increased later as it saw offensive combat. Lieutenant Johnson's infirmary and aid stations took care of all types of casualties. While in the Marbache sector on October 14, 1918, he received a memo requiring him to report daily to the division's surgeon on numbers of casualties broken down by wounded, gassed, sick and neuroses. In a handwritten response on October 21, 1918, he wrote, "There has been no evacuation of casualties from this

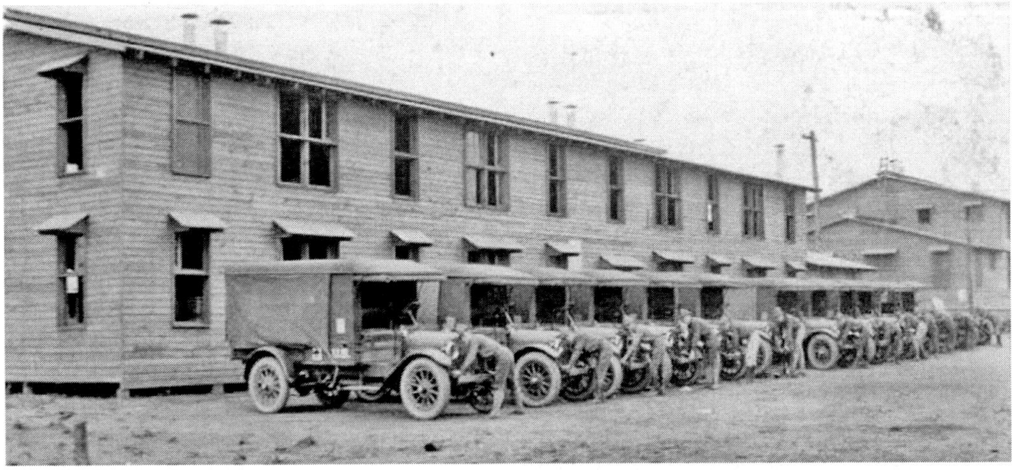

Motor ambulances at Camp Upton, New York (National Archives).

infirmary since October 14, 1918. When companies of this battalion are on the line, all casualties ... are sent to hospital through the Battalion Aid Station of the infantry to which they are attached.... All cases evacuated from this infirmary to hospital will be reported by name and number as requested by you." Even as the war ended with the Armistice on November 11, 1918, there were numerous lingering medical cases requiring treatment before Lieutenant Johnson returned home. In February 1919, the 92nd Division returned to the United States. By the time of his discharge, Dr. Johnson had served in the army more than one and a half years.

Career

After returning to New York from France in 1919, Dr. Johnson was attracted to opportunities in New York City. A large and thriving African American community was developing there with a heavy concentration in Harlem. In 1920 Dr. Johnson married Myrtle Lillian Capehart of Raleigh, North Carolina. She was the daughter of a prominent Raleigh physician, Dr. Lovelace B. Capehart. They lived in Harlem at 221 West 138th Street not far from Harlem Hospital. At that time the hospital only employed white doctors and nurses.

Dr. Johnson joined the local North Harlem Medical, Dental and Pharmaceutical Association. In the early 1920s, he became involved with a broad coalition of African American medical doctors and political activists seeking to secure hospital and municipal appointments for black physicians and jobs for black nurses. The activists won a victory in 1923 when black nurses were hired.[3]

In early 1924, the *Journal of the National Medical Association* published a lengthy article written by Dr. Johnson about the timing and advisability of surgery to treat certain pelvic conditions.[4] His peers were recognizing him for his professional skill and knowledge.

Then in 1925, black leaders agreed to a temporary measure in which five black physicians would be hired as assistant visiting surgeons and physicians at Harlem Hospital. Their positions were considered provisional until they had demonstrated their competence to the white staff. Dr. Johnson was one of the five pioneers. Their goal was to achieve full staff recognition, and they continued to apply political pressure to make that happen. Unfortunately, Dr. Johnson did not survive long enough to see that day come. He died prematurely from complications following appendicitis surgery at Harlem Hospital in November 1925.[5] In fact, it wasn't until 1928 that his friend and associate, Dr. Louis T. Wright, was hired to the staff at Harlem Hospital following years of political wrangling and pressure. That opened the door for other African American doctors and is a legacy that Dr. Johnson would have treasured.

Dr. Johnson was survived by his wife and their two-year-old daughter, Marie. His wife was pregnant at the time of his death. That child, Myrtle Douglas Johnson, followed in her father's footsteps through the Medical College at the University of Vermont and enjoyed a long career in medicine as an anesthesiologist. Myrtle's older sister, Marie, was also quite accomplished studying mathematics at Hunter College in New York City and Radcliffe College at Harvard in Cambridge, Massachusetts. Many of Marie's six children pursued careers in science and mathematics.

A continuing tradition of family academic accomplishment and community service is reflected in Dr. Johnson's grandsons. The eldest, Dr. David Douglas Newstein (named in honor of his grandfather), earned a PhD in epidemiology from Columbia University. Another grandson, Dr. Michael Charles Newstein, earned his M.D. from the Alpert Medical School at Brown University and specializes in infectious diseases. Dr. Johnson would most certainly have been extremely proud of all of them.[6]

Dr. Johnson was buried in Bronx, New York, in the Woodlawn Cemetery, a beautiful and still active 400-acre, non-sectarian cemetery since 1863. He rests in good company. The cemetery is a National Historic Landmark with many notable citizens interred there including author Herman Melville, publisher Joseph Pulitzer, mayor Fiorello LaGuardia, salsa singer and performer Celia Cruz, pianist and bandleader Duke Ellington, composer and lyricist Irving Berlin, and women's rights activist Elizabeth Cady Stanton.[7]

Notes

1. NAACP, *The Crisis*, Vol. 23, November 1921, 28.
2. John L. Thompson, *History and Views of Colored Officers Training Camp for 1917 at Fort Des Moines, Iowa* (Des Moines: The Bystander, 1917) 65.
3. Vanessa Northington Gamble, *Making a Place for Ourselves: The Black Hospital Movement, 1920–1945* (New York: Oxford University Press, 1995) 58.
4. "Pelvic Surgery," *Journal of the National Medical Association (JNMA)*, January–March 1924, Vol. 16, 14.
5. Vanessa Northington Gamble, *Making a Place for Ourselves: The Black Hospital Movement, 1920–1945* (New York: Oxford University Press, 1995) 58.
6. Dr. Michael C. Newstein, grandson, correspondence with authors in 2014.
7. Woodlawn Cemetery, thewoodlawncemetery.org.

George Wesley Patrick JOHNSON

1 March 1886–10 September 1949
Meharry Medical College, 1911

Roots and Education

George W. P. Johnson was born in Savannah, Georgia, to Ed and Ella Johnson. He had an older brother, Ulysses G. Johnson, who was called "Euly." In 1900, when he was 14, the family was living at Hog Wallow in Tattnall County, Georgia, a rural area about 70 miles west of Savannah.[1] He graduated from nearby Swainsboro High School with a certificate as a medical student and was an AME church member.[2]

Johnson trained at Fisk University in Nashville, and later attended Meharry Medical College from 1907 to 1911. Following graduation he first came to Gainesville, Florida, in 1911 where his mother and brother were living. From there he moved to Key West, Florida, and practiced medicine there for several years.[3]

On January 8, 1913, "at a quiet wedding" he was married at the home of his bride's family in Key West.[4] A marriage announcement appearing in *The Crisis* in March 1913 said Dr. George W. P. Johnson, a leading colored physician of Key West, married Miss Bloneva W. Terry.[5] His wife soon became seriously ill. A news report in February 1914 said her condition was improving.[6] She did not survive.

By 1915 he had returned to Gainesville and lived at 205 East Union Street. His office was located at 912 North Pleasant Street.[7] He did not practice long. By the fall, Dr. Johnson was back in school, this time in Detroit. He earned a doctor of public health degree from the Detroit College of Medicine and Surgery (now part of Wayne State University) in June 1916.[8] He then returned to his Gainesville practice.

Military Service

In 1917, as America entered the First World War, Dr. Johnson, now 31, registered for the draft. His registration shows him married then to Elizabeth (Lizzie) Johnson and practicing medicine at 504 North Pleasant, Gainesville.[9] He entered the U.S. Army in September 1917 as a first lieutenant in the Medical Reserve Corps and reported to Fort Des Moines, Iowa, for training.

He successfully completed his training in early November 1917 and was sent to Camp Funston, Kansas, to the 92nd Division. From there he was honorably discharged at the end of November 1917 as being "physically disqualified." Although his active service was brief, he received two months of intense military training, and he was proud of his service.

Career

After his military service, Dr. Johnson and Lizzie settled in Tampa, Florida, where he practiced for more than 30 years. According to the 1920 Census, they rented a house at 1108 Ashley Street. The family now included a two-year-old daughter named Yvonne and a baby named Mercedes. Daughter Imogene would join the family later. His mother Ella and a nephew lived with them. Dr. Johnson's office in the early 1920s was at 1404½ Central Avenue and his residence was now at 1518 Nebraska Avenue.

It appears he separated from Elizabeth in the mid 1920s because by 1927 he was married to June C. Johnson. His former wife, Elizabeth, was a public school teacher, and she and their children remained in Tampa. At this time Dr. Johnson maintained his medical office in his home at 1606 Mitchell Avenue.

In May 1928, he and Dr. J. A. Parker traveled to Tallahassee to attend the Grand Lodge Convention of the Order of Knights Pythians and Calanthes of Florida. They were both medical directors for the fraternal orders.[10] Both organizations were devoted to charitable activities. By 1932, he had been grand medical director for the Florida Court of Calanthes for 15 years. He was also health director for the African American schools of Tampa, and president of the Booker Washington High School PTA.[11]

In February 1932, Dr. Johnson was made superintendent of the Clara Frye Tampa Municipal Negro Hospital.[12] In 1907 Nurse Clara Frye (1872–1936) had established a hospital for African Americans in her home. In 1923 she moved to a small 17-bed hospital at 1615 Lamar Avenue, where she relied heavily on donations to alleviate the financial struggles of running a hospital. In 1928, the City of Tampa purchased the hospital on Lamar Avenue. It then became known as the Tampa Negro Hospital. Dr. Johnson held the Superintendent post for almost 20 years during the 1930s and 1940s. In 1933 the hospital was visited by Dr. Cutter, a representative of the American Medical Association. As a result of his investigation, the hospital was placed on the AMA register of hospitals, a quality assurance vote for any facility.[13]

For more than 50 years, the hospital served thousands of African Americans until it closed in 1967 following integration. According to the book *African American Sites in Florida*, "Segregation became a way of life for Tampa blacks in the 20th century. Even when they became sick they had to go to segregated facilities ... for example the Clara Frye Memorial Hospital."[14]

As early as March 25, 1933, the American Medical Association determined the hospital under Dr. Johnson's leadership had greatly increased its equipment and status and was now worthy of a place in the AMA published register of hospitals.[15] There were about eight nurses there, and doctors would come from other Tampa hospitals to perform tonsillectomies, tracheotomies, and other procedures that required hospitalization.[16]

In 1934, in an example of his personal courage, the newspaper reported Dr. Johnson had "won the approval of his superiors, friends and all law abiding citizens of the city by the fearless manner in which he wounded and captured a marauder who had been prowling the various properties owned by the doctor." He encountered the intruder in his house on Nebraska Avenue and shot him in the left thigh and right wrist, subdued him and called the police and had the man arrested.[17]

Dr. Johnson was an active member of the Tampa Negro Chamber of Commerce.[18] At its annual meeting in July 1938 he was recognized as one of four physicians who made civic contributions by giving health talks.

That same year Dr. Johnson was able to move his staff into an entirely new hospital facility that had been made possible by an investment of $117,404 by the Federal Works Progress Administration. The new 40-bed hospital replaced the "congested and dilapidated quarters" on Lamar Avenue. It was brick and concrete, and virtually fireproof. The two-story structure contained nurse quarters, and one story wings had private rooms and wards. New equipment had been provided by the city and through private donations. It was modern with an operating room, laboratories, x-ray, drug and obstetrical departments, children's department and electrical kitchens and steam heat.[19] It is a testimonial to Dr. Johnson that he championed and was medical director of this project serving Tampa's large African American community.

Dr. Johnson continued to serve his community and the hospital for many more years until he became seriously ill himself. He went for extended care to the Tuskegee Veterans Hospital for African Americans in Tuskegee, Alabama. He passed away there in 1949 at age 63. He was buried in Tampa at Rest Haven Memorial Park Cemetery under a bronze marker supplied in 1950 by the U.S. Army quartermaster general to his oldest daughter, Yvonne E. Johnson.[20]

NOTES

1. 1900 U.S. Federal Census.
2. Meharry Archives Report dated July 17, 2012, Meharry Medical College, Nashville, TN.
3. *Catalogue of 1911–1912, Meharry Medical College, Walden University*, Nashville, TN, 50.
4. "Key West News," *The New York Age*, January 16, 1913, 7.
5. "Along the Color Line," *The Crisis*, March 1913, Vol. 5, No. 5, Whole No. 29, 219.
6. "Key West News," *The New York Age*, February 19, 1914.
7. *Gainesville, Florida City Directory, 1915*, ancestry.com.
8. AMA Deceased Physician Card, National Library of Medicine, Bethesda, MD.
9. World War I Draft Registration Car, ancestry.com.
10. "Tampa, Fla., by Elva," *Pittsburgh Courier*, May 26, 1928, Second Section, 7.
11. "Pick Meharry Grad to Head Hospital," *Chicago Defender*, February 27, 1932, 2.
12. *Ibid.*
13. "Tampa," *Pittsburgh Courier*, April 1, 1933, 10.
14. Kevin M. McCarthy, *African American Sites in Florida* (Sarasota: Pineapple Press, 2007) 102.
15. "Key West News," *Pittsburgh Courier*, April 1, 1933, 10.
16. University of South Florida Oral History Program "Interview with Coreen Glover, 2009," http://digital.lib.usf.edu/SFS0022452/00001 (accessed August 2, 2014).
17. "Medic Commended for Capture of Burglar," *Atlanta Daily World*, January 19, 1934, 1.
18. "C. of C. Cites Members for Achievement," *Chicago Defender*, July 23, 1938 10.
19. "Open New Municipal Hospital in Tampa, Fla.," *Chicago Defender*, December 24, 1938, 3.
20. Application for Headstone or Marker to Office of the Quartermaster General, December 14, 1949, Johnson, George W.P., ancestry.com.

Romeo Asburn JOHNSTON

21 November 1882–11 October 1931
Starling Medical College, 1909

Roots and Education

Romeo A. Johnston was born to Louis and Jane Hull Johnston in Bath County, in the mountains of western Virginia. Bath County is named for the English resort city of Bath. The county is comprised of a number of villages including Hot Springs, Warm Springs, Millboro and Mountain Grove. Hot Springs and Warm Springs are the most well known of the villages. The county's population in 1900 was 5,595.

The Reconstruction Constitutional Convention of 1867–68 mandated a statewide system of free, state-funded schools for black children. The public schools were racially segregated, and the focus was primary education. Virginia had only a handful of true black high schools before 1906. None appear to have been in Bath County. The quality of teaching and level of funding were inadequate, and black schools received the least of both. There is no evidence that Romeo Johnston attended anything other than Bath County public schools, but it was from this educational foundation that he was able to be pursue a medical degree.

About 1905, he entered Starling Medical College in Columbus, Ohio. The presence of medical colleges in Columbus provided the community with a cross section of established physicians as faculty members, and the yearly graduating classes meant a continuing supply of new, young doctors for the region.[1]

The first private hospitals established in Columbus were associated with the existing medical colleges and were organized by physicians and responsible citizens. While Romeo Johnston was in Columbus, St. Francis Hospital existed in the Starling Medical College building. It functioned as a training ground for the physicians-in-training. In later years Starling became Ohio State University College of Medicine.[2]

After graduation from Starling in 1909, Dr. Johnston was awarded an internship at Freedmen's Hospital in Washington, D.C.[3] He completed his training and set up his medical practice in Nelsonville in Coshocton County, Ohio. The town is halfway between Columbus and Parkersburg, West Virginia. There he met Martha "Mattie" I. Lett.

Mattie was the daughter of Edward Thomas and Elizabeth Norman Lett of Nelsonville. Her father was a well-respected citizen there who for many years worked as a coal miner for the C. L. Poston Coal Company. He was active in the local Republican Party, at one time serving as president of the local Republican McKinley Club.[4] Her mother had six children by a previous marriage. The Letts had two daughters of their own, Martha (Mattie) and Grace May. Ed Lett also raised three girls from her first marriage—Isa, Henrietta, and Islita. All of the girls received educations. Mattie worked as a servant in Athens, Ohio, about the time she met Dr. Johnston.

Mattie and Romeo married in Coshocton County, Ohio, on July 7, 1913. She was 27 and he was 30 at the time of the marriage. There would be no children. The couple was living at 200 Lexington Avenue in Columbus when Dr. Johnston enlisted.

Military Service

Johnston (military records list him as Johnson) responded to the call for African Americans to volunteer for service for the First World War. He left his wife Mattie and his practice to report to the medical officers training camp at Fort Des Moines on August 2, 1917. After three months of training he was sent to Camp Funston at Fort Riley, Kansas, where he was assigned to the 92nd Division's 368th Field Hospital. After he arrived in France in August 1918, he was billeted at the home of Madame Antoine at #19 Rue D'Elopes in the village of Jarmenil in the Vosges Mountains.[5] His unit was en route to the St. Dié sector for training and its first exposure to actual combat. Officers often stayed in the homes of residents. Housing was in short supply, and residents were happy to have the money.

By September 6, 1918, First Lieutenant Johnston was transferred to the 366th Ambulance Company. His ambulance company was with reserve troops in the Meuse-Argonne sector offensive. About this time the Spanish Flu pandemic struck the troops in terrific numbers, and the medical units became focused on treating the sick.

During the American Expeditionary Forces' campaign in the Meuse-Argonne, the epidemic diverted urgently needed resources from combat support to transporting and caring for the sick and the dead. Influenza and pneumonia killed

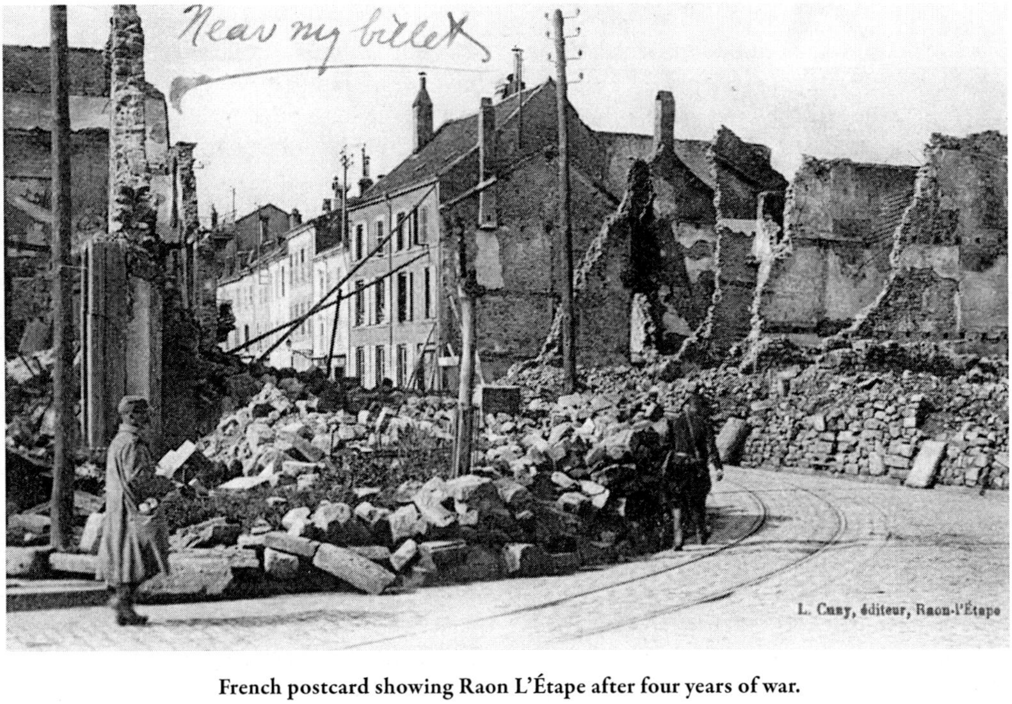

French postcard showing Raon L'Étape after four years of war.

more American soldiers and sailors during the war than did enemy weapons.[6]

The 366th was then moved to the Marbache sector (Lorraine) on October 8 and saw action in the battle of Metz just before the end of the war. Here the men of the 366th were front line troops.

Casualties were significant. The men of the ambulance companies supplied litter bearers to carry sick and wounded from front line positions to battalion aid stations and to ambulance dressing stations. Once there doctors and medics provided first aid to the sick and injured, as well as cared for the lightly gassed patients. The medical care provided allowed troops to return to their units. More serious illness and wounds were treated and then transported to divisional field hospitals.

Treatment could include dressing wounds, immobilizing fractures, or providing pain relief before transporting the wounded to field hospitals. The ambulance companies also transported medical and other supplies from the field hospital forward to the dressing stations and aid stations. Ambulance company physicians continued to treat the wounded and gassed well after the war ended on November 11.[7]

Career

After he was honorably discharged on March 13, 1919, Dr. Johnston returned to Ohio to Nelsonville and his practice in Athens. In the 1920s he and Mattie moved to Columbus and set up his office at 202 East Fourth Street. They lived at 200 Lexington Avenue in the Bronzeville community.

The presence of The Ohio State University drew college educated African Americans to the city. The Bronzeville community was flourishing.[8] Development escalated. By the 1920s, in the Jefferson-Garfield blocks on East Long Street, there were ten black physicians, six dentists, ten churches, two drug stores, two undertakers, and more than 100 African American owned homes. Toward the end of the 1920s, the Johnsons bought a house at 1506 Mt. Vernon Avenue.

Unfortunately, Dr. Johnston died soon afterward, shortly before his 49th birthday. He had served his local community for less than 10 years when he passed away. The cause of death was toxic myocarditis that brought on heart failure. Contributing factors were diabetes and his pulmonary tuberculosis. Mattie applied for and received a military headstone for his grave in Union Cemetery in Athens, Ohio. Mattie stayed in the house in Columbus after his death and continued her work as a social worker with the Columbus Urban League.

Notes

1. https://hsl.osu.edu/mhc/15-columbus-medical-and-health-1880–1914 (accessed September 20, 2013).
2. u.osu.edu (accessed March 6, 2015).
3. "This Week in Society," *Washington Bee*, November 19, 1910, 5.
4. Edward Thomas Lett, ancestry.com.
5. RG 120, Records of the American Expeditionary Forces (World War I), 92nd Division, 317th Sanitary Train, National Archives, College Park, MD.
6. ncbi.nim.nih.gov (accessed March 6, 2015).
7. U.S. Army Medical Department, Office of Medical History, Vol. VIII Field Operations, Chapter IV, Medical Service of the Division in Combat (Washington, D.C.: GPO, 1925) history.amedd.army.mil (accessed April 23, 2015).
8. u.osu.edu (accessed March 6, 2015).

Elisha Henry JONES

20 February 1883–6 February 1963
University of West Tennessee, 1907

Roots and Education

Elisha Jones was born at Talladega, Alabama. His father, Henry Clay Jones, was a farmer and his mother Jane (Doone) Jones was a nurse. He was one of four children and the oldest son. His older sisters became teachers. Jones was schooled in Talladega and graduated from Talladega College in 1904. The college is Alabama's oldest private historically black liberal arts college. He became president of the college's Alumni Association in 1905.[1] Jones went to work in education and was the principal of the Lauderdale College elementary school in Birmingham, Alabama, for two years. He then enrolled in medical school at the University of West Tennessee in Memphis where he worked to help pay for his education by teaching Latin and algebra. He earned his M.D. in 1909.

Dr. Jones returned home to Alabama and passed the Alabama State Medical examination that same year. He opened his medical practice in Talladega and continued it for 50-plus years. He started practicing medicine from his home, a simple one-story frame house, before the erection of his office building on West Battle Street. He was also connected to the New Era Pharmacy in 1909–1910, and subsequently with the Highland Drug Co. It was common for physicians to be associated with pharmacies to earn additional income and better serve their patients.

Even as a young physician, he was quite active in civic, fraternal and political organizations. As early as 1914, he was a member of the Executive Committee of the Talladega NAACP branch[2] and chairman of the Congregational Laymen's Missionary Movement for Alabama. He was a Republican, a member of the Social Settlement Club, and served as secretary for the Living Endowment Association of his alma mater, Talladega College.[3]

He married Effie May Murphy of Montgomery, Alabama, on July 29, 1910.[4] They had a daughter and five sons and were married 52 years. They lived for many years at 114 Pulliam Street in Talladega and later at 720 Pulliam Street. His medical office was at 236 West Battle Street.

The city of Talladega is small and the county seat of Talladega County. The county is in the north central part of the state about 50 miles east of Birmingham. It experienced very slow steady population growth throughout the 20th century, from 35,000 in 1900 to 74,000 by 1990. The African Americans in the community made up roughly 40 percent of the population Talladega College has been an important institution there since it was founded in 1867.

Military Career

When the United States first entered the First World War in 1917, Dr. Jones volunteered and received a commission as a first lieutenant in the Army Medical Reserve Corps. He was 34 years old when he reported for military training at Fort Des Moines, Iowa, in October 1917. He successfully completed a month of training and was assigned to the 92nd Division's Sanitary (Medical) Train at Camp Funston, Kansas. He was assigned first with the

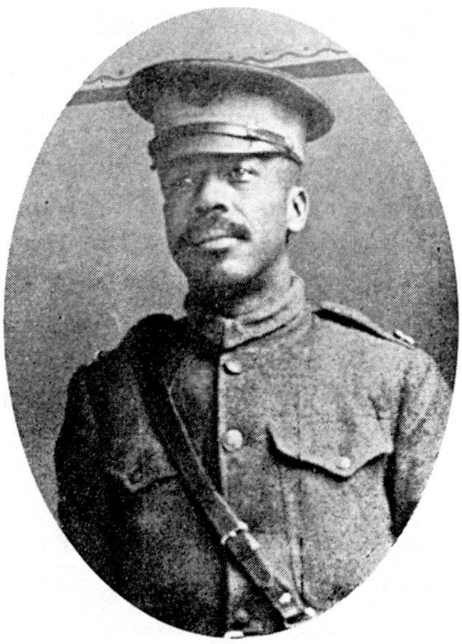

Capt. Elisha H. Jones (courtesy General Research & Reference Division, Schomburg Center for Research in Black Culture, New York Public Library Astor, Lenox and Tilden Foundations).

365th Ambulance Company and was later reassigned as surgeon to the 349th Machine Gun Battalion. It was Jones' job to help oversee the medical care of the roughly 750 officers and men in the battalion. Sanitation was always an issue and many suffered illnesses brought on by wet and often cold conditions, as well as "cooties," infestations of lice. Influenza and pneumonia were common problems, as was "trench foot." Casualties resulting from enemy action, artillery, gas, and air attacks were all part of the mix.

Jones served in France in combat with that unit and was promoted to the rank of captain. After the war ended he returned home in 1919 and was honorably discharged April 9th. He returned to Talladega to rejoin his family and resumed his practice after serving his country on active duty for more than 18 months.

Career

Dr. Jones' life in Talladega was busy and his impact on the lives of African Americans in Alabama went well beyond that city. In 1933, he was the Sunday morning speaker at the Adult Department of the Sixteenth Street Baptist Church in Anniston. In 1939, he was a speaker at the NAACP's Birmingham Branch banquet.[5] In 1943, he was an examining physician for the summer Boy Scout Camp for Negro Youths that was held in the Choccolocco region. Troops with 105 scouts and leaders participated from more than eight towns, including Brewtonville, Anniston, Hobson City, Jacksonville, Talladega, Sycamore, Gadsden, and Sylacauga.[6]

He was very involved with the Alabama State Medical Society and was honored with a certificate of merit at the group's annual meeting in 1950 at Tuskegee,[7] and he became historian of the organization.[8] He served as editor of the National Alumni Association for his medical school, the University of West Tennessee, and addressed that group in Memphis in 1950.[9]

There are numerous examples of Dr. Jones' role in his community. In February 1953, he spoke on behalf of the Talladega College community at a memorial service for a revered community teacher and minister's wife.[10] In June 1954, Jones was one of four Talladega College graduates of the class of 1904 who were honored at their 50th Reunion Alumni Dinner.[11] In February 1962, he received a 25-year award from the Alpha Phi Alpha fraternity chapter in Talladega.[12] In 1995, more than 30 years after his death, a Memorial Medical Scholarship in his name, with two of his sons, was established at Talladega College to "benefit a promising graduating senior who is accepted to an accredited United States Medical School."[13]

After he died of a heart attack in 1963, shortly before his 80th birthday, the U.S. Army provided Captain Jones with a granite grave marker recognizing his service in the First World War. He had received the Victory Medal that was awarded to World War I veterans who had served honorably.[14] He is buried in Talladega at the Westview Cemetery alongside his wife Effie, who passed away 13 years later, in 1976. Some of his medical instruments have been on display in the Heritage Hall Museum in Talladega.[15]

NOTES

1. *Talladega College Catalogue, 1905.*
2. "The Annual Conference of the National Association for the Advancement of Colored People—Notes from the Branches-Talladega," *The Crisis*, April 1914, 48 pages, 289–290.
3. Frank L. Mather, Editor, *Who's Who of the Colored Race* (Chicago: 1915) Vol. One, 160.
4. *Ibid.*
5. "Alabama," *The Crisis*, December 1939, 373.
6. "Colored Youths Enjoy Week of Outdoor Life," *The Anniston Star*, August 17, 1943, 5.
7. "Alabama Medics Honored," *Pittsburgh Courier*, June 24, 1950, 11.
8. "Birmingham, Ala.," *Pittsburgh Courier*, June 23, 1956, 17.
9. "Medical Grads of West Tenn. Univ. to Hear Dr. E. H. Jones," *Memphis World*, Tuesday, April 18, 1950, Front Page, www.crossroadstofreedom.org.
10. "Final Rites for Mrs. Hamilton at Talladega College," *Atlanta Daily World*, February 12, 1953, 3.
11. "Photo Standalone 3—No Title," *Atlanta Daily World*, June 16, 1954, 2.
12. "Founders' Day, Epsilon Delta Lambda and Alpha Beta," *The Sphinx*, February 1962, Vol. 48, No. 1, 27.
13. Talladega College Scholarships, www.talladega.edu/students/scholarships.asp.
14. Application for Headstone or Marker, U.S. Army Quartermaster General, ancestry.com.
15. Amos Wright, *Hidden Legacies: I. African-American Physicians in Alabama*, www.uab.edu (accessed March 21, 2015).

Thomas Edward JONES

26 May 1880–4 April 1958
Howard Medical College, 1912

Roots and Education

Thomas Edward Jones was born to Campbell and Emma (Glenn) Jones in Lynchburg, Virginia. His father was a merchant. Jones attended public grammar school and graduated from Lynchburg High School in 1896. He went on to Howard University in Washington, D.C., for his undergraduate education and medical school.

While still in school, he married Leonie Annette Sinkler (1879–1939) on April 3, 1901. She was the daughter of Edward and Mary Sinkler of Charleston, South Carolina. Leonie was an accomplished teacher before her marriage.

While in school, Jones worked at different times as a newsboy, waiter, messenger, laborer, and watchman in government service. It was hard work, but he was cheerful and determined. And he succeeded.[1] He entered the Howard University Medical School as a "special student" in 1908 and completed all of his freshman work except histology and physiologic chemistry. During the 1909–10 sessions he completed all his sophomore year and also the deficiencies of his freshman year. Jones graduated with his M.D. degree in 1912 and interned at Freedmen's Hospital until October 1, 1913.[2] Following his training, he was appointed anesthetist at the hospital, a position he held until 1917. In June 1917 he delivered a paper entitled "Anesthesia" at meeting of the Medico-Chirurgical (Surgical) Society of the District of Columbia.[3]

Military Service

As early as 1914, he was serving as a citizen soldier in the District of Columbia as a member of the D.C. National Guard. He was a lieutenant in Company C of the First Separate Battalion. That battalion was an African American component of the District National Guard.[4]

In 1917, when America entered the First World War, Jones volunteered for the Army Medical Reserve Corps and entered the Medical Officers' Training Camp (MOTC) at Fort Des Moines, Iowa. He received 60 days of training and on November 3, he was sent to Camp Meade, Maryland, near Washington, D.C., to join the 368th Infantry Regiment of the 92d Division. First Lieutenant Jones served throughout the First World War with the 368th Infantry. His unit was stationed at St. Dié in the Vosges mountains, the Meuse-Argonne and the Marbache sector near Pont-à-Mousson on the Moselle River.

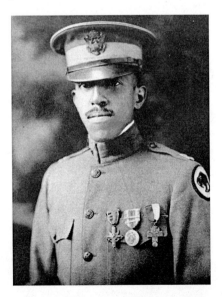

Captain T. E. Jones, with Distinguished Service Cross, Croix de Guerre, and Meuse-Argonne campaign medals (Yenser, *Who's Who in Colored America*, 6th ed. [1940–44]).

Lieutenant Jones was awarded the Distinguished Service Cross and the French Croix de Guerre when he displayed extraordinary heroism in the Argonne Forest campaign in action near Binarville, France. He was promoted to captain for attending the wounded in an open area while under machine gun fire. The U.S. Army notation on Jones' Medal No. 1844 says, "While dressing a wounded runner, a machine-gun bullet passed between his arms and his chest and a man was killed within a few yards of him."[5] Another account reads, "Under falling shell and machine gun fire ... the boys say he walked out and got wounded men with the same coolness that was his when he was putting a patient to sleep for an operation."[6]

Career

Following the war, Dr. Jones returned to Washington, D.C., to Freedmen's Hospital as Resident Assistant Surgeon from 1919 to 1921. He was then appointed assistant surgeon-in-chief. In 1936, he was promoted to the top job and became surgeon-in-chief, a position he held until his retirement in 1942, after a total of 27 years of service to the hospital. Dr. Jones also taught gynecology at Howard University Medical School.

The Smithsonian Institution holds a formal photograph of Dr. Jones standing next the U.S. president's wife, Eleanor Roosevelt, and interior secretary, Harold L. Ickes. He was clearly recognized as a leader in the African American community.[7]

His commitment to his community is remarkable. He was active in benevolent societies including the Masons, Odd Fellows, and Pythians. He belonged to and was a steward in the Methodist Episcopal Church and was a member of the John F. Cook Lodge of the Freemasons in D.C. (FAAM). In 1919 he was the Washington, D.C., leader of the Methodist Church campaign commemorating the 100th anniversary of Methodist missions.[8]

Jones's professional organizations included the Medico-Chirurgical of the District and the National Medical Association (NMA). He was active in the NAACP, the YMCA, the presti-

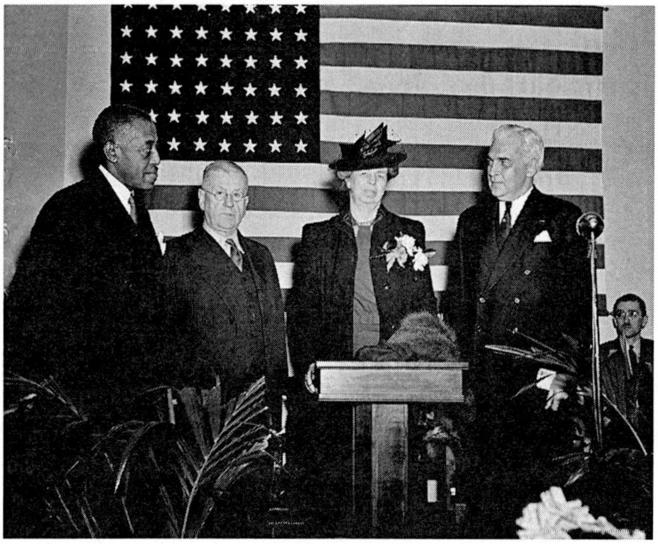

Dr. T. E. Jones with Secretary Harold Ickes, Mrs. Eleanor Roosevelt and Secretary Paul McNutt (Scurlock Studio Records, Archives Center, National Museum of American History, Smithsonian Institution).

gious Alpha Phi Alpha fraternity and the Chi Delta Mu medical fraternity. In 1925 he was elected grand sergeant-at-arms for Chi Delta Mu at its fourth annual convention in New York City.[9]

His military memberships included the Legion of Valor, whose members include Medal of Honor winners and recipients of the Army Distinguished Service Cross, the second ranking army decoration for extraordinary heroism. In 1934, he was mentioned as American Legion post surgeon in a news report headlined "DC Legionnaires Adopt Resolution Deploring Segregation in Civil Service; Urge Passing of Anti-Lynch Bill."[10] In 1941 he represented the medical world in the second selective service drawing in Washington, D.C. He was then surgeon-in-chief of Freedmen's Hospital and a member of the James E. Walker Post of the American Legion.[11] He would later become president of that post.[12]

By 1950, at the age of 70, Dr. Jones was in semi-retirement at his home at 1505 12th Street, NW, Washington, D.C., a four-story elegant brick townhome located near Logan Circle in downtown D.C. He kept his medical office open downstairs where he saw patients. After a long illness, he died of a coronary thrombosis on April 4, 1958, just before his 78th birthday. He was survived by his second wife, Minerva Jenkins Jones, and three children, Jeanette M., Emma Jane and Thomas E. Jr. He was buried with full military honors at Arlington National Cemetery next to his first wife, Leonie Annette Sinkler Jones (1879–1939).[13]

Dr. Jones believed that the best interests of his race would be promoted "by acting for the good of the masses rather than by the accumulation of property and by manifesting a financial interest in the projects of the community in which we live."[14] He lived a long and very productive life serving his country and community. He was a patriotic, courageous and hard-working physician who was well known and respected for many years.

Notes

1. Arthur Bunyan Caldwell, *History of the American Negro*, Vol. 6 (Atlanta, 1922), 99.
2. AMA Deceased Physicians Card, National Library of Medicine, Bethesda, MD.
3. "The Town Crier," *The Washington Herald*, June 28, 1917, 7.

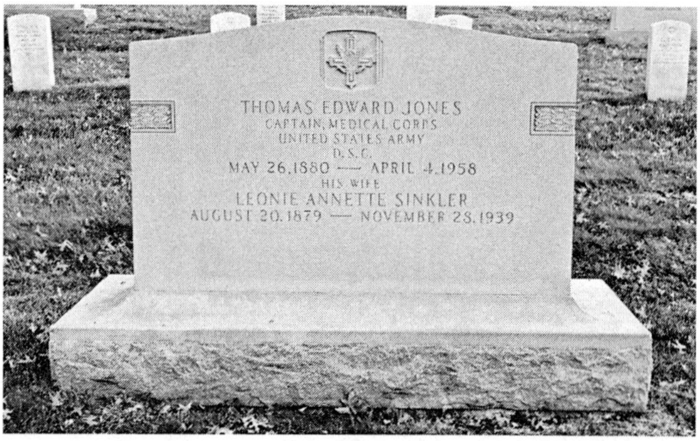
THOMAS EDWARD JONES
CAPTAIN, MEDICAL CORPS
UNITED STATES ARMY
D.S.C.
MAY 26, 1880 — APRIL 4, 1958
HIS WIFE
LEONIE ANNETTE SINKLER
AUGUST 20, 1879 — NOVEMBER 28, 1939

Captain T. E. Jones headstone, Arlington National Cemetery (photograph by W. Douglas Fisher).

4. "Citizen Soldiers of District Ready to Begin Great War Game," *The Washington Post*, July 26, 1914, E3.
5. Thomas Yenser, ed. and pub, *Who's Who in Colored America, 1941–1944* (New York, 1944), 300.
6. Professors G. M. Lightfoot, A. L. Locke, M. Maclear, *Howard University in the War* (Washington, D.C.: Howard University, 1919).
7. Photographs—1930–40—Black and White Negatives, Scurlock Studio (Washington, D.C.), Smithsonian Institution, National Museum of American History, Archives Center, Washington, D.C.
8. "Methodists Ready to Begin Drive for Big Reconstruction Fund," *Harrisburg Telegraph*, May 16, 1919, 20.
9. "Chi Delta Mu Medical Fraternity in Session," *The New York Age*, April 25, 1925, 2.
10. "DC Legionnaires Adopt Resolution Deploring Segregation in Civil Service; Urge Passing of Anti-Lynch Bill," *Pittsburgh Courier*, August 25, 1934, 5.
11. "Race Leaders Participate in Second Annual Selective Service Drawing," *Pittsburgh Courier*, July 26, 1941, 2.
12. G. James Fleming & Christian Burckel, *Who's Who in Colored America*, 1950 (Seventh Edition), 318.
13. "Professional News," *Journal of the National Medical Association (JNMA)*, September 1958, Vol. 50, No. 5, 399.
14. Caldwell, *History of the American Negro*, 100.

James Arthur (Jack) KENNEDY

10 October 1882–1 September 1966
Meharry Medical College, 1914

Roots and Education

Jack Kennedy was born to John H. and Mary Cowan Kennedy in Cotton Plant, Arkansas. The town was originally called Richmond, but there was another "Richmond" nearby. Cotton had been introduced in 1846, and it thrived so the town fathers changed the name to honor its most important crop. Cotton Plant's first post office opened in 1852. With the advent of the railroad, cotton gins, warehouses and cotton presses, the town became a bustling economic and culture center of Woodruff County in the later part of the 19th century.[1] It is somewhat diminished now, but it's still a nice small town. Following his public school education, Jack attended Branch Normal Institute in Pine Bluff. The school is now a branch of the University of Arkansas.

Kennedy was only 22 and at Branch Institute when he married his first wife, Tempy E. Holly. The couple separated when he went to Nashville's Fisk University. After Fisk, he stayed in Nashville and entered Meharry Medical College. In 1914, Kennedy graduated from both the Pharmaceutical *and* Medical departments of Meharry Medical College. He moved to Chicago and set up a surgery practice. He continued to apply for credentials in various states until his reciprocity in medicine covered 40 states, and he was certified in pharmacy in 32 states.[2]

Military Service

In 1917, Dr. Kennedy lived at the YMCA in Chicago when his application for the Army Medical Reserve Corps was accepted.[3] There he showed his true mettle. From the Meharry Annual we learn:

"Captain J. Arthur Kennedy, Surgeon of the 2nd Battalion, 366th Infantry, received the Distinguished Service Cross from General John J. Pershing for exceptional valor and meritorious service under fire at Norray, France, Nov. 10–11, 1918.

"It was during the last hours of the war when the Germans threw great clouds of gas and shrapnel upon the 92nd Division that Kennedy voluntarily moved his Aid Station from a bomb proof dugout 500 yards behind the front lines to the front line, out in the open in a partially wrecked shack. With the assistance of four of his hospital corpsmen, he personally attended and evacuated 360 severely gassed and wounded men. It was his friend and fellow physician First Lieutenant Edward W. Bates and 20 of his ambulance corpsmen who were evacuating the wounded and dying from Kennedy's station. These wounded soldiers were carried on litters two miles from the Aid Station under fire, through narrow, muddy trenches to horse-drawn ambulances. They were then taken four miles back to the 368th Ambulance Company's Station under the command of another friend and fellow physician captain H. H. Walker.

"Captain Kennedy worked until late in the evening of November 11, the final day of the war, identifying, wrapping in blankets and tagging for burial the many dead left upon the battlefield."

Kennedy survived and the following day (November 12, 1918) recommended Lieutenant Bates for the Distinguished Service Cross (DSC) and had his 20 men "cited in general orders" long before he knew that he himself was recommended by Major Sawkins for the Distinguished Service Cross.[4]

The friendships he made during the war would continue throughout his life. One larger-than-life friend from the war years would have an enormous influence: Dr. Joseph Ward of Indianapolis.

Career

After the war, Dr. Kennedy returned to Chicago. In 1919 he was initiated into the prestigious Omega Psi Phi. The fraternity's stated purpose was to attract and build a strong and effective force of men dedicated to its cardinal principles of manhood, scholarship, perseverance, and uplift. Its membership includes many recognized leaders in the arts, academics, athletics, entertainment, business, civil rights, education, government, and science fields.[5] He would remain active with this group for the rest of his life. The 1920 U.S. Census reports he was boarding with Mrs. Mattie Meyer at 3139 Calumet Avenue.

In the biography of her great-grandmother, Madam C. J. Walker (the wealthiest African American woman in the United States at this time), A'Lelia Bundles talks about Dr. Joseph Ward's affection for Dr. Kennedy. In fact, she refers to him as Ward's "protégé." He was the preferred choice among daughter A'Lelia's suitors. "Gentleman Jack," as he was affectionately known to his friends, was lean and handsome and had an agreeable manner. In May 1919, he was summoned from his home in Chicago to New York as Madam Walker lay dying. She wanted to be sure he knew she approved of the marriage to her daughter A'Lelia. Kennedy was there with Ward at her deathbed. A'Lelia was in Panama when Walker died. She was not able to return until after the funeral. Kennedy was at Grand Central Station to comfort her and her adopted daughter Mae. Kennedy was not yet divorced from his first wife Tempy. Impulsively, A'Lelia turned to another suitor, Dr. Wiley Wilson. It was a decision she would regret.[6]

By the fall of 1921, Wiley and A'Lelia separated. A'Lelia went on an extended tour of Europe. While there she wrote Kennedy, and he responded with some affectionate letters. When she got to Paris, he urged her to enjoy the city as he had in the final days there after the war. She returned to the United States in 1922, and over the next several years they saw one another in Chicago and New York, and they divorced their spouses.

The New York headline read, "A'Lelia Walker Is Married to Fiancé of Youthful Days." A'Lelia and Jack were married in Indianapolis in May 1926.[7] Their agreement was that they

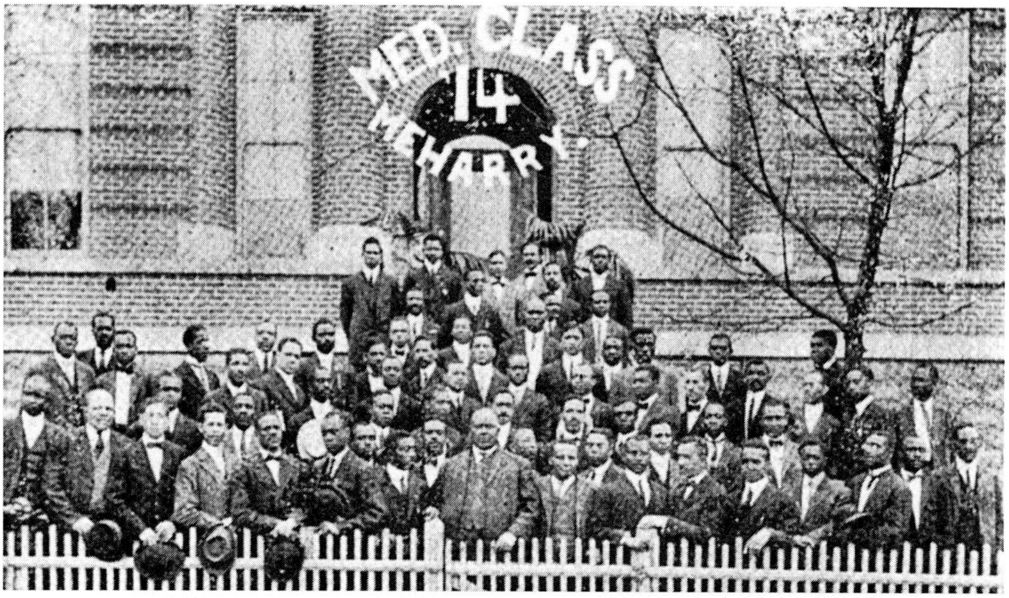

Meharry Medical School class of 1914 (courtesy Meharry Medical College Archives).

would live in New York and Chicago and take turns commuting.

In 1926, Dr. Joseph Ward was taking charge of the U.S. Veterans Hospital at Tuskegee. He invited several of the doctors he had worked with during the war to join him. That December, Dr. Kennedy, who had passed the civil service exam with excellent marks,[8] reported to Tuskegee as Ward's assistant medical officer in charge.[9] Kennedy had experienced a series of financial setbacks and didn't want to take A'Lelia's money and so he accepted Ward's offer.[10]

As second in command, he was responsible for the clinical records of thousands of patients, the sanitation of the enormous institution, the adjustment of complaints by staff and patients, and the disposal of all bodies. He also began his study of treatments for tuberculosis and would become an authority in its treatment.[11] The job required long hours and didn't leave much time for commuting to New York to see A'Lelia. While she was willing to commute to Chicago, Tuskegee, Alabama, was another thing. The marriage failed. They were divorced by 1931.

By 1936, white Southern Democrats were seeking to regain control of the administration of the veterans' hospital. Indictments were issued against 15 African American healthcare workers at the hospital. Dr. Kennedy was one of them. In his position he was one of two physicians in charge of sanitation, including caring for the dead. William Gover, the undertaker under contract with the hospital was fired for supplying inferior caskets. Then Dr. Kennedy was charged with "failing to properly inspect the corpses or to observe the quality of the equipment given them. Because Kennedy is known to be a scrupulously careful officer, charges against him have created deep resentment."[12] Kennedy did not survive when Ward was ousted in 1936, but he did stay in Tuskegee on the staff of the Tuskegee Institute's hospital.

Tuskegee was home to several important African American institutions, The Tuskegee Institute, the Veterans Hospital and the John Andrews Hospital. Many highly educated, professional African American men were drawn to the city each year to learn, teach and hone their skills.

During the 1930s, Kennedy, who was quite a sports enthusiast, took time to be the physician for the Tuskegee Institute football squad. He accompanied the team to games as far away as Soldiers Field in Chicago in 1938.[13] He also had an opportunity to visit with many of his Chicago friends when they came to Tuskegee for the Tuskegee-Wilberforce game.

He was one of the "crack golfers" who participated in the 1939 Tuskegee Golf Tournament organized by Dr. Edwin H. Lee. Lee had been with Kennedy in France during World War I. The event became annual the following year, and Dr. Kennedy was a regular participant. He was also an avid tennis player. In 1941, he was president of the Tuskegee Tennis Club and chairman of the local tournament.

Kennedy never lost his interest in the military and the Army Medical Corps. In 1943, he was elected first vice commander of the local Tuskegee American Legion Post.[14]

His friends from various parts of the country would come to Tuskegee for programs and special events. In 1945, a party of his Arkansas friends came to Tuskegee for commencement exercises at the Institute and Kennedy, still on the faculty of the Institute, took them on a tour of the facilities.

Dr. Kennedy remarried. His marriage to Phala was his final one. He continued to practice on the staff of the famed John A. Andrew Memorial Hospital, part of the Tuskegee Institute.

He and Phala lived in Tuskegee for the rest of his life. In 1961, at the age of 79, Dr. Kennedy was still practicing at the Tuskegee Institute where he had served for more than 25 years, and he was still involved in his fraternity. That year, he and Phala again attended its local annual banquet.[15]

Dr. Kennedy lived a long, productive life. Phala was with him when he died of pneumonia at the age of 83. He was buried in Tuskegee's Greenwood Cemetery with a military headstone.

Notes

1. http://en.wikipedia.org/wiki/Cotton_Plant,_Arkansas (accessed October 20, 2014).
2. *Meharry Annual, Military Review 1919*, Harold D. West Collection, Meharry Medical College Archives, Nashville, TN, 42.

3. "Draft Catches Many Members of the Race," *Chicago Defender*, July 28, 1917, 7.
4. *Meharry Annual, Military Review 1919*, 41.
5. http://en.wikipedia.org/wiki/Omega_Psi_Phi (accessed October 20, 2014).
6. A'Lelia Bundles, *On Her Own Ground: The Life and Times of Madam C. J. Walker* (New York: Simon & Shuster, 2001) 268.
7. "A'Lelia Walker Is Married to Finance of Youthful Days," *The New York Age*, May 8, 1926, 1.
8. "Through the Lorgnette of Geraldyn Dismond," *Pittsburgh Courier*, September 10, 1927, 8.
9. "Order Reigns at Veterans' Hospital; Threat Rumor Unfounded: Ward Place in Charge. Race War Over. Director Hines Acts," *Pittsburgh Courier*, July 19, 1924, 1.
10. Bundles, *On Her Own Ground*, 280.
11. "Returns to Post at Hospital," *Metropolitan Post*, October 29, 1938, 16.
12. "Charge Southern Democrats Seek Control of Veterans" *The New York Age*, October 3, 1936, 1.
13. *Metropolitan Post*, Chicago, October 29, 1938, 33.
14. "Johnson Heads Mckenzie Post," *Pittsburgh Courier*, July 24, 1943, 16.
15. "Types," *Pittsburgh Courier*, February 18, 1961, 20.

Oliver Willard LANDRY

12 November 1886–14 October 1969
Meharry Medical College, 1911

Roots and Education

Oliver Landry was born into a large, well-known and well-respected African American family in Louisiana. Its patriarch, Pierre Landry, was a clergyman, builder, lawyer, and politician. According to a 1915 "Who's Who of the Colored Race" he was married twice (both wives died) and had 11 children, 7 sons and 4 daughters. All were educated, and many had professional titles. In addition to three physicians, his children became pharmacists, educators and clergy. One daughter was married to a professor, one to a doctor, and another to a clergyman. One daughter was a public school teacher.[1] Another source credits Pierre Landry with 14 children, 12 with his first wife and 2 by his second wife.[2]

The Landry home was at 5215 Constance Street in New Orleans. Oliver was the youngest of Pierre's three sons to graduate from medical school. His oldest brother, Lord Beaconsfield Landry, was a 1908 graduate of Meharry Medical College in Nashville. The L.B. Landry Senior High School in New Orleans was named for him. Another brother, Eldridge P. Landry, graduated in pharmacy from Flint Medical College in New Orleans. He became a Georgia state food inspector.

Oliver studied at Flint Medical College in New Orleans for three years before that college was forced to close its doors in 1911. The students from Flint were then transferred to Meharry Medical College in Nashville, Tennessee. Landry graduated in 1911 and returned to New Orleans to practice medicine.

A 1912 New Orleans city directory lists Dr. Landry as a physician with offices in his residence at 1419 Burdette Street. Subsequent New Orleans city directories for 1913–1917 and 1919 have him at different addresses, but still in town.

On June 19, 1916, he married Cecelia N. Marshall, age 30, in New Orleans.

Military Service

In 1917, at age 30, Dr. Landry registered for the World War I Draft and listed his home address as 2225 Valence Street and his office as 1832 Dryades Street. He gave as a reason for draft exemption that he had a wife who de-

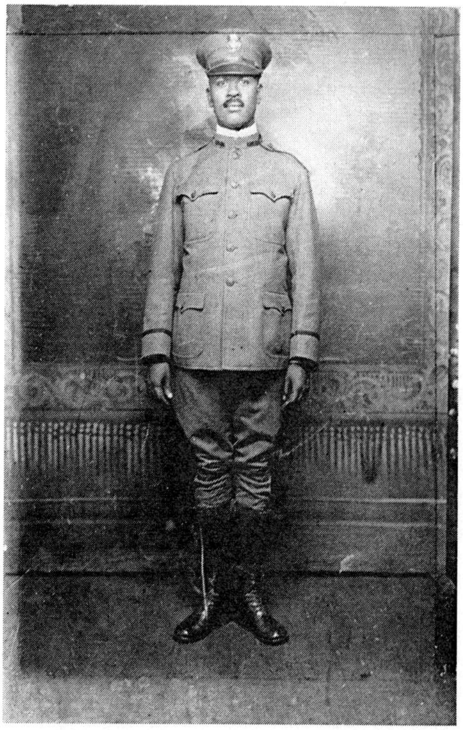

Lt. Oliver W. Landry (courtesy Amistad Research Center, Tulane University, New Orleans, Louisiana).

pended on him for support, saying "my profession demands my attention." (The draft registrar described him as tall and stout.)

He expected the draft exemption might be declined so he volunteered for the U.S. Army Medical Reserve Corps.

On August 12, 1917, First Lieutenant Landry reported to the Medical Officers Training Camp at Fort Des Moines, Iowa. He was there for 11 weeks. He completed his training and was assigned to the 92nd Division, 317th Sanitary (Medical) Train at Camp Funston, Kansas.[3] His division was sent to France in June 1918. The division's medical teams consisted of medical detachments, ambulance companies and field hospitals. Lieutenant Landry was one of five physicians assigned to the 92nd Division's 367th Field Hospital.

Shortly after his arrival at Brest, France, he encountered problems with the army. A complaint was filed against him on July 3, 1918, by the commanding officer of the Pontanezen Barracks. Those old barracks were a stopping off point for many thousands of soldiers awaiting transport inland from the coast for further training and combat. He was detained there for investigation of "drunkenness on duty." He was returned to duty on July 8, then on July 23 he was removed from duty to "Absent in Arrest" for trial. Unit records show he was dismissed from the service per Special Order #209 on September 29, 1918.[4] His name does not appear on later unit records so it is assumed he was then returned to the United States.

Career

During the early 1900s, Chicago had become America's second largest and most flourishing metropolis. There were a large number of highly respected, competent African American surgeons, dentists and lawyers. In addition to these professionals, there were many successful black businessmen.[5] In 1920, seeking to share in this opportunity, Dr. Landry and his wife, Cecilia, chose to move there. Initially, they lived just north of Washington Park in a rented room at 4847 Langley Avenue. He would spend the rest of his life on the South Side neighborhood.

In March 1921, W.E.B. DuBois' *The Crisis* magazine reported that "Dr. Willard Landry, a Negro Surgeon in Chicago, had performed four successful Caesarian operations."[6] Unlike today, a Caesarian operation was a surgical procedure only used in extremis to try to save the lives of mothers and babies. It was used when complications from labor and/or delivery occurred. Sometimes it was even performed after the mother had died in order to try to save the infant. In those years, the incidence of these procedures was low and the mortality rate was high. With the advent of penicillin and other antibiotics in the 1930s and 1940s, the mortality rate declined and the use of the procedure increased.

A biography published in 1985 about an eminent African American scientist, Ernest Everett Just, mentions names of a number of notable African American professionals in Chicago in the early 1900s, including Willard Landry, who he credited as the surgeon who standardized the method of childbirth by caesarean section.[7] Prior to that time physicians had been experimenting for years with different procedures with varying degrees of success.

Late in 1921 Dr. Landry suffered the loss of his young wife. Cook County death records show she died in Chicago at Provident Hospital on November 30, 1921. She was buried in New Orleans. One can only speculate about the impact this had on Dr. Landry, but later in the 1920s and 1930s Landry's professional life and personal life became complicated, to say the least.

By 1930, Dr. Landry now 42 was married to a much younger woman named Barbara Landry (23). She and Dr. Landry lived at 3535 Calumet Avenue in Chicago with her stepfather and stepmother, Omar F. Magee (46) and Myrtle Magee (42). Her stepfather was an embalmer and owned an undertaking business.

When he wasn't working Dr. Landry's favorite activity was bridge. He was considered an expert. In 1938, he was among a "caravan of bridge experts from all sections of the country" to converge on Washington, D.C., to participate in the national championships of the American Bridge Association.[8] In 1943, the newspaper column "How to Play Contract Bridge" featured a hand that Mr. and Mrs. Landry won.[9]

In late December 1938, a Chicago newspaper reported a bizarre story entitled "Woman Is Held for Crime."

"Another questionable milestone in the hectic life of Dr. Willard Landry, 55, was uncovered Thursday morning when police carried the physician to Provident hospital with a knife wound below the heart inflicted by a woman. Dr. Landry, whose license was revoked several years ago following charges of malpractice, was stabbed by Miss Hazel Battle, 34, in her room at 4748 Vincennes Avenue in the course of a fight.

"Miss Battle, at the point of hysteria, was taken to Fifth District police station where she revealed that she and the physician had been living together as man and wife for the past six months. Questioned about the wounding of her suitor, Miss Battle charged that Dr. Landry came home about 6 o'clock Thursday morning and began abusing and beating her. Substantiating this, the woman exhibited numerous bruises and contusions about her face and head. "I simply became desperate. I don't know where I got the knife; I just grabbed it and struck at him after he had knocked me down several times.

"Miss Battle was later taken to Eleventh street police station where she will be arraigned Friday morning in Women's Court on a charge of assault with a deadly weapon. Dr. Landry's condition was reported as fair by Provident hospital Thursday night."[10]

He recovered and by 1942, he had moved once again. According to his World War II draft registration, his residence address was 62 East 36th Place, Chicago. His business address was 65 East 43rd Street. It appears he was living with Mrs. Louise Paris because he wrote her name in the space for "the person who will always know your address."

Further news of Dr. Landry is lacking until we learn that his sister, Georgia Landry Gibson, died Saturday, September 14, 1957, and her death notice said she was survived by two brothers, Dr. O. Willard Landry of Chicago and Dr. E.P. Landry of West Palm Beach, FL.[11]

Lacking further information about the latter part of Dr. Landry's life, one can only speculate it was unsettled. His unfortunate experience in France suggests he could be somewhat reckless, but he had been a competent, and innovative surgeon. The news report of his stabbing in 1938 indicates a troubled life. One can only guess at the nature and quality of his life during his latter years.

Finally, a death notice appeared in Louisiana saying Dr. Landry died at the age of 83 at the Michael Reese Hospital in Chicago. He was buried at Lincoln Park Cemetery, Chicago, on October 20, 1969.[12]

NOTES

1. F. L. Mather, editor, *Who's Who of the Colored Race*, Vol. 1, 1915, Memento Edition, Half-Century Anniversary of Negro Freedom in U.S., Chicago, IL.
2. "Dunn-Landry Family Papers Collection, 1872–2003," Amistad Research Center, Tulane University, New Orleans, LA, www.amistadresearchcenter.org (accessed September 30, 2012).
3. Table of Medical Reserve Corps—Colored—Receiving Instruction, Medical Training Camp, Fort Des Moines, Iowa, RG-112, Records of the Army Surgeon General, National Archives, College Park, Maryland.
4. RG -120, 92d Division, Records of the 317th Sanitary Train, National Archives, College Park, Maryland.
5. Kenneth R. Manning, *Black Apollo of Science: The Life of Ernest Everett Just* (New York: Oxford University Press, 1983) 56.
6. "*The Crisis*," March 1921, Vol. 21 No. 5, Whole No. 125, 226.
7. Kenneth R. Manning, *The Life of Ernest Everett Just*, 57.
8. "Common Sense Bridge," *Chicago Defender*, August 13 1938, 15.
9. "How to Play Contract Bridge," *Pittsburgh Courier*, July 10, 1943, 22.
10. "Woman Is Held for Crime," *Pittsburgh Courier*, December 31, 1938, 8.
11. "Rites Arranged for Mrs. Gibson," *The Times-Picayune*, Sept 17, 1957, 2.
12. "Death Notice," *The Times-Picayune*, October 21, 1969.

Charles Henry LAWS

23 June 1883–7 March 1962
Leonard Medical School, 1911

Roots and Education

Charles was born in Phoebus in the Tidewater region of Virginia. He was one of seven children in the Frank and Matilda (Washington) Laws family. Phoebus is a small town located in Elizabeth City County in eastern Virginia. Upon incorporation in 1900, it was named in honor of local businessman Harrison Phoebus (1840–1886), who is credited with convincing the Chesapeake and Ohio Railway (C&O) to extend its tracks to the town from

Newport News. The town was consolidated with the city of Hampton in 1952. Phoebus is now an important historic neighborhood of Hampton and is listed on the National Register of Historic Places. While "Charlie" Laws (as he was listed on the 1900 U.S. Census) was still young, the family moved to nearby Chesapeake.

He attended the Hampton Normal & Agricultural Institute in Hampton, Virginia, but did not graduate. The school's most famous graduate was Booker T. Washington. Hampton Institute was founded in 1868 by Northern philanthropists for African Americans. The school's founding principal was General Samuel Chapman Armstrong, who led the school until his death in 1893. It was neither a government nor a state school but was chartered by a special act of the General Assembly of Virginia and was controlled by a board representing different regions of the country as well as various religious groups.

On August 26, 1899, Laws married Lula Pearl Slaughter in Plumerville, Arkansas. The details of further college study are not known, but Laws entered the four-year program at Leonard Medical School of Shaw University in Raleigh, North Carolina, around 1907. Graduation requirements stated "every candidate for graduation must be at least 21 years of age, and furnish satisfactory evidence of good moral character. He shall have attended the four-years' course or its equivalent. He shall be required to dissect the entire cadaver. Satisfactory examinations must be passed in all branches of medicine with ... an average of not less than 80 percent."[1]

While the catalog describes quite a stringent program, Leonard did not fare so well compared with other African American medical schools or students around the country. Failure rates on state licensure exams had become the measure of a school's worth. "Leonard always received C ratings, compared with Howard's and Meharry's A's and B's." There was no library, no museum and only a small amount of equipment in the chemical library for pathology.[2]

Dr. Laws graduated from Leonard in 1911. He had to take the West Virginia state medical exam twice before passing it on April 21, 1914. He then set up his medical practice in Elkins, West Virginia.

Military Service

Dr. Laws volunteered for World War I and reported to training camp at Fort Des Moines on July 31, 1917. He was 35 at the time. Upon completion of his training he was initially assigned to the 365th Ambulance Company of the 92nd Division at Camp Funston[3] and subsequently reassigned to the 372nd Infantry Regiment of the 93rd Division at Camp Stuart, Newport News, Virginia.

The 372nd sailed on the SS *Susquehanna* from Newport News, Virginia, on March 30, 1918. It arrived at St. Nazaire in France in early April 1918, where it was attached to the French 63rd Infantry for training. The soldiers traded in their American equipment for French helmets, gas masks and guns. "For 7 months Dr. Laws was with the 372nd Infantry Regiment. The 372nd was brigaded with a crack French regiment, with its insignia the 'Red Hand,' an emblem which has been in the French Army for more than 200 years."[4]

His regiment fought alongside the American 371st Infantry and saw significant combat from July to September 1918 in the Verdun Sector. Late in 1918, as the war was nearing its end, Lieutenant Laws was reassigned to the 366th Infantry Regiment of the 92nd Division. He rejoined two doctors there with whom he had trained at Fort Des Moines—William H. Bryant and Ulysses G. B. Martin. In February 1919 Laws returned to the United States with the 92nd Division. He was honorably discharged on March 14, 1919.

Career

Right after the war, Dr. Laws returned to practice again in Elkins, West Virginia. He and his wife Lula lived at 309 First Street with their 10-year-old daughter, Edna B., and his father-in-law, Albert Slaughter, a barber. He moved the family and his medical practice from Elkins to Hinton, West Virginia. Hinton was then a thriving railroad town on the New River. African Americans moved to the area to construct and later inspect the miles of track that transported ore from the mines of West Virginia to the rest of the country. These were the "Gandy Dancers" who were known for their rhythmic chants as they drove spikes into cross ties or lifted heavy loads. After the numbers needed for railroad work declined, many of the men stayed in the area to work the mines.[5] The railroad and mine workers kept Dr. Laws busy.

When the West Virginia Medical Society met in Beckley in 1927, Dr. Laws was elected president. In addition to the usual duties of a convention delegate, he sang a solo with the Beckley Chambers Quartette.[6] The next year he was elected to Hinton's City Council. He served three terms. The 1930 Census has the Laws' address at 119 Main Street in Hinton, West Virginia. The family still lived there in 1942 when he completed his draft registration card for World War II.

In 1937, Dr. Law's wife, Lula Pearl Slaughter Laws, suffered a heart attack and ten minutes later died. During her 12 years in Hinton, Mrs. Laws had written a column for the local paper on the black community. She also devoted her time "to worthwhile civic and religious enterprises."[7] She was buried at Esquire Cemetery, an African American cemetery in Summers County, West Virginia.

Five years later, Dr. Laws married a second time on August 19, 1942. His marriage to Alfreda Pierce Smithers was held at the bride's home at 111 Pleasant Street in Hinton. The Reverend R. J. Watson, pastor of the Second Street Baptist, officiated. The bride was born in Middleport, Ohio, on July 21, 1887, and she had taught for a number of years in the Hinton public schools. At the time of their marriage, she was principal of Hinton's Lincoln Elementary School. The Laws were both prominent members of the African American community.[8]

Laws was a member of the highly-regarded Kappa Alpha Psi fraternity, and in 1954 he received the "coveted Achievement Award" at its annual meeting in Winston-Salem, North Carolina.[9] He was also a lifelong member of the National Medical Association (NMA). In 1954 he was appointed to the position of state vice president for West Virginia.[10] The next year at NMA's 60th convention, he was "one of 199 physicians who received an award for 40 years or more of service to the medical profession."[11]

At the 1961 commencement exercises at Shaw University in Raleigh, North Carolina, Golden Anniversary (50-year) Awards were presented to the class of 1911. Dr. Laws received a citation, but did not attend the ceremony.

The idea of integration of Hinton public schools had long been debated, but the school board refused to consider it. A local chapter of the NAACP was formed in 1961 and the state NAACP soon began an investigation of the school board's method of hiring teachers. "On February 8, 1962, the state president of the NAACP, Rev. C. Anderson Davis, appeared before the board, along with Everett Crawford and Dr. Charles Laws. By the end of that meeting, the board said it would consider hiring teachers on the basis of merit. Everett Crawford applied as a science teacher. He was hired by the board on May 1, 1962. Headlines in the newspaper announced 'Crawford First Negro Teacher at High School.'"[12] Dr. Laws did not live to see it.

He died on March 7, 1962, at the Memorial Hospital in Beckley, West Virginia. He was survived by his second wife Alfreda and her daughters.

His funeral included pallbearers from among the leadership in the Hinton African American community. Honorary pallbearers came from the West Virginia Medical Association, Bachelor Benedict Club of Charleston, American Legion, Kappa Alpha Psi fraternity and the Hinton Chamber of Commerce.[13]

He was buried at Hilltop Cemetery in Hinton. When his wife Alfreda died in 1967, she joined him there.

NOTES

1. "*Examinations and Graduations*," Leonard Schools of Medicine and Pharmacy, Shaw University, 1912, 19.
2. Savitt, Todd L., *Race & Medicine in Nineteenth- and Early-Twentieth-Century America* (Kent, OH: Kent State University Press, 2007) 166.
3. "Unit Records Morning Report, 365th Ambulance Co, 317 Supply Train, November 1917," National Personnel Records Center, National Archives, St. Louis, MO.
4. "Graduates and Ex-Students," *The Southern Workman*, Vol. 48, Jan—Dec 1919 (The Press of The Hampton Normal & Agricultural Institute, 1919) 253.
5. "*C & O Historical Society Photo, Heritage and History 2014 Calendar*," Veterans Museum, Hinton.
6. "West Virginia Doctors Meet in Beckley Is Fine," *Pittsburgh Courier*, July 9, 1927.
7. "Sudden Death of Mrs. C. H. Laws Is Shock to Friends," *Pittsburgh Courier*, November 13, 1937, 22.

8. "Hinton Activities," *Beckley Post-Herald*, August 20, 1942, 12.
9. "Achievement Award," *Pittsburgh Courier*, June 26, 1954, 20.
10. "NMA Activities," *Journal of the National Medical Association (JNMA)*, March 1954, Vol. 46, No. 2, 146.
11. *Ibid.*, The Forty Year Practitioners, November 1955, Vol. 47, No. 6, 414.
12. "Black History Month Lincoln School: The Rest of the Story," *Hinton News*, February 27, 1996, 1.
13. "Services Saturday for Dr. C. H. Laws," *Beckley Post-Herald*, March 9, 1962, 12.

Jesse Leonidas LEACH

23 December 1892–26 February 1981
Meharry Medical College, 1914

Roots and Education

Leach was born in Nashville, Tennessee, to John H. and Delia Leach. He received his early education there. Orphaned at the age of seven, he was taken into the home of his mother's former employers, Dr. Paul F. Eve and his wife. "The encouragement and guidance I received from this fine family," said Dr. Leach, "motivated me to consider medicine as a career."[1]

He earned his A.B. at Walden University in Nashville in 1910. In the fall of 1910, Dr. Eve accompanied young Jesse to the Dean's office at Meharry Medical College in Nashville and helped him enroll as a freshman. To help pay his tuition expenses, Jesse took a job as monitor of the freshman class and worked part-time as custodian at the college. To provide for his room and board, he served meals at a resident boarding house.[2]

Later, as a result of schooling he received during summer vacation at the Cincinnati College of Embalming in Ohio, he was placed in charge of anatomical material at Meharry and Vanderbilt Colleges of Medicine. This position afforded him additional funds for his college education.[3]

Dr. Leach graduated from Meharry Medical College in 1914 and interned at the Hubbard Hospital there. During his internship he served as first surgical assistant to Dr. J. H. Hale, the South's most prominent African American surgeon. He then accepted a teaching position at Meharry College. While teaching, he also served as medical inspector on the staff of the Nashville City Board of Education.[4]

On June 28, 1916, he married Frances R. Pipes at Natchez, Mississippi. He and a fellow Meharry graduate and his close friend Dr. Jonathan N. Rucker were married on the same day at the same place. Rucker married Miss Fannie Ross of Natchez.[5] In May 1917, Leach was elected secretary and treasurer of the "Volunteer State Funeral Directors and Embalmers' Association" at its first annual meeting in Nashville.[6] Also in 1917, Drs. Leach and Rucker volunteered to serve this country as army medical officers.

Military Service

Leach trained for 95 days at the MOTC at Fort Des Moines, Iowa, from August 1 to November 3, 1917. He was well regarded and recommended for command. He was sent to Camp Funston where he joined the 317th Sanitary (Medical) Train of the 92nd Division. The camp newspaper in a YMCA report in March 1918 notes that First Lieutenant Leach was one of eight officers engaged in religious work there.[7] Leach was a member of the African Methodist Episcopalian (AME) Church.

He was first assigned as surgeon of the 349th Machine Gun Battalion, then transferred to the 365th Field Hospital, and finally assigned as surgeon with the 317th Ammunition Train. He sailed with the Train for France aboard the USS *Covington* on June 15, 1918,

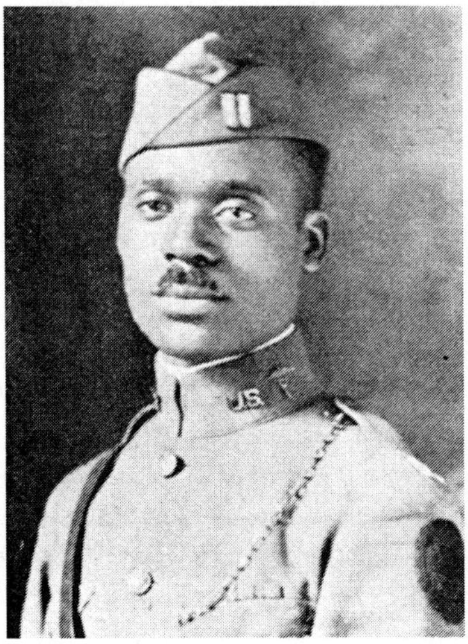

Dr. James L. Leach (courtesy Meharry Medical College Archives).

and served with that unit throughout the war. Only days after delivering him and his fellow troops to Brest, the *Covington* was sunk by a German U-boat on July 2, 1918.

Lieutenant Leach served in France in the 317th Ammunition Train alongside another notable MOTC graduate, Lieutenant William H. Dyer. The Dyer biographic entry in this book includes vivid excerpts of their shared experiences.

In 1919 Leach's commanding officer, Major M. T. Dean wrote a very strong recommendation for Leach thanking him for his "thoroughly efficient and at all times loyal service and your energy and devotion to duty." He added that his "efficient service has contributed to dispel the assertion of many that the Colored officers did not possess the qualities required in a commander of troops."[8] Leach rose to the rank of captain in the Medical Corps before his discharge in 1919.

Career

After the War, Dr. Leach returned to Nashville to practice medicine. He is remembered for his flat refusal to lead a black military unit in a Jim Crow parade. He told the white commander, "We were not behind in France, and I will be damned if I will put my men behind over here."[9]

In 1920 he moved to Flint in Genesee County, Michigan, where he opened his practice. Buick was a major presence and during the 1920s automobile production in Flint began to rival Detroit. The black population tripled and Flint became Michigan's second largest city. The *Flint Journal* tells us Leach "is credited as a pioneer of civil rights in Flint." His list of achievements show he was a leader in many other fields: medicine, government, social welfare, religion and education.[10]

His record of public service in Flint is extensive. He organized the first African American Legion Post in Michigan, was the first African American to serve on the staff of the city physicians and was the first elected to serve on the Flint Board of Supervisors. He was also the first African American to serve as chairman of the Genesee County Board of Health. Dr. Leach served on the Flint Welfare Committee for 25 years. He pioneered an improved program of medical aid for the indigent in 1959. He was also Flint's first African American medical examiner.

Dr. Leach was president of Flint's unit of the NAACP shortly after it was organized in 1919. He then served 10 years (1941–1951) as head of the Michigan Conference of NAACP branches and 18 years on the NAACP national board of directors.[11]

Leach was described by Melvin Banner, a black historian, author and teacher in Flint, as "the most important black person in Flint history" because of his work in the national Civil Rights Movement. He said Leach kept the relationship between blacks and whites on an even keel. And, more importantly, he helped build a sense of unity among black people. "He encouraged blacks to go to school and become educated. He was revered in the black community because he could talk to anyone. And he wouldn't forget your name. He had an excellent memory for names and faces."[12]

Dr. Leach was a member of the Elks and served as state president in 1932. The group, formed in 1898, was a large, predominantly black, fraternal organization with a tradition of benevolence and charitable service to their surrounding communities.[13] In July 1933, he was re-elected to its presidency.[14]

He was also a very active member of the Republican Party, and as early as 1932 he was Michigan's member of the committee established for planning campaign strategies for work among African Americans.[15] In November 1932 he spoke at the Union Memorial AME Church in Benton Harbor at a Republican Rally. He issued a challenge to an open debate to a Detroit Democrat speaker named Bledsoe.[16] No record was found of such a debate.

In November 1932, as principal speaker at the same AME church, he gave a patriotic speech that was described as electrifying.[17]

In May 1937, Dr. Leach, always a trailblazer, became the first African American member of the Genesee County Board of Supervisors and secretary of its Educational and Health Committee. He was there to welcome Charles

Robinson, the second African American member to the board.[18] Leach served 20 years, until 1949, when he was forced to resign because of his health.[19]

The *Flint Journal* reported Leach was "the first to invoke the Civil Rights Act in Flint when, in December 1937, a restaurant and gasoline station operator was arrested for refusing to serve him."

He found time for play. In March 1938, he was a visitor at a winter resort in Hot Springs, Arkansas, where bathing, horseback riding, and other social activities were prominent.[20]

Dr. Leach was president of the Flint Southside Development Company, a group of black businessmen who proposed in 1943 to build a 105-unit housing project to upgrade living conditions for blacks in Flint.

In 1947, he was a delegate at the five day 37th annual meeting of the Kappa Alpha Psi fraternity in Los Angeles.[21] This African American fraternity was founded in 1911 at Indiana University and its national membership includes many distinguished African Americans.

In 1950, Leach was among political leaders who met with the governor of Michigan to discuss renewing attempts to secure fair employment practices legislation for Michigan. He represented the Michigan NAACP as its president.[22] That same year he was a delegate to the mid-century White House Conference on Children and Youth. In 1953, he attended the presidential inauguration in Washington, D.C., for Dwight D. Eisenhower.

In 1960, he organized about 25 African Americans who collectively pledged $25,000 to Flint's College and Cultural Development.

"Dr. Leach was a very inspirational man for young people. He pushed us to the last degree and encouraged us to be our best. If I had to name any one person from back in those days who most impacted lives of young people, it would be Dr. Leach," said Mary Towner, a former educator.

In May 1966, he was featured on the cover of the Bulletin of the county medical society. He had been a member since 1922. When he was honored for a half century of distinguished service, Dr. Leach stressed, "A doctor's got to love people. His service has to be put above financial return."

Leach was the first black to be elevated to the presidency of the Michigan Academy of General Practice. He was also president, not without drama, of the National Medical Association (NMA), the pre-eminent medical organization for black physicians. The *Chicago Defender* reported Leach, president-elect of the association, was ousted (impeached) from the position after a spirited battle at the 1939 convention in New York. It seems it became known Leach had been involved in a 1928 bootlegging case during prohibition. In fact he had been convicted of selling and transporting liquor. He actually bought two cases of Sandy MacDonald whiskey in Canada without a license and then delivered them to a friend and received $45. He was convicted on both counts. Ultimately, he pled guilty and Judge Tuttle sentenced him to pay a fine of $500.

The entire affair came to light as a result of Dr. Olin West, official of the American Medical Association (white), "throwing it in the faces of Dr. Giles, Dr. Roberts and Dr. Bowles, the fact that the NMA had elevated a man who had been convicted of a crime to the presidency-elect of the NMA. This happened when the three doctors went to the AMA con-

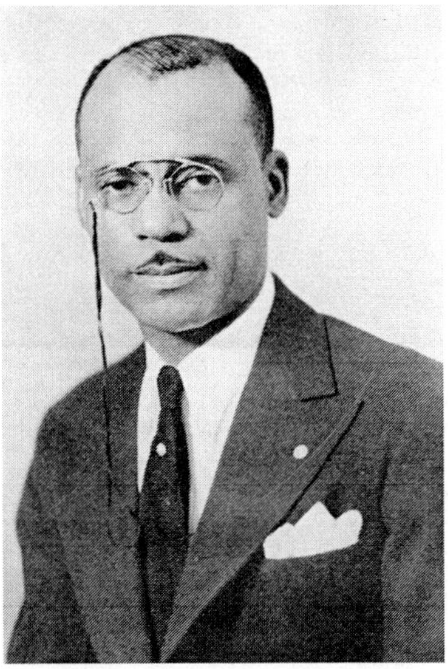

Dr. J. Leonidas Leach, president-elect, National Medical Association (courtesy U.S. National Library of Medicine).

vention to protest that organizations putting 'COL' after all black doctors names in the AMA journal and against discrimination against Negro doctors and nurses generally."

There was already a serious rift in the NMA with the black doctors in the west and south usually joining forces against those in the north. Finally, Dr. Leach, a consummate politician, rallied other Meharry Medical School graduates. After five hours of furious debate in a locked room from which the press was excluded, Dr. Leach was vindicated by a block of the delegates and was allowed to take his place as NMA president in 1939. Then in 1940, in a highly political move, he was removed by action of the NMA Executive Board.

In 1967 Dr. Leach was honored by the medical society in Flint at a dinner and presented with a gold wristwatch in recognition of his 52 years in medicine.[23] The next year, he was honored, along with five national NAACP board members, including UAW president Walter Reuther, at the NAACP annual state convention.[24]

His service to his community and his nation for more than 65 years was extraordinary. He died in Flint in 1981 at the age of 89, and was survived by his second wife Louise and his son J. Leonidas (Leon) Leach, Jr. He was eulogized as a "God-given genius who made this world a better place because he lived and did not just exist."[25]

NOTES

1. "In Memoriam," Jesse L. Leach, M.D., *Genesee County Medical Society Bulletin*, April 1981, 118.
2. *Ibid.*
3. *Ibid.*
4. *Ibid.*
5. "Marriages," *The Meharry News*, July, 1916, Vol. 14 No. 3.
6. *The New York Age*, May 31, 1917, 7.
7. Russell S. Brown, *YMCA No. 11 (Colored Service)* March 9, 1918, Jesse Moorland Papers, Box 126–72, Howard University Manuscript Archives, Washington, D.C.
8. *Meharry Annual, Military Review 1919*, 59, Harold D. West Collection, Meharry Medical College Archives, Nashville, TN.
9. "In Memoriam," Jesse L. Leach, M.D., *Genesee County Medical Society Bulletin*, April 1981, 118.
10. "Dr. Jesse Leach: A Man of Firsts," *The Flint Journal*, February 13, 1952, A3.
11. *Ibid.*
12. Melvin E. Banner, *A Short Negro History of Flint* (M. E. Banner:1964).
13. "Grand Rapids, Mich.," *Pittsburgh Courier*, June 9, 1932, 5.
14. "Elks in State Meet," *Pittsburgh Courier*, June 8, 1933, 4.
15. "Republicans and Democrats Name Advisory Committees for Work Among Negroes," *The New York Age*, October 1, 1932, 3.
16. "Issues Challenge to A.M.E. Debate," *The News-Palladium*, November 5, 1932, 5.
17. "Dr. Williams to Talk Upon "Americanism," *The News-Palladium*, November 7, 1932, 9.
18. "Dr. J. L. Leach Photo and Caption," *Pittsburgh Courier*, May 8, 1937, 22.
19. "Negro Supervisor Resigns," *The News-Palladium*, March 17, 1949, 15.
20. "Hot Springs, Ark.," *Pittsburgh Courier*, March 26, 1938, 23.
21. "Kappas Hold 'Blue Ribbon' Confab in Los Angeles," *Pittsburgh Courier*, August 23, 1947, 11.
22. "Governor Seeks New FEPC Bill," *The News-Palladium*, March 9, 1950, 6.
23. "Honor Michigan Medic for Half Century of Service," *Jet Magazine*, December 21, 1967, 47.
24. "Reuther Will Give Talk Here," *The St. Joseph Herald-Press*, September 17, 1968, 1.
25. "In Memoriam," Jesse L. Leach, M.D., *Genesee County Medical Society Bulletin*, April 1981, 118.

Edwin Henry LEE

3 March 1886–2 February 1952
Howard Medical College, 1916

Roots and Education

Edwin Henry Lee was born 35 miles east of San Antonio in Seguin, Texas. His father was a teacher. By 1900, the family had moved to Tuskegee, Alabama, where his father taught at the famous Tuskegee Normal & Industrial Institute. Young Edwin was the second eldest of six children, and the oldest son. He and his older sister Birdie were educated at the Tuskegee Institute and became teachers.[1] Edwin went on to earn a B.S. degree at the Teacher's College of Columbia University in New York City in 1909. The degree was awarded after completion of a two-year professional curriculum including educational psychology, the history and principles of education, a major subject of professional and academic work, and elective courses.

In 1910, at age 24, Edwin was a teacher at Tuskegee Institute. A year later Edwin enrolled at the Howard University Medical School in Washington, D.C. He graduated in 1915 with his M.D.[2] Dr. Lee stayed in Washington for his internship at Freemen's Hospital. Then in 1916 he moved to Kansas City, Missouri. There he lived at 2460A Flora Avenue, not far from the city's General Hospital No. 2 for African Americans.[3] When the United States entered the First World War, he volunteered to serve in the U.S. Army Medical Corps.

Military Service

First Lieutenant Lee was sent for military training to Fort Des Moines, Iowa, to the Medical Officers Training Camp for Colored officers. He was one of the early arrivals at camp on August 17, 1917. After 79 days of training, he was one of 12 graduates who were recommended by Lieutenant Colonel Bingham, the camp commander, for promotion to Captain. They were cited for "their exceptional abilities and qualifications, their ability to command men and loyalty to their superiors." He was identified as having the ability to command an ambulance company. Upon graduation he was sent to Camp Funston at Fort Riley, Kansas, where he was assigned to the 317th Sanitary Train of the 92nd Division.[4]

Captain Lee was in command of the 366th Ambulance Company of the 317th Sanitary Train. There were four other MOTC doctors who served under Captain Lee—lieutenants McLaughlin, Felder, Gloster and Brown. He remained in command of that unit at Camp Funston and in France until September 1918, when he was assigned to the 367th Infantry Regiment. Clearly, Dr. Lee performed well. He became the senior African American officer in that 367th Infantry Regiment medical detachment and became the assistant regimental surgeon. He reported to a Major Robert Conard, a white officer, who was the regimental surgeon. Captain Lee returned home and was discharged on March 1, 1919. He returned to Kansas City.[5]

Career

Dr. Lee worked at the Kansas City General Hospital No. 2. This hospital holds special significance to many African American physicians who interned and worked there. It was established as a Negro hospital by the city when public hospitalization for the non-white population was very limited. Years earlier, when a new white hospital was built, the old City Hospital became General Hospital No. 2. It was used to care for Negro and Mexican patients. In addition to treating that population, it was designed to train men and women in medicine and nursing. By 1914, an African American staff took over the supervisory duties of the hospital. It became the first municipal hospital and school of nursing to be completely managed by African Americans.[6] He remained at General Hospital No. 2 as a staff surgeon until 1931. He did special tubercular work there for seven years and took charge of its tuberculosis clinic, the only one for African Americans in the city.[7]

In 1925, Dr. Lee was 39 and living at 1201 East 18th Street when he married Jennie C. McCampbell, age 35, of 2744 Woodland Avenue in Kansas City.[8] She was originally from South Carolina and was a longtime librarian for the Kansas City school and public library system. Jennie was also the widow of another African American physician, Dr. Ernest James McCampbell. He was on the General Hospital No. 2 staff until he died of pneumonia in March 1918. She was left with three small children, and had been a widow for seven years when she remarried. Dr. Lee moved into her home, and they remained there until 1931.

In 1931 the family left Kansas City for Veterans Hospital No. 91 in Tuskegee. One of his World War I army colleagues, Dr. Joseph A. Ward, had been hired as director of the hospital. Dr. Ward chose Dr. Lee to be his medical director.

Dr. and Mrs. Lee lived and worked in Tuskegee for another 21 years. Their lives were not all work. Dr. Lee was a golfer. In July 1939, he was the chairman of the Tournament Committee for the First Open Golf Tournament of the Tuskegee Golf Club. He was actually listed among the "crack golfers" participating in the event that attracted men from Chicago, North Carolina, South Carolina, Louisiana, Georgia, and Alabama.[9] His colleague at the hospital, and fellow World War I veteran, Dr. James A. Kennedy, was mentioned as another great golfer. By 1940, the tournament became an annual event in Tuskegee.

Dr. Lee participated in community medical programs. In 1941, he was one of eight specialists at the 15th annual clinic in Tallahassee at Florida A&M College Hospital. He was the neurologist. Free examination clinics for operations were provided over the course of three days to candidates who were admitted to the hospital the prior weekend. The medical specialists all came from different hospitals and Lee represented the Veteran's Hospital in Tuskegee.[10]

Dr. Lee continued to work until he fell ill with cancer of the liver. He passed away February 2, 1952. Nine months after his death the *Journal of the National Medical Association* published a medical research article written by Dr. Lee and Dr. Charles N. Pitts. It concerned "present day" therapy for myasthenia gravis, a chronic autoimmune neuromuscular disease characterized by varying degrees of weakness of the skeletal muscles of the body.[11]

Dr. Lee was a natural leader who served his country for more than 20 years in war and peace. He cared for its soldiers in France and its veterans in Alabama. He also cared for the African American community in Kansas City for almost 15 years. He was a skilled physician, teacher and administrator whose service was of the highest order.

NOTES

1. 1900 U.S. Federal Census.
2. AMA Deceased Physician Card, National Library of Medicine, Bethesda, MD.
3. Soldiers' Records: War of 1812—World War I, Missouri Digital Heritage Collection, LEE, EDWIN HENRY, www.sos.mo.gov/archives/soldiers.
4. Table of Medical Reserve Corps—Colored—Receiving Instruction, Medical Training Camp, Fort Des Moines, Iowa, RG-112, Records of the Surgeon General, National Archives, College Park, MD.
5. Record Group 120, Records of the American Expeditionary Forces (World War I), 92nd Division, 317th Sanitary Train, National Archives, College Park, MD.
6. "Kansas City General Hospital No. 2," *Journal of the National Medical Association (JNMA)*, September 1962, Vol. 54, No. 5, 525–530.
7. "Howard U. Grad Gets Tuskegee Hospital Post," *Baltimore Afro-American*, February 14, 1931, 1.
8. Marriage License, Edwin H. Lee and Jennie C. McCampbell, June 6, 1925, ancestry.com.
9. "Tuskegee Golf Open on July 7," *Chicago Defender*, July 8, 1939, 16.
10. "Medical Specialists to Conduct Clinic at Fla. College Hospital," *The New York Age*, February 8, 1941, 2.
11. "Myasthenia Gravis," *Journal of the National Medical Association (JNMA)*, Nov, 1952 Vol. 34(6), 426–434.

George Ignatius LYTHCOTT

27 May 1887–1 May 1938
Boston University, 1913

Roots and Education

Lythcott was born in Guyana on the Caribbean coast of South America. It was a British colony, and his father, the Honorable William Lythcott, was in the consular service in Guyana at the time of his birth. His mother, Mary Peroune, was also born in British Guyana.

His education in Guyana included preparatory study at Queen's College. The school had been established in 1844 as the Queen's College Grammar School for boys by William Percy Austin, D.D., bishop of the Anglican diocese of then British Guiana. It continues to operate as a secondary school in Georgetown, the capital city. Lythcott successfully completed his prep school work there.[1]

According to research by grandson Michael Lythcott, his grandfather arrived at Ellis Island on July 29, 1906, aboard the SS *Parima*. He was one of nine young men brought to the United States to be educated under the auspices of the African Methodist Episcopal (AME) Church Missionary Service. According to the ship manifest, each had $30 in his pocket. The manifest also tells us their U.S. contact was a "friend," Dr. H. B. Parks at 61 Bible House in New York City. Bible House was a famous institution and in addition to producing bibles in several languages, it was considered to be the headquarters for American Christian missionary work worldwide.[2]

From Michael Lythcott we learn, "Dr. H. B. Parks (later appointed Bishop) was at that time the 'Secretary of Missions' for the AME Church. He was credited with a great and successful expansion of their missionary efforts in South America. The Methodists had taken an early stand that freed slaves had to be prepared for leadership in order to improve the lives of their people. There was some question within the church hierarchy as to whether African Americans were capable of great education or great societal achievement. Many of the first efforts of the Methodist church in education and preparation of American Africans were considered to be a great social experiment."

On the ship's manifest, George Lythcott is described as a "Demerara African." Demerara was a region in South America in what is now

Guyana that was colonized by the Dutch in 1611. The British invaded and captured the area in 1796. It is located on the lower courses of the Demerara River, and its main town was Georgetown, now Guyana's capital. The "African" in the manifest likely refers to his father's family heritage.

Lythcott attended Claflin College. Claflin (now a university) is a private school in Orangeburg, South Carolina, founded in 1869 by the United Methodist Church. Granddaughter Ngina Lythcott remembered hearing that originally he was to go back to Guyana as a Methodist minister. During college, he decided to stay in the United States. He determined to become a doctor and likely appealed to the college and church to help him. He married while still in college. The 1910 Census tells us his wife Bertha was from Charleston, South Carolina.

Michael Lythcott says, "I am sure that grandfather was an excellent student at Claflin and that his progress was watched closely by those monitoring the great social experiment." From Claflin, Lythcott was accepted at Boston University Medical School. It may well have been the same Claflin family that supported the university (and for whom it was named) that brought him to Boston. The family was certainly wealthy and well connected in the city of Boston, as well as with the Methodist Church and Boston University. There is no way that he could have afforded the transportation, room, board, tuition and lab fees at Boston University Medical School without financial support.

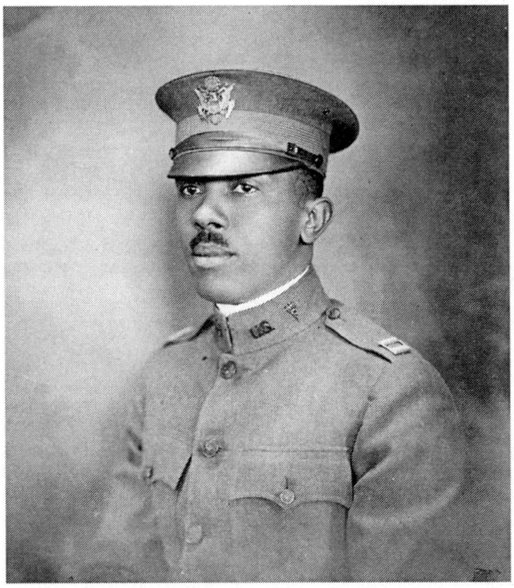

Lt. George I. Lythcott (courtesy Michael J. Lythcott).

When the couple moved to Boston, they lodged with a family named Harrison on Sawyer Street while he attended medical school. He spent some Sundays preaching in Boston's Methodist churches.

Soon after he was awarded his medical degree in 1913, he registered to practice medicine in Massachusetts and New Jersey. He and his wife Bertha had no children, and the marriage soon ended in divorce.

Dr. Lythcott was registered to practice medicine in Massachusetts and New Jersey. Then, on September 14, 1916, Lythcott (now 29) married Evelyn Hortense Wilson. She was 21 and the daughter of the late Reverend Joshua E. Wilson, a minister and the postmaster of Florence, South Carolina, for 20 years. Her older brother was Dr. Roscoe J. Wilson, a Claflin college friend and an ear, nose and throat specialist in Florence.

Dr. and Mrs. Lythcott moved to Darlington, South Carolina (close to Florence).[3] He became involved in community organizations in Florence—the Masons, the Pythians and the Elks. He was also active in the Palmetto Medical Association, the South Carolina state medical association for African American physicians. In 1916, he was elected its vice president.

Military Service

In 1917, Dr. Lythcott and his brother-in-law Roscoe J. Wilson joined the army. On August 17, 1917, the two men reported to the Medical Officers Training Camp (MOTC) at Fort Des Moines. While there, First Lieutenant Lythcott joined the newly formed war chapter of Omega Psi Phi fraternity. He trained at Des Moines until November 3, when he was promoted and sent to Camp Upton, Long Island, New York.

In the spring of 1918, Captain Lythcott left Camp Upton and the army. The Omega Psi Phi fraternity's publication *The Oracle* reported that he would be engaged in continuing service at home because a "prolonged illness" prevented him from continuing service with his country.[4] His illness was also noted in his military file. In 1919 he sought the advice of W. E. B. Dubois regarding his discharge papers and membership in the state organization of the Veterans of World's War. In a letter to Lythcott, Dubois wrote, "get [it] in writing. Do not rest satisfied with a verbal answer which they can easily deny." It was good advice. Later Lythcott received his honorable discharge papers reflecting his eight months of army service.

Career

In 1918, Dr. Lythcott's young wife Evelyn was pregnant and ill. The couple's son, George I. Lythcott, Jr., was born on April 29, 1918. On March 7, 1920, before the child's second birthday, Evelyn died from bilateral pulmonary tuberculosis.

During his career, Dr. Lythcott gave special attention to bacteriology and the treatment of tuberculosis in his practice, perhaps because of his wife's death. Today she could have survived with antibiotic treatment. These drugs did not exist in the early 20th century.

The 1920 U.S. Census lists his son George as living with his Wilson grandmother. That household included his friend and fellow MOTC graduate, Dr. Roscoe J. Wilson, and Wilson's wife Lillian.

In 1923 Dr. Lythcott went to Kansas City General Hospital No. 2 for an internship program. He returned in 1924. By the late 1920s Lythcott and his son moved to Tulsa, Oklahoma. Tulsa was an oil boomtown in the 1920s and 30s. It was also a place of tremendous racism. The Greenwood Historical District was once one of the most affluent African American communities in the United States and referred to as Black Wall Street. In 1921, 35 blocks of businesses and residences were burned in this district during the infamous Tulsa Race Riot, the bloodiest racial riot in the history of the United States.

The Tulsa Race Riot was a large-scale racially motivated conflict on May 31 and June 1, 1921, in which whites attacked the black community of Tulsa, Oklahoma. It resulted in the Greenwood District being burned to the ground. During the 16 hours of the assault, more than 800 people were admitted to local hospitals with injuries, and more than 6,000 Greenwood residents were arrested and detained at three local facilities. An estimated 10,000 blacks were left homeless, and 35 city blocks composed of 1,256 residences were destroyed by fire. The official count of the dead by the Oklahoma Department of Vital Statistics was 39, but other estimates of black fatalities have been up to about 300.[5]

The events of the riot were long omitted from local and state history: "The Tulsa race riot of 1921 was rarely mentioned in history books, classrooms or even in private. Blacks and whites alike grew into middle age unaware of what had taken place."[6] In 1996 the state legislature commissioned a report, completed in 2001, to establish the historical record. It has approved some compensatory actions, such as scholarships for descendants of survivors, and economic development to help rebuild Greenwood.[7]

Clifford A. Lythcott, George's brother who was a dentist, joined them in Tulsa. Lythcott married for a third time to Corinne. According to the 1930 U.S. Census, the four lived at 2102 Peoria Avenue in Tulsa. The doctor's office was at 696 North Archer Street. His brother Clifford later married Julia and moved nearby to 1121 North Greenwood.

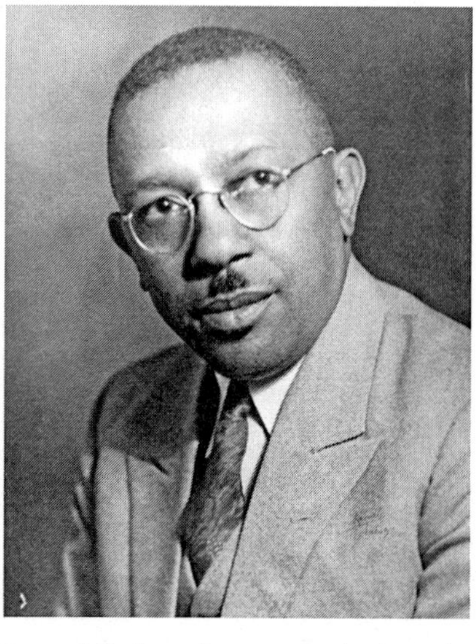

Dr. George I. Lythcott (courtesy Michael J. Lythcott).

The Lythcott brothers arrived after the riots, but the city's stigma was there. Many other professional African Americans had left Tulsa by the time they arrived. In addition to his practice, Dr. Lythcott became director of health in the Tulsa school system and surgeon-in-chief at Tulsa Municipal Hospital #2. He was also active in the Oklahoma State Medical Society.

In 1934 he was appointed head of the new state hospital named the Oklahoma State Hospital for Negro Insane. The *New York Age* called him "one of the most outstanding members of the medical profession in the entire state of Oklahoma."[8] That August Leslie Beck, a hospital engineer, was on the hospital grounds and followed Dr. Lythcott. "The doctor realized he was being followed and turned just in time to ward off a blow from the pistol Beck was carrying. In the ensuing scuffle, the doctor got possession of the gun after one shot had been fired." After Beck had been taken by authorities, Dr. Lythcott showed off a hat pierced by the bullet.[9]

On December 4, 1937, the *New York Age* reported Dr. Lythcott's appointment for a second term as physician in charge of the hospital.[10] He did not live to serve out that term. He died in Tulsa on May 1, 1938. His wife Corrine lived 30 years after his death and passed away at age 90 in 1969.

Lythcott's son George did very well in school. Sadly, his father did not live long enough to see him follow in his footsteps and choose a career in medicine. George enrolled at his father's alma mater, Boston University School of Medicine. He graduated and specialized in pediatrics and then, as his father had done before him, he accomplished a lot more.

In 1956 Dr. George I. Lythcott II was the first African American to be appointed to the faculty of the University of Oklahoma. He was brought in because of his work in children's diseases and was appointed "clinical assistant in pediatrics in the university's school of medicine." Part of his job was to present demonstrations and lectures to the medical students.[11]

His son Michael tells a bit more of his father's story. "Dad was recruited in 1965 to lead a massive smallpox eradication effort in the twenty countries of west and central Africa. Against all odds, the teams did it. They eradicated the disease from that enormous area, and they did it a year and a half ahead of schedule."

A World Health Organization publication on smallpox includes this description of him: "An able and diplomatic administrator, Lythcott played an important role in sustaining the momentum of the program through many political and logistical crises."[12]

During the Carter Administration, he was appointed the assistant surgeon general of the United States (1977–81). As Administrator of the Health Services Administration, he oversaw the largest budget and portfolio in the Department of Health and Human Services. He was a two-star admiral in the U.S. Public Health Service, the highest-ranking African American in the public health service. Every year the Black Commissioned Officers Advisory Group of the United States Public Health Service awards the "George I. Lythcott Award" to exceptional young officers. Michael says, "Grandfather would have loved that." Indeed, that's quite a legacy.

Admiral George I. Lythcott died at the age of 77 on October 7, 1995, in Vineyard Haven, Martha's Vineyard, Massachusetts. Admiral Lythcott's son Michael is a successful entrepreneur living in Marlboro, New Jersey.

NOTES

1. en.wikipedia.org/wiki/Queen%27s_College,_Guyana (accessed January 5, 2013).
2. Research and written material throughout the biography provided by grandson Michael Lythcott.
3. Arthur Bunyan Caldwell, *History of the American Negro, South Carolina Edition* (Atlanta: A. B. Caldwell Publishing Co., 1918) 616–618.
4. "The War Chapter," *The Oracle*, semi-annual publications of the Grand Chapter of The Omega Psi Phi Fraternity, June 1919, 16.
5. www.wikipedia.org/wiki/Tulsa_race_riot (accessed January 20, 2013).
6. en.wikipedia.org/wiki/Tulsa_Race_Riot (accessed January 6, 2013).
7. *Ibid.*
8. "Oklahoma Physician Shot by Hospital Attendant," *The New York Age*, August 18, 1934, 1.
9. "Attack on Negro Physician Probed," *Miami (OK) News Record*, August 9, 1934, 6.
10. *Ibid.*, "Installed as Hospital Head," December 4, 1937, 1.
11. "Oklahoma U. Adds Negro to Faculty," *Pittsburgh Courier*, November 3, 1956, 2.
12. F. Fenner, D. A. Henderson, I. Arita, Z. Jezek and I. D. Ladnyi, *Smallpox and Its Eradication*, World Health Organization, Geneva, 1988, 873.

James L. MARTIN

2 November 1882–25 January 1974
Leonard Medical School, 1906

Roots and Education

Martin was born in Jonesville, Virginia, to Alexander and Amanda (Allen) Martin. Jonesville was a small but thriving center of local commerce in the Appalachian region at very tip of southwestern Virginia. As the coal boom ebbed in the early 20th century, so did the town's economy.[1]

Martin had his earliest education in Jonesville and went on to receive his B. S. degree from Swift Memorial College in 1902. Swift was a historically Black college that operated in East Tennessee from 1883 to 1952. The school was founded in Rogersville, Tennessee, by the Reverend William H. Franklin, the African American pastor of a local Presbyterian church. It focused on high school and normal school (teacher education).[2] Martin earned his medical degree from Shaw University's Leonard Medical School in 1906. He went on to practice medicine in Staunton, Virginia. The 1910 Census reports him there, single and living with the M. W. Parnell family at 613 Augusta Street.

Military Service

He was still in Staunton in 1917 when he volunteered for service in the Army Medical Reserve Corps. He reported to the Medical Officers Training Camp, and after completing his training in November 1917, he went to Camp Upton, New York. He was assigned to the medical detachment of the 367th Infantry Regiment. Once in France, he was reassigned to the 365th Ambulance Company of the 317th Sanitary (Medical) Train, 92nd Division. The 365th was made up largely of men from Chicago and other parts of Illinois. He served with this unit throughout the war.

In the fall of 1918 all medical officers in U.S. camps and in France had to deal with the worst flu epidemic in American history, twenty-six percent of the army was struck. The arms race brought new weapons that generated new, horrible injuries that took life or limbs in a moment. Poison gases burned and suffocated. "Trench foot" was a new disease caused by the sodden boots and standing water in the trenches.[3] As a member of the Medical Corps, Martin treated much of it.

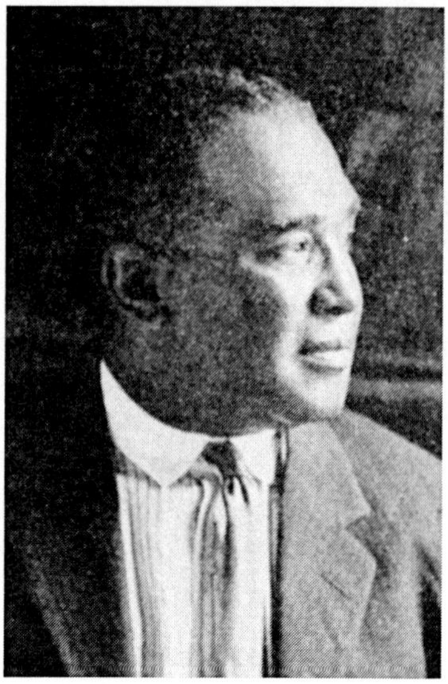

Dr. James L. Martin (national pictorial, members of the National Medical Association, 1925, courtesy Kansas City Public Library).

Ambulance companies were established to care for and transport ill and injured soldiers. For each of the four infantry regiments in the 92nd Division, there was an ambulance company and a field hospital. Each ambulance company consisted of 12 ambulances and was staffed with several physicians and medical support troops. While in combat situations, they treated and transported wounded and gassed soldiers from aid stations to field hospitals, where they were triaged. Soldiers who were unable to walk were carried or transported on litters to the ambulances.[4]

During the drive toward Metz, in the action on November 10 and 11, the 365th Infantry lost 43 men killed in action or dying from their wounds. About 200 others were wounded or gassed. Another 32 were thought missing in action, but were later found to have been killed or died from their wounds. The doctors and medics were frantically busy.[5]

Martin performed well and before the end of the war he was promoted to the rank of captain. In April 1919 he returned to Philadelphia.

Career

On June 25, 1919, Dr. Martin married Martha Oliver in Manhattan, New York. They bought a home at 2027 Catherine Street, Philadelphia, Pennsylvania, and lived there the rest of their lives. They would have no children. He opened a medical practice while attending the Graduate School of Medicine, University of Pennsylvania (1921–23) and specializing in radiology. He is listed as a roentgenologist, a physician dealing with diagnosis and therapy through x-rays. Soon after graduate school, he was appointed chief of the x-ray department at Mercy Hospital in Philadelphia.

Mercy Hospital and School of Nurses opened at 17th and Fitzwater Street in 1907. The Hospital instituted a training school for nursing that same year. It continued after the hospital moved to 50th Street and Woodland Avenue in Southwest Philadelphia in 1919.[6] In 1948 Mercy merged with Frederick Douglass Hospital. Its nursing school was active until it graduated its last class in 1960. Mercy-Douglass Hospital closed in 1973.

Other doctors who had volunteered for service in World War I and who trained with Dr. Martin at Fort Des Moines worked with him at Mercy Hospital. Drs. Egbert T. Scott, F. E. Boston and DeHaven Hinkson were given the same "pioneer" status as Martin in the field of surgery.[7]

Dr. Martin became a staff member at the Graduate School of Medicine at the University of Pennsylvania. He was one of the authors of Experimental Studies of the Combined Effects of X-ray and Ultraviolet Rays on the Skin, and he authored a report to the National Medical Association (NMA) on hyperthyroidism.[8] At NMA's 1926 annual meeting in Philadelphia, Dr. Martin led x-ray clinics held at Polyclinic Hospital. He also participated in a symposium on diseases of the pituitary gland by presenting the x-ray findings.[9]

Philadelphia's Mayor Wilson came to Mercy Hospital on an inspection in May of 1936. One of the things that impressed him was Dr. Martin's demonstration of x-ray technique. He was also interested in the explanation of the workings of the outpatient department from Martin's longtime friend Dr. Egbert Scott. Newspaper coverage spoke of the Mayor's praise of Mercy as comparing favorably with any other hospital in the city.[10]

Dr. Martin's membership in professional organizations included the American Medical Association, the National Medical Association, the Philadelphia County Medical Society, the Clinical Pathological Society, and the Academy of Medicine.[11] He was equally active in his community where he was a member of the Elks, Pythians, and Alpha Phi Alpha. He was also an active Republican and a Presbyterian.

In a May 1951 issue of the *Journal of the National Medical Association*, Dr. Martin is called a pioneer in the field of radiology.[12] He died in Philadelphia at the age of 92.

NOTES

1. en.wikipedia.org/wiki/Jonesville,_Virginia (accessed March 12, 2015).
2. tennesseeencyclopedia.net/entry.php?rc=1682 (accessed July 31, 2013).
3. *The U.S. Military and the Influenza Pandemic of 1918–1919*, www.ncbi.nih.gov/pmc/articles/PMC28623 371 (accessed February 4, 2013).
4. U.S. Army Medical Department, Office of Medical History, Vol. VIII Field Operations, Chapter IV, Medical Service of the Division in Combat (Washington, D.C.: GPO, 1925) history.amedd.army.mil (accessed April 23, 2015).
5. W. Allison Sweeney, *History of the American Negro in the Great War* (New York: Negro Universities Press, 1919) 212.
6. www.nursing.openn.edu/history/documents/Merc Dougweb.pdf (accessed July 30, 1913).
7. Russell F. Minton, MD, "The History of Mercy-Douglass Hospital," *Journal of the National Medical Association (JNMA)*, May 1951, 158.
8. Thomas Yenser, ed. and pub., *Who's Who in Colored America* (New York, 1941–1944), 359.
9. "NMA Activities," *Journal of the National Medical Association (JNMA)*, July–September 1926, 144–145.
10. "Mayor Wilson Praises Mercy Hospital," *Philadelphia Tribune*, May 7, 1936, 3.
11. AMA Deceased Physicians, National Library of Medicine, Bethesda, MD.
12. Russell F. Minton, MD, "The History of Mercy-Douglass Hospital," *Journal of the National Medical Association (JNMA)*, May 1951; 43 (3): 153–159.

Ulysses Grant Baldwin MARTIN

12 February 1887–22 May 1964
Howard Medical College, 1908

Roots and Education

Ulysses Martin was born in the District of Columbia, one of seven children. His parents, George and Elizabeth Baldwin Martin, believed in the importance of education. In 1870 his father held a U.S. government job as a messenger in the Treasury Department. As early as July 21, 1871, he had established an account with the Freedman's Bank, most unusual for many African Americans at that time in history.

The family lived in the District at 308 New York Avenue, NW. Next door at 310 was the Joseph Martin family. Joseph's brother Thomas, a physician, lived with them. Thomas was 32 years older than Ulysses, and was a role model for his career choice. All of the children in both homes went to school. Ulysses' older sister, Rosia, became a schoolteacher, as did two of the Joseph Martin children next door.

Dr. Martin was a 1908 graduate of Howard University Medical School and interned for one year at Freedmen's Hospital. He received his District of Columbia medical license in 1909, giving his parent's home address at 308 New York Avenue, NW. He traveled to Chicago in 1910 and while in Chicago he lived at 5106 State Street, according to American Medical Association (AMA) records. Then he returned to the District of Columbia in 1911 where he practiced for the rest of his life. He was a member of the Methodist Episcopal Church.

Military Service

In 1917 Martin was single when he volunteered and received his commission in the Army Medical Reserve Corps.[1] He completed 79 days of military medical training at Fort Des Moines and was then assigned to the 92nd Division at Camp Funston at Fort Riley, Kansas. By the time he reached Camp Funston, Martin had already been promoted to the rank of captain and made commanding officer of the 367th Ambulance Company. His early promotion was no doubt related to his prior military training and experience. He had been a high school military science cadet and as early as 1902, Martin had been a member of the competitive cadet drill team, winning a competition at his high school in D.C.[2] A D.C. newspaper report in June 1918 mentioned Captain Martin's name among high school military science cadets from Dunbar High School who were serving in World War I.[3]

Soon after arriving in Kansas, Captain Martin was joined by his sweetheart from D.C., Rosa Elizabeth Williams. They were married on Christmas Day, 1917, in nearby Junction City, Kansas.[4] She was born in the District of Columbia on June 10, 1889, and became a public school home economics teacher.

In early 1918, prior to being shipped to France, he filed reports for the 367th Ambulance Company. He identified sick soldiers who should not accompany the command overseas, determined soldiers who were unfit for service, and recommended actions on arrests. His leadership qualities were recognized, and he was one of only a dozen African American doctors promoted to higher grade early in their service.

One military report in France in October 1918 states that Captain Martin was himself ill in a hospital in France for some days. He was not the only physician who fell ill, which was not surprising given the harsh conditions and diseases prevalent among the troops.

As Captain of the Ambulance Company, Martin had to deal with a variety of normal medical and unusual soldier screw-ups. One of his odd reports from France in January 1919, said a soldier who was an orderly was being returned to the ranks because "the orderly claims to have lost the reports thru [*sic*] pulling his gloves out of his pocket to put the glove on his hands." One can almost visualize Captain Martin throwing up his hands as he sent the orderly back into the ranks.

Many of the unit's monetary accounts also came to Captain Martin for review and signature before going on to Lieutenant Colonel David B. Downing, MC for final approval. As the end of the war approached, several of his fellow physicians from their basic training days at Fort Des Moines were sending certificates to him for his approval and signature, including Frederick A. Stokes, Charles H. Laws, Charles C. Buford, and William H. Bryant. By December 1918, lieutenants Vanderbilt Brown and Clarence Janifer were reporting to him as well.

In February 1919 Captain Martin returned with the 92nd Division to the United States and spent some time out-processing at Camp Upton, Long Island, before being discharged.

Career

The American Medical Association records indicate Dr. Martin was in Ohio in 1919. The 1920 Census lists Dr. Martin living with the Laws family in Columbus, Ohio, as a "lodger." One of his compatriots in the army was Dr. Charles H. Laws, which may be a link to his time in Columbus. Ultimately, he returned to the District of Columbia where he resumed his medical practice.

In the late 1920s Dr. and Mrs. Martin bought a house at 2409 M Street, NW, where they lived and he maintained an office. It was quite close to the Columbia Hospital for Women located in a nice area near Rock Creek, Georgetown, and not far from Washington Circle. Columbia Hospital pioneered the use of innovative obstetrical and gynecological techniques. Martin and his wife had no children but in the 1930s, her 14-year-old nephew Edward Williams lived with them. The Martins lived there for the rest of their lives.[5]

The Martins must have been a fun-loving couple. During the 1930s, Dr. Martin was vice president of New York's Union Club. At one spring formal dance, "Leon Gross and his Club Danceland Orchestra played the music for dancing. On the program was the floor show from the Ubangi Club and such headliners as Miss Pearl Baines, vocalist; Roland Holder, Tap dancer, Drusilla Drew, Hot-cha singer and dancer ... and Edna Mae Holly, torso dancer."[6] Certainly a good time must have been enjoyed by all.

Martin served the medical needs of African Americans in Washington for many years. He died from lung cancer in 1964 in the Veterans Administration Hospital at age 78.[7] His wife Rosa had predeceased him in 1950. They are now resting together beneath a large granite headstone in Arlington National Cemetery, Section 8, Grave Site 5496.

NOTES

1. John L. Thompson, *History and Views of Colored Officers Training Camp for 1917 at Fort Des Moines, Iowa* (Des Moines: *The Bystander*, 1917) 71.
2. "Company B a Winner. Competitive Drill of the High School Cadets," *Colored American Newspaper*, Washington, D.C., May 24, 1902, Vol. X Issue 7, 9, 1.
3. "High School Cadets Military Science. Our High School Cadets—What They Have Accomplished," *Washington Bee*, June 8, 1918, 1.
4. "Officers Wed at Camp Funston, Sweethearts Prove True—Some Came from the East—Others Came from the South to Wed Brave Officers," *Advocate Newspaper*, Kansas City, Kansas, January 4, 1918, 1.
5. DC Archives, Office of Public Records, Washington, D.C., 1943,1944,1945 & 1946, Registration Cards of Persons Licensed to Practice the Healing Art in the District of Columbia.
6. "Union Club Has Spring Revelry," *New York Amsterdam News*, May 16, 1936, 7.
7. AMA Deceased Physicians Card, National Library of Medicine, Bethesda, MD.

Allen Augustus McDONALD

12 October 1892–19 February 1928
Meharry Medical College, 1915

Roots and Education

Allen McDonald's father, Hero "Hal" McDonald, was born in Steward County, Georgia. He moved to Russell County, Alabama, where he was very active in the AME Church for five years. He married Ella Reed and began a family. In 1880 the family moved to East Texas and settled in Mexia, a small city 90 miles south of Dallas. His father owned and operated a grocery store there for the rest of his life. The couple reared their nine children in the AME Church. When his father died in 1919, there was an outpouring of sympathy for the family with nearly a full page of messages in the local African American newspaper, the *Dallas Express*.[1]

Prairie View Normal School was the first state-supported college in Texas for African Americans. It was also the second oldest public institution of higher education in Texas.[2] It is likely that his father's active role in the AME Church helped Allen McDonald secure a place in the school. It was his own efforts that got him the certificate of graduation and enrollment at Meharry Medical School in Nashville, Tennessee. He earned his medical degree in 1915.

After medical school, Dr. McDonald passed the Texas state boards, married Inez Lewis (the principal of an African American school) and opened his practice in Calvert, a small city 35 miles north east of College Station, home of Texas A&M University. After the Civil War, cotton was still the big crop in this area of Texas and the location of the railroad through Calvert brought it prosperity. In fact, Calvert claimed to have the world's largest cotton gin. Dr. McDonald was active in the Lone Star State Medical, Dental, and Pharmaceutical Association, an organization of African Americans in the health field. Throughout its history the association emphasized discussion of medical practice and public health education.[3]

Military Service

When McDonald registered for the draft, he was married and operated a medical practice. He volunteered to serve in the army's Medical Reserve Corps and reported rather late to the Medical Officers Training Camp at Fort Des Moines, on October 5, 1917. He received slightly less than one month of basic training. While in camp, the doctors and medics were trained in camp-making sanitation, administration (army paperwork), bearer work and fieldwork in general. Some of the doctors did not see the need for the practice marches or the nights spent learning the various army forms they would be expected to use.[4]

From Fort Des Moines, First Lieutenant McDonald was assigned to the 92nd Division at Camp Funston, Kansas, with the 368th Ambulance Company, before leaving for France in June 1918. He served with this unit throughout the war.

The U.S. Army description of the medical field operations for ambulance companies said they would be "established at the farthest point forward that ambulances can reach with reasonable safety. Patients were to be disturbed as little as possible and were not to be removed from the litter." Dressings and splints were to be applied at battalion aid stations, but would be checked and redressed here if needed. "Warmth will be constantly maintained and hot drink given to those able to take them but withheld in abdominal cases." Cases were distributed from here to the various hospitals.[5] In battles like the Meuse-Argonne, it would have been a chaotic, dangerous job.

Career

After the war, Dr. McDonald returned to Calvert, Texas. By 1920, he and his wife Inez were living at 22 Kezee Street with their two children, Ruth and Allan, and his 15-year-old sister Ella. The town never really recovered from a flood in the late 19th century or a fire in 1900. The population steadily declined until

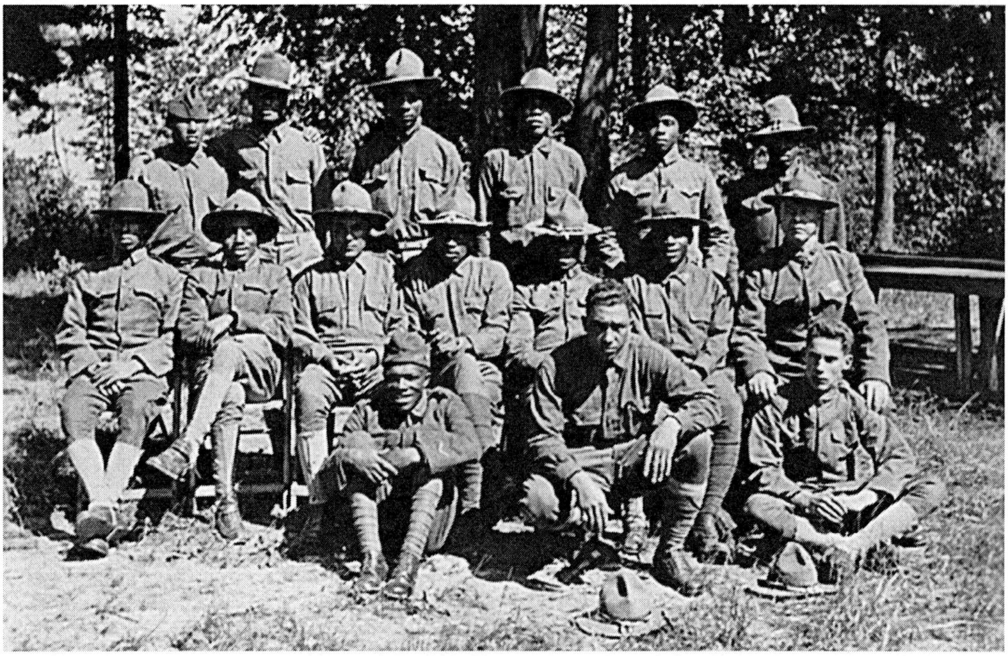

Medics at Fort Des Moines (National Archives).

it was only about 2,000 when the McDonald family made the move to Phoenix, Arizona, in 1924. They were only in Phoenix for three years.

Finally, by December 1927, Dr. McDonald and his family settled in Pueblo, Colorado, where he had his office on East Evans Avenue. Two years later at the age of 35, Dr. McDonald died of lobar pneumonia. Inez raised the children and lived in Pueblo another 37 years.

"There is no passion to be found in playing small—settling for a life that is less than the one you are capable of living," Nelson Mandela once said. Dr. McDonald brought his passion for life and healing to his patients and his community. Sadly, he died too young to see the fruits of his labors.

NOTES

1. "Biography of H. J. Mcdonald," *Dallas Express*, May 17, 1919, 4.
2. www.pvamu.edu/discover-pvamu/history-of-prairie-view-am-university/ (accessed August 30, 2014).
3. www.tshaonline.org/handbook (accessed August 30, 2014).
4. The Medical Department of the U.S. Army in the World War, Vol. VII, Training, 268, National Archives, College Park, MD.
5. history.amedd.army.mil/booksdocs/wwi/field operations/chapter4.html (accessed August 30, 2014).

Andrew Battle McKENZIE

4 January 1887–17 December 1951
Leonard Medical School, 1912

Roots and Education

McKenzie was born and raised in Tallassee, Alabama. He was the oldest of five children born to John Thomas DeLoach and Ellen McKenzie. He studied at the Tuskegee Institute, St. Augustine's College in Raleigh, and earned his medical degree in 1912 at the Leonard Medical School of Shaw University in Raleigh. Then he returned to Alabama and interned at the John A. Andrew Memorial Hospital at Tuskegee Institute until July 1913.

After Tuskegee he moved to Tuscaloosa and opened his medical practice. Located in western Alabama, the city had a population of about 10,000. It is the home of the University of Alabama and Stillman College. McKenzie was the first African American physician in Tuscaloosa. His community involvement began early. In May 1916 he gave a presentation at the eighth annual meeting of the Alabama State Negro Business League in Tuscaloosa entitled "Health Topics: The House Fly."[1]

Military Service

When America entered the First World War in 1917, Dr. McKenzie volunteered for service in the U.S. Army and was awarded a commission as a first lieutenant in the Medical Reserve Corps. He trained at Fort Des Moines at a special Medical Officers Training Camp (MOTC) for Colored doctors. When he completed his training he was assigned to the 317th Sanitary (Medical) Train of the 92nd "Buffalo" Division at Camp Funston, Fort Riley, Kansas. The 92nd was a black combat division with 27,000 men. Lieutenant McKenzie was assigned to the headquarters of the medical train and he continued to serve with it in France during the war. He was the adjutant for the headquarters unit, and because of his intelligence and effectiveness, he was promoted to the rank of captain in October 1918.

Captain McKenzie's assignment in the headquarters provided him with quite a different experience from the doctors who served with the infantry and other line units. At the headquarters he had access and exposure to all the activities of the division's medical units and

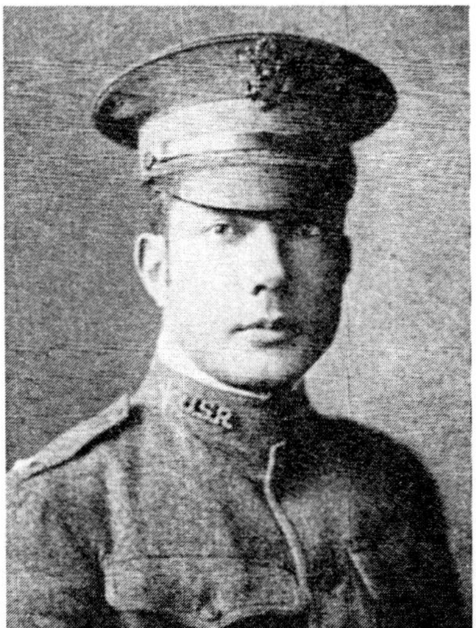

Lt. Andrew B. McKenzie (Emmett J. Scott, *Scott's Official History of the American Negro in World War I*, 1919).

the performance of its personnel. He was responsible for many personnel field assignments. In early November he was reassigned to the division's 365th Field Hospital in direct support of major combat operations. Here he was responsible for overseeing care of soldiers with a wide variety of injuries, including gassing and shell shock.

World War I was the first conflict to see the use of deadly gases as a weapon. Gas burned skin and irritated noses, throats, and lungs. It could cause death or paralysis within minutes, killing by asphyxiation. As soon as troops learned that gas was in their area, they had to put on masks. Even having the fumes in their clothing could cause blisters, sores, and other health problems. Hospital medics bathed and changed the clothes on gassed patients immediately upon their arrival, but that arrival could be hours after the gas attack. Many thousands of gas victims suffered the painful effects of damaged lungs throughout their lives.

Some injuries were not physical. Most soldiers got used to living in muddy areas filled with rats, rotting corpses, and exploding shells, but others could not. As the war progressed, a mental illness caused by these conditions became known as shell shock. Sufferers could be hysterical, disoriented, paralyzed, and unable to obey orders. These soldiers were evaluated and either sent back to their units or sent to base hospitals for treatment before evacuation.

McKenzie's assignment with the 365th Field Hospital got him out from behind a desk and into the trenches at the height of this most bloody of wars. When the war ended he returned to Tuscaloosa to resume his medical practice.

Career

Dr. McKenzie practiced in Tuscaloosa for the rest of his life. He married Marie Sanford McKenzie, whom he had met at St. Augustine College in Raleigh. They had two children: son Sanford, who became an educator, and daughter Dorothy.

He was widely known and respected as a leader in the city's African American community. He had a reputation as a hard-working man who devoted himself to numerous civic and religious affairs.

McKenzie was chairman of the board of trustees of the Hunter's Chapel AME Zion Church, a 33rd degree Mason and the State Grand Medical Director for the Masonic Lodge. He was the first president of the Beta Pi Sigma Chapter of the Phi Beta Sigma fraternity. He was an I.B.P.O.E. member, and the only African American member of the Tuscaloosa Chamber of Commerce. In 1927 he was elected one of three lay delegates to the North Alabama Conference of the AME Church during its six-day meeting in Birmingham.[2]

He was also active in professional medical organizations. In 1930 McKenzie was re-elected secretary of surgical clinics for the renowned John A. Andrew Clinical Society at its annual clinics held at the Tuskegee Institute.[3] Then in 1931 he was elected vice president, and by 1933 he had been elected president.[4]

Dr. McKenzie was on the medical staff at Tuscaloosa's city hospital (known as Druid City Hospital), a trustee of Stillman College, an advisory board member of the Alabama Federation of Colored Women's Clubs, a Khedive Temple Shriner, and a member of the Veterans of Foreign Wars and the American Legion.

In 1936 he served as grand medical registrar at the annual meeting of the Grand Lodge of the Knights of Pythias in Birmingham, where he gave an address. He was popular and a good speaker, and was re-elected to serve at the 50th Anniversary meeting. In 1937 he delivered the 50th oration and made "an earnest eloquent and historic expression of the Order of the Knights of Pythias in Alabama. The address was well delivered and briskly applauded by the hundreds of people who filled the spacious church auditorium."[5]

In 1940 McKenzie was invited to address the 62nd annual meeting of the Masons. More than seven hundred people attended this meeting in Huntsville, Alabama.[6]

Dr. McKenzie had a very light-skinned complexion and might have passed as white, but he always chose to care for and act as an advocate and leader of his African American community. A church history written in 1976 reports "very few people knew he was a black man. He used this rather advantageously to promulgate the economic and social advancement of the black race."[7] He owned large real estate holdings in Tuscaloosa, including an office building, apartment buildings and rental houses, a cemetery and two poolrooms.

He was a sought after public speaker and was described as a pillar of wisdom, service and quite often sacrifice among the African Americans of Tuscaloosa. In a telephone interview in March 2014, his granddaughter, Adrienne Coleman of Rockville, Maryland, said he often saw patients in his office who could not afford to pay him.

When he died of a heart attack while working in his office in 1951, local newspapers wrote articles about his many contributions. The Tuscaloosa Rotary Club, a white organization, offered a memorial tribute to Dr. McKenzie, saying, "There was no man in the medical profession here greater respected by its members. He was the arbitrator of his race. No man in our community could be greater missed by his people."[8]

In 1952, shortly after his death, the City of Tuscaloosa built its largest public housing development, a 340-unit housing project. It was built for African Americans and represented the best housing available for the population—either public or private sector. It was named "McKenzie Court" in his honor.

Dr. McKenzie was buried in the West Highland Cemetery of his beloved Tuscaloosa, next to Stillman College where he had served as a trustee.

Notes

1. "Alabama Business League in Session," *The New York Age*, May 4, 1916, 5.
2. "Delegates Elected to General Body," *Pittsburgh Courier*, December 17, 1927, 4.
3. "13th Annual Meeting of the John A. Andrew Clinical Society to Be Attended by Many Notable Medics," *The New York Age*, April 5, 1930, 10.
4. "Notables to Attend Tuskegee Clinic," *Pittsburgh Courier*, April 8, 1933, 13.
5. "Alabama Pythians Re-Elect O. Adams," *The New York Age*, August 21, 1937, 11.
6. "Alabama Masons Hold 62nd Annual Meeting in Huntsville, Ala," *The New York Age*, August 3, 1940, 8.
7. Robert L. Glynn, *How Firm a Foundation: A History of the First Black Church in Tuscaloosa County, Alabama* (Tuscaloosa: Friends of the Hunter's Chapel African Methodist Episcopal Zion Church and the City of Tuscaloosa, Alabama Bicentennial Committee, 1976).
8. "Dr. Mckenzie Dies in Office of Heart Attack," *Tuscaloosa News*, December 18, 1951.

English Newton McLAUGHLIN

10 September 1892–July 1970
Boston University, 1916

Roots and Education

McLaughlin was born in Camden, South Carolina, the county seat of Kershaw County. Kershaw County was a rural agrarian area in the central part of the state. Camden is about 35 miles northeast of the state capital at Columbia. The town was segregated with a large population of African Americans. Camden has a long history going back to pre-revolutionary times, and it was the site of an important Revolutionary War battle.

English's father was Charles McLaughlin and his mother was Jennie English. His father died in his early 40s, but his mother lived to almost 90.[1]

Young English left South Carolina and moved to New Haven, Connecticut, in the early 1900s. He lived there with his older sisters and mother while he attended school. He graduated from the New Haven High School in 1911. When he entered Boston University, he moved to West Newton, Massachusetts, and lived with his sister, Annie E. McLaughlin, a hairdresser. McLaughlin graduated from the Boston University Medical School earning his M.D. in June 1916. He joined the American Institute of Homeopathy that same year. Homeopathic medicine was still popular and had not yet been supplanted by allopathic medicine.

Dr. McLaughlin continued to live in Newton with his older sister and opened a medical practice in his sister's home at 265 Adams Street. He was still there when he registered for the draft in 1917. He was one of the early African American volunteers to join the Army Medical Reserve Corps. The United States had entered the First World War, and he responded to the call for soldiers.

Military Career

First Lieutenant McLaughlin was accepted into the Medical Officers Reserve Corps. He was called on active duty and was sent to Fort Des Moines where he attended the Medical Officers Training Camp (MOTC). He arrived in early August 1917 and completed 85 days of training

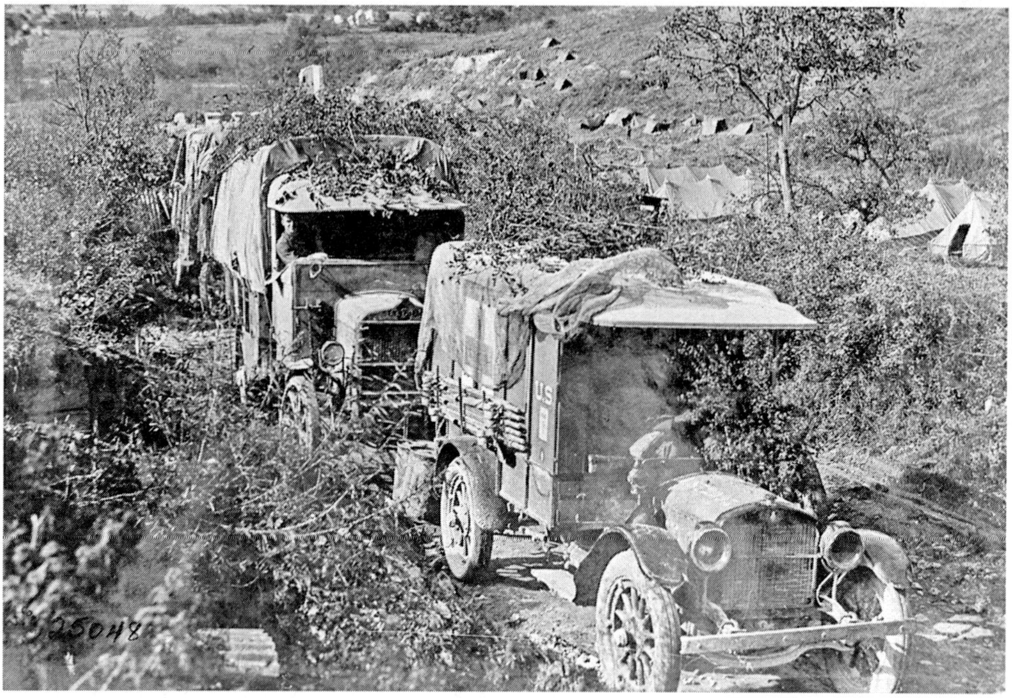

Division convoy on the move (National Archives).

in early November. He was ordered to the 92nd Division's 317th Sanitary (Medical) Train at Camp Funston at Fort Riley, Kansas. There he joined the Train's 366th Ambulance Company and served with that unit for more than eight months.

During January 1918, he was detailed for duty as an Assistant Medical Officer at the Infirmary. After the division arrived in France in mid–1918, he was reassigned to the 365th Field Hospital on August 1, 1918.[2] He was a member of the surgical team at the division's triage hospital at Millery in the Marbache sector during the last months of the war, where he reported to Dr. Louis T. Wright.[3] He served with that unit for the remainder of the war.

In 1919 *The New York Age* published part of a letter written by Dr. McLaughlin from France to his friend, Mr. Walter Lewis in New Haven. In it he wrote, "Previous to the present time we have established hospitals all along the line in various sectors endeavoring to aid the brave soldiers of the 'Allied Nations.' Our work is constant, day and night, and necessitates efficiency and willingness for one to do his bit. Nevertheless through all of the seeming disadvantages, every man goes about doing his duty with a smile on his face. Sometimes things seem to get serious, the atmosphere seems to change, and it is then that the grave and serious countenance takes the place of the smile.... I believe that all the 'world knows by this time the material that the 'American Youngsters' are made of. Once upon a time it was 'German Kultur,' now it is 'American Efficiency and Dash.'"[4]

Career

Upon his discharge from service in 1919, Lieutenant McLaughlin returned to Boston. By 1920, his sister, Annie E. had married William McKnight and given birth to two children. They all lived together over a restaurant at 470 Brookline Avenue in Roxbury. McKnight was "chef-cook" for the restaurant.[5]

The 1930 U.S. Census lists Dr. McLaughlin still living there with McKnight and his sister Annie, as well as his elderly mother, Jennie Lang, and McLaughlin's wife Eva.[6] Boston University records show his address (presumably his office) as 28 Claremont Park in South Boston from 1927 to 1935.

In March 1932 Dr. McLaughlin was struck

by a hit-and-run driver's car while crossing Northampton Street in Roxbury. He suffered fractured ribs after being thrown several feet in the air.[7] It appears he fully recovered.

The Great Depression of the 1930s must have been challenging financially for the family. In 1940 the McKnight/McLaughlin family was still living together and his brother-in-law McKnight was working as a cook at a rectory. Dr. McLaughlin was working as a research editor at the WPA (Works Projects Administration),[8] a governmental jobs program that was started during the Depression.

Boston city directories continue to show him working as a WPA researcher in 1943. In 1942, when Dr. McLaughlin completed a World War II draft registration card, he described himself as a doctor, his age as 49, and his home and mailing address at 75 Monroe Street, Roxbury. His sister Annie McKnight and his mother Jennie Lang were living with him. He may well have held two jobs to help support his family. In 1946 he had an office at 6 Worcester Place and during 1954 two other addresses are listed for him, 1845 Washington Street, Boston and 86 Walnut Avenue in Roxbury. By the 1960s his home and office address was at 220 Northampton Street in Boston. In his later years he suffered from poor health, and he died in July 1970 at the age of 77.

A descendent of the McKnight family referred to him as "Uncle Doc" and described his later years. "He was confined to a wheel chair and his eyesight gone due to glaucoma. A condition that each of his siblings and grandnieces/nephews developed in their aging process." While discussing family history she learned "Doc" had a small independent practice in the Roxbury neighborhood of south Boston servicing the African American community. In his early years if his patients needed to be hospitalized they were transferred to white doctors because of Jim Crow practices.[9]

Discrimination and segregation was a problem in hospitals throughout the first half of the 20th century. This was also true in New York City and other cities in the northeast. By the mid–1950s hospital integration was becoming more common in the North with 83 percent of the hospitals reporting they provided "some degree" of integrated services. Nevertheless a report from 2004 states, "Discrimination existed in overt patterns in hospitals throughout the North and South until the mid–1960s. These discriminatory policies and practices barred black professionals from the medical staffs of hospitals and black patients from beds and services, and they denied black students access to nursing and residency training programs. While actions taken by Congress and the federal government helped eliminate overt racial discrimination in hospital staff privileging, patient admissions, and education programs, without strong court rulings these advances would have fallen short of their intended outcomes."[10] For institutions in the South, real integration took several more decades.

McLaughlin was a quiet, hardworking man who was dedicated to his profession and the African American community. Before his death, Dr. McLaughlin had served that community in Boston for more than 50 years.

NOTES

1. "Application for Registration of Birth, State of South Carolina," English Newton McLaughlin, April 13, 1954, ancestry.com.
2. RG-120, 92d Division, 317th Sanitary Train, Headquarters, Special Orders No. 6, 1 August 1918, National Archives, College Park, MD.
3. Wright, Louis T. "I Remember," (unpublished autobiographical typescript) Moorland Spingarn Research Center, Howard University, Washington, D.C., undated, 90.
4. "AMERICAN EFFICIENCY Vs. GERMAN KULTUR, New Haven, Conn.," *The New York Age*, April 5, 1919, 4.
5. 1920 U.S. Federal Census.
6. 1930 U.S. Federal Census.
7. "Boston Physician Hurt," *Afro-American*, March 19, 1932, 9.
8. 1940 U.S. Federal Census.
9. Source: Great niece Annie M. McKnight, Boston, MA via www.ancestry.com, July 30, 2012.
10. P. Preston Reynolds, MD, PhD, FACP, "Professional and Hospital DISCRIMINATION and the U.S. Court of Appeals Fourth Circuit 1956–1967," American Journal of Public Health, 2004 May; 94(5): 710–720.

Charles Clayton MIDDLETON

16 November 1886–15 March 1955
University of Michigan, 1912

Roots and Education

Middleton was the older of two sons born to Louis G. and Amanda Curley Middleton in

Savannah, Georgia. His father was a barber, and his mother was a schoolteacher. The family lived at 505 Charlton Street. The boys were reared and educated in Savannah. Charles went on to school at Knoxville College in Tennessee. Both brothers entered the field of medicine. Charles became a physician, and his younger brother Louis became a dentist.

In 1907 Charles entered the University of Michigan Medical School. He earned his degree in 1912. Dr. Middleton returned to Savannah to practice medicine and received an appointment as a city physician. He was one of four such physicians and served the "Eastern District," the African American community. His activity and financial reports appear in Savannah's annual mayor's reports for 1913 and 1914. They included detailed monthly data about numbers and types of treatments provided, outcomes, and receipts and disbursements.[1]

On December 29, 1914, he married Jennie Belle Bugg from Lynchburg, Virginia. She had been a teacher in the Lynchburg public schools. Jennie and Charles moved into the family home at 505 Charlton Street. They were there in 1917 as the United States entered the First World War. Dr. Middleton volunteered, and was appointed first lieutenant in the Medical Reserve Corps.

Military Career

Middleton was called to active duty in early August 1917. He reported for training at Fort Des Moines, Iowa. After successfully completing 82 days of training he was ordered to Camp Dix, New Jersey. He was assigned to the Medical Detachment of the 349th Field Artillery of the 92nd Division and served with that unit throughout the war. They were engaged in combat operations near Metz with the 92nd Division for a short period in November 1918 before the Armistice was declared on November 11. His unit suffered only a handful of casualties with none killed. Artillery units were not front line units such as the infantry. They sustained battle casualties primarily from air attacks and enemy artillery fire with high explosive and gas weapons. Most of Middleton's time in service would have been spent treating the sick and injured, rather than dealing with front-line battle casualties.

Career

At the end of the war, Captain Middleton was honorably discharged March 18, 1919, and returned home to Savannah. In 1920 and 1921 Dr. Middleton, his wife Jennie and two young daughters, Catherine, age 4, and Amanda, age 2, lived in the family home on Charlton Street. His wife had a job as a bookkeeper at an insurance company and they had several boarders living with them. Their financial circumstances must have been improving because by 1922 they had moved from the family home into their own home at 611 36th Street West. In 1928 Dr. Middleton had an office at 467 West Broad Street.

It was during the mid–1920s that Dr. Middleton was attracted to New York City. His brother was working there. After the death of his father in 1915, his mother remarried in 1917 and moved to New York. The "Great Migration" to the northern cities, particularly to Harlem, was in full swing. His younger brother, Dr. Louis R. Middleton, a dentist, graduated from Howard University in 1917 and the University of Illinois in 1922. He had taken a job as a dental surgeon with the Bureau of Child Hygiene, New York Health Department. He was the only African American dentist in the dental department of New York City,[2] and he became president of the North Harlem Dental Society.

During the late 1920s, Dr. Middleton moved to New York City and moved in with his brother. In early 1930 Dr. Middleton and his brother relocated their home and office, announcing their move "for the practice of Medicine and Dentistry" into larger and more convenient quarters at 148 West 118th Street. Their offices formerly were at 115th Street and Seventh Avenue in New York.[3] The 1930 Census confirms Dr. Middleton lived at West 118th Street along with his brother, his mother, Amanda C. Spaulding, and his stepfather, Francis M. Spaulding. He stepfather was a Pullman porter for the railroad.[4] It appears Dr. Middleton's wife and children chose not to move to New York.

He was elected president of the Knoxville College Club in New York in May 1930.[5] Dr. Middleton also maintained ties to his home state of Georgia. In 1931 and 1932 he served as president of New York's United Sons of Georgia Association. In fact he was re-elected to that position in 1938.[6] He continued to serve as a director of the club in the 1940s.

Dr. Middleton became very active in Harlem's African American medical community. He was vice president and president of the North Harlem Medical Society during extremely contentious times in 1930. He and fellow supporters ultimately withdrew from the organization to form the Manhattan Medical Society. Dr. Louis T. Wright, former president of the North Harlem Medical Association, joined the new group, and its president was Dr. James L. Wilson. Dr. Middleton was vice president.

Interestingly, all three of these men had trained together at Fort Des Moines and served in the army during the First World War. Their objective at this time was to open Harlem Hospital to black physicians and nurses on an equal footing basis and to work with the political leaders of New York to accomplish this. The actions of Drs. Wright, Middleton, Wilson, and others were opposed by some white and black doctors who feared for their positions. Ultimately, Dr. Wright and his group prevailed and succeeded in opening more doors for black medical professionals to compete on an equal basis with whites.

By 1935, he was a member of the executive committee of the Central Harlem Medical Society. It was created in 1934 with the reconciliation and merger of the former North Harlem Medical Society and the Manhattan Medical Society, which had split in 1930. He served as toastmaster at its annual banquet.[7] In 1941 he retired as president of the Society.

When the National Medical Association held its large 1939 annual convention in New York, Middleton was a member of the New York host committee and chairman for the President's Ball.

He was active in civic matters as well. In 1940 he was a speaker at a men's day celebration at a church discussing the poor state of housing and health conditions in Harlem.[8] That same year he was in charge of a group of physicians and dentists who strategized for the election of Municipal Court Justice Charles Toney,[9] and he was appointed as one of 11 Harlem physicians to be examining physicians for the New York City draft boards. There were 120,000 men in Harlem subject to the new draft law.

Dr. Middleton lived at 160 West 119th Street in 1940, where he resided with two boarders, one was a teacher with W.P.A. Recreation.[10] From as early as 1938, he was a member and executive secretary of the Tri-State Bridge Club.[11] The club members played in national tournaments and had a number of distinguished New York professionals in its membership.[12] As late as 1950–51, he served as the association's president.

When he registered for the World War II draft in 1942, he gave his age as 55. His address was still 160 West 119th Street. As an examining physician for the draft boards, he won the Congressional Selective Service Merit for outstanding service during the Second World War.

Dr. Middleton continued to practice medicine in New York for the rest of his life. He died in 1955 at age 68 and was buried in the Long Island National Cemetery in Farmingdale.

Middleton helped break down the color line in the hospital and health care system. He also sought help for the poorer citizens of Harlem by engaging with city leaders and bringing their attention to important matters of health care and housing.

His obituary states he was survived by his wife, Mrs. J. B. Middleton and two children, Mrs. Millard Williams of Washington, D.C., and Dr. Catherine B. Middleton of Raleigh, North Carolina, and granddaughter Margaret Williams, as well as his brother, Dr. Louis R. Middleton.[13] Military interment records indicate that his widow, Jimmie B. Middleton, was to be interred there as well,[14] but when she passed away almost 12 years later, her oldest daughter, Catherine, had her mother buried in Raleigh.[15]

NOTES

1. *Reports of the City Officers of Savannah, Georgia for the Years Ended December 31, 1913 (p 450) and December 31, 1914 (p 413)*, University of Georgia Library.
2. Thomas Yenser, ed. and pub., *Who's Who in Colored America* (Sixth Edition), 1941–1944 (New York, 1944), 365.
3. "Drs. Middleton Move Offices to 118th Street," *The New York Age*, April 19, 1930, 2.

4. 1930 U.S. Federal Census.
5. "Knoxville College Club," *The New York Age*, May 10, 1930, 2.
6. "C.C. Middle Heads Ga. Club," *New York Amsterdam News*, January 1, 1938, 9.
7. "Dr. Wiley M. Wilson Installed Head of Harlem Medical Soc.," *The New York Age*, February 15, 1935, 2.
8. "Harlem Housing Worst in City," *New York Amsterdam News*, November 11, 1939, 12.
9. "Harlem Heads Back Watson," *New York Amsterdam News*, August 24, 1940, 4.
10. 1940 U.S. Federal Census.
11. "Bridge Tourney Begins Tuesday," *New York Amsterdam News*, January 21, 1939, 5.
12. "Social Snapshots," *The New York Age*, October 5, 1940, 6.
13. "Services for Dr. Middleton Held Last Week," *New York Amsterdam News*, April 2, 1955, 4.
14. "Report of Interment, April 8, 1955, the Quartermaster General, Washington 22, D.C." Middleton, Charles Clayton, ancestry.com.
15. North Carolina Death Certificates, 1909–1975 for Jimmie Bugg Middleton, ancestry.com.

Thomas Ezekiel MILLER, Jr.

26 July 1880–16 January 1954
College of Physicians and Surgeons (Chicago), 1913

Roots and Education

Miller came from a large and distinguished African American political family in South Carolina. His father was a successful attorney, educator and a well-known and seasoned local and state politician. Following the Civil War, his father earned a scholarship to Lincoln University, a school for African American students near Philadelphia. He graduated in 1872. He married Anna Marie Hume in 1874, and they had nine children; one was Thomas Jr. The family lived in various cities in South Carolina, including Beaufort, Columbia, Charleston, and Orangeburg.

His father served in the U.S. Congress in 1890–1891 and eventually served as the president of the State Negro College (later South Carolina State University) for 15 years from 1896 to 1911. From 1923 to 1934, Miller Sr. and his wife lived in Philadelphia, Pennsylvania, and then returned to South Carolina.[1] His wife passed away in 1936 at age 83, and he passed away in 1938 at age 88. They are buried in Charleston at the Brotherly Association Cemetery.

In stark contrast to his father, Thomas Jr. appears to have lived a long and relatively quiet professional life. He was born in Grahamville, South Carolina, and educated in the state until he went away to medical school. In the early 1900s he lived and studied at the State Negro College in Orangeburg where his father was president. He went to Chicago in 1910 to study medicine, graduating in 1913 from the Chicago College of Medicine and Surgery, which later became part of Loyola University. He returned to South Carolina and passed his South Carolina state boards in November of 1913. He established a medical practice and was single and living in Anderson, South Carolina. When America entered the First World War he became one of the first men in South Carolina to volunteer for military service. He wrote that he was a member of the Knights of Pythias and the Presbyterian Church.[2]

Military Service

He received a commission in the U.S. Army Medical Reserve Corps as a first lieutenant and was ordered to Fort Des Moines for military training. He was 37 years old when he left home and he received 42 days of training at the Medical Officers Training Camp between September 23 and November 3, 1917. He was assigned to Camp Funston, Kansas, to the 317th Sanitary (Medical) Train of the 92d "Buffalo" Division.[3]

While at Funston, he was assigned to various medical units of the Sanitary Train during the first half of 1918. Initially, he was one of several physicians assigned to the 365th Ambulance Company. On March 3, 1918, he was detailed for duty to contagious barracks at Building 1935. He returned home briefly from Fort Des Moines to Charleston and married Harriet (Hattie) E. Chambers on March 30, 1918, at St. Mark's Church, while he was serving in the Army Medical Corps.[4] Following the war, the couple would go on to live and work in Charleston for the rest of their lives.

A Fort Des Moines roster of officers dated May 27, 1918, lists him among 39 MOTC officers who had completed a gas course at the School of Arms. He was assigned then to the 367th Field Hospital. His name appears on a company fund accounting book for the 366th Field Hospital in June 1918, shortly before he was sent to France with the 92nd Division.

Once in France, First Lieutenant Miller is listed in August and September 1918 as a member of 367th Field Hospital. By November 1918, he had been promoted to Captain, an indication of his competence and leadership skills.[5]

His field hospital provided early care for many battle casualties. Stretcher-bearers carried wounded soldiers from the front lines to a doctor's care at the battalion aid station, where bandages and splints were applied. No resources were available there for additional care. From the battalion aid station, other stretcher-bearers and ambulances carried the wounded back to a triage point at one of an infantry division's field hospitals, a few miles from the front lines.

At triage, the wounded were sorted into "light" and "serious" cases, sick men were sent to a designated field hospital, and those suffering from poison gas went to another hospital. (The line between light and serious wounds varied, and gas casualties often had other wounds as well.) Some additional care was available at the triage point, but field hospitals had limited equipment and could only treat the lightly wounded.

From triage, wounded men were taken by ambulance to the evacuation hospitals for surgical care. They stayed there several days to stabilize and begin recovery. They were then taken by hospital train to base hospitals, where they could receive complicated procedures and recuperate.

Miller was also commanding officer of the 92nd Division, Sanitary Squad No. 31. Sanitary Squads were established to prevent disease through vigorous sanitation efforts. His report on Sanitary Squad No. 31 became Chapter 3 of the U.S. Army Medical Department's history of the 92nd Division. In it Captain Miller tells of the French towns' affliction with polluted water. "Manure was piled high in front of nearly every house, all of which threatened the health of the soldiers." Sanitary squads were employed to educate troops in measures necessary to maintain health, the construction of bathing and disinfesting plants, supervision of disposal of sewage, garbage, and refuse, sanitary inspections and cognate duties. There were only two Sanitary Squads for each division. Each squad consisted of an officer (usually a physician), four non-commissioned officers, 20 privates and two drivers plus one mobile laboratory consisting of one officer and five enlisted personnel.[6]

The army training and responsibility Dr. Miller shouldered undoubtedly served his community well after he returned to Charleston in 1919.

Career

Dr. Miller returned to Charleston and resumed his medical practice. By 1920, he and his wife Hattie were still living at his parent's home at 78 Radcliffe Street in Charleston. By January 1923, his professional and home address was 150 Spring Street in Charleston which would remain their home for the rest of their lives.

The practice was made up of Dr. Miller along with his brother Dr. John Hume Miller, his brother-in-law Dr. Charles Wendell Maxwell, and Dr. Lawrence A. Earle were active members of the Palmetto Medical Association (PMA).[7] Dr. Earle was one of its founders. The PMA was established in 1896 for African American physicians in South Carolina and was part of the National Medical Association (NMA). In 1936 the PMA held its first free clinic for the public in connection with its annual meeting. It proved to be a boon to countless numbers of sick and afflicted needing expert professional care. At a postgraduate seminar, the PMA drew upon the physicians of South Carolina and other states throughout the nation to broaden their perspectives. The PMA, which was later renamed the Palmetto Medical, Dental, Pharmaceutical Association, helped keep members abreast of advances made in medicine, dentistry and pharmacy.

Dr. Miller practiced medicine in Charleston's large local African American community for more than 30 years. He was well regarded and prominent in the local medical establishment. After Dr. Miller retired from his medical practice, his wife, Hattie, died of breast cancer in October 1951. Slightly more than two years later he died of esophageal cancer at the age of 73 at Charleston's esteemed Roper Hospital. Three weeks before his death, he donated a pipe organ to St. Mark's Protestant Episcopal Church. It was to have been dedicated the Sunday just after his death.[8] He and Hattie are buried in the same Charleston cemetery, Brotherly Association Cemetery with his parents.[9]

NOTES

1. "Thomas Ezekiel Miller, Republican from South Carolina," Black Americans in Congress, baic.house.gov/member-profiles/profile.html?intID-20 (accessed August 1, 2012).
2. John L. Thompson, *History and Views of Colored Officers Training Camp for 1917 at Fort Des Moines, Iowa* (Des Moines: *The Bystander*, 1917) 73.
3. Table of Medical Reserve Corps—Colored—Receiving Instruction, Medical Training Camp, Fort Des Moines, Iowa, RG-112, Records of the Army Surgeon General, National Archives, College Park, MD.
4. Sarah Nesnow, Genealogist and historian in Charleston, South Carolina, correspondence August 7, 2014.
5. Record Group 120, Records of the 92d Division, 317th Sanitary Train, Memoranda 1918, National Archives, College Park, MD.
6. U.S. Army Medical Department, Office of Medical History, Chapter 3, World War I, The Sanitary Corps history.amedd.army.mil/booksdocs/HistoryofUSArmyMSC/chapter3.html (accessed January 3, 2013).
7. Sarah Nesnow, genealogist and historian in Charleston, South Carolina, correspondence August 7, 2014.
8. "Final Rites Held for Dr. Miller, Negro Physician," *Charleston News & Courier*, January 19, 1954, 7.
9. South Carolina Death Records, 1821–1955, ancestry.com.

Daniel Miller MOORE

2 May 1888–12 July 1958
University of West Tennessee, 1912

Roots and Education

Dan Moore was born in Grambling, Louisiana. Nothing could be found about his family or his early life. Early records in this very small North Louisiana town are no longer available. There was no Grambling State University there during his childhood. And, the farmers that pushed for a school to better educate their children didn't begin to organize or gather funds until 1896. That's when Booker T. Washington of the Tuskegee Institute was approached for help and sent Charles P. Adams to help those farmers get the school underway.

Even Grambling's predecessor, The North Louisiana Colored Industrial and Agricultural School, didn't open until November 1, 1901. Moore would have been 13 so it is possible that he was able to study there, but no paperwork exists.

Somehow, Moore received enough education to gain admittance to the Flint Medical College in New Orleans. When it closed after losing its American Medical Association accreditation in 1911, he transferred to the University of West Tennessee Medical School in Memphis graduating in 1912. That December, he married Essie Gipson of Stamps, Arkansas. He was 23, and she was only 18. The couple settled in central Oklahoma. He initially opened medical offices in 1913 in the town of Kingfisher, and then in 1916 they moved to El Reno, 30 miles west of Oklahoma City.

Military Service

When American entered the First World War in 1917, Dr. Moore volunteered for the U.S. Army Medical Reserve Corps. He left his wife Essie with his family in Grambling and reported to Fort Des Moines on October 12, 1917. First Lieutenant Moore trained there for 30 days before his transfer to the 370th Infantry Regiment of the 93rd Division, where he was attached to the medical unit of its Supply Company. The 370th was formerly the 8th Illinois National Guard.

After a brief period of training at Camp Logan near Houston, Texas, the regiment was shipped to Camp Stuart in Virginia and sailed for France aboard the SS *Susquehanna* from Newport News, Virginia, on March 30, 1918. After arriving in France, the officer in charge of the regiment, Colonel Denison, was told they would be turned over to the French army and be attached to its 73rd Infantry Division. American equipment and arms were switched for French, and the men were moved to a quiet sector in the Vosges for some training before moving to the action.

By June 1918, they had moved into the trenches in the St. Mihiel sector with the French army. Fortunately, there was light combat action initially. The men then moved to other sectors, gaining competence and confidence.[1]

In late September 1918, the 370th was part of the attacks at Canal de l'Oise-l'Aisne where the Germans were finally pushed back across the canal on October 3. For the next month, the 370th pushed the Germans further back, continually suffering casualties. Reconnaissance patrols were sent out at night to find German machine guns and to map German positions. By November 9, they were finding abandoned posts.

The medical detachment was composed of 23 men. They treated approximately 560 officers and men who were wounded and the 105 killed in action or who died of their wounds.[2]

"Black Devils" was the name they were given by the Germans. In December 1919 French general Vincendon illustrated the high regard the country had for the 370th in his special order praising them which closed with "The blood of your comrades who fell on the soil of France mixed with the blood of our soldiers, renders indissoluble the bonds of affection that unite us. We have, besides, the pride of having worked together at the magnificent task, and the pride of bearing on our foreheads the ray of a common grandeur."[3]

Career

After the war, Dr. Moore returned to the United States and decided to build a practice in the state capital, Oklahoma City. By the end of 1919, he and Essie owned their own home at 828 East Third Street. He advertised his medical office as "over Bethel's drug store, 330 East Second Street." That early ad in the local *Black Dispatch* also contained notice of the availability of a furnished room in his home." By the 1920 U.S. Census, James Wooden was boarding with them.[4]

Essie must have died because by the next year he was married to Venus and living in the same house. By 1925 the couple bought and moved into a home at 1235 East Seventh Street. His office remained on East Second Street. A daughter Doleeta was born in 1926.

In 1929 Dr. Moore moved his offices into the heart of the downtown community to the second floor of the well-known Slaughter Building. Located at the northwest corner of Northeast Second and Stiles Streets, the mixed-use building housed a variety of endeavors. Randolph Drug Store and soda fountain was located on the first floor. On the second floor there were professional offices (lawyers, dentists, doctors) and the first black library, the Dunbar. The top floor "Slaughter's Hall" was for jazz, dancing and community meetings. The building was the center of the downtown community.[5]

Most of the doctors on the second floor were connected to the nearby African American hospital. It was the first black hospital west of the Mississippi and was built in Oklahoma City by Dr. William L. Haywood. He opened it in 1908 and initially he named it Utopia Hospital.[6] Sometime around 1920, the hospital's name was changed to Great Western Hospital.

Dr. Moore served with the hospital's founder, Dr. Haywood, as administrator of the Great Western until it closed in 1947.[7] Undoubtedly, his World War I army training and experience served him well in that capacity. He moved his office upstairs at 429 Northeast Fourth Street. He later went on to practice at the new Edwards Memorial Hospital. The hospital was dedicated on April 18, 1948. It was a 105-bed, three-story modern institution built at a cost of $431,000, totally financed by black entrepreneur W. J. Edwards.

Edwards Memorial Hospital had two operating rooms, a delivery room and a light, airy nursery, a general examination room, eye, ear, nose and throat clinic, x-ray room and modern laboratory, diet kitchens, pediatric ward and physical therapy room.

The hospital offered great opportunity for the training of African American doctors, nurses and laboratory technicians. Twenty-six of Oklahoma City's leading white doctors joined 13 Negro doctors to help with training and instruction. They gave the hospital its first interracial staff.[8]

Ten years later, Dr. Moore, suffering from atherosclerotic heart disease, died in the Veterans Administration Hospital in Oklahoma City at the age of 69.

Dan Moore rose from the poverty of a very small north Louisiana town to become a physician, a well-regarded medical officer, and then the chief administrator of an African American hospital. He took care of the residents of Oklahoma City in his own practice, trained new doctors and saw to it the city's citizens got the best care available at its African American hospital facility.

NOTES

1. Frank E. Roberts, *The American Foreign Legion* (Annapolis, MD: Naval Institute Press), 2004, 147–150.
2. *Ibid.*, 370–372.
3. W. Allison, Sweeney, *History of the American Negro in the Great World War* (New York: Negro Universities Press), 1919, 155.
4. gateway.okhistory.org (accessed September 9, 2014).
5. www.dougloudenback.com/maps/vintage_slaughter.htm (accessed Sept 9, 2014).
6. ndepth.newsok.com/black-history (accessed September 9, 2014).
7. www.dougloudenback.com (accessed September 8, 2014).
8. wjedwards.net/History%20by%20Ruth.htm (accessed September 9, 2014).

Isaac Edward MOORE

28 September 1890–16 March 1931
University of West Tennessee, 1915

Roots and Education

Moore was born in Vicksburg on the banks of the Mississippi River. He grew up living in the working part of town near a great bend in the river at 708 Bowman Street. His father William Moore worked as a porter. His mother, Annie Moore, raised several children. Isaac was their oldest son. He had two younger brothers, Henry and William.[1] By 1910 his family had moved a few blocks further inland to larger quarters at 1118 Locust Street.[2] Later that same year Isaac graduated from Carmel Academy.

Moore entered medical school in 1911 at the University of West Tennessee College of Medicine and Surgery in Memphis, upriver from Vicksburg.[3] He was one of 26 physicians who graduated in 1915.[4] From there he chose Jefferson City, Missouri, to practice his craft. Jefferson City was a busy place on the Missouri River with an established African American community. An article from 1915 described the city as having 15,000 people with 1,100 new homes having been built between 1910 and 1915. Modern school buildings for the high school and two other schools had been built, and the city had a fine hospital. The community had a strong German influence and most residences were brick and moderate in size and cost.[5]

His World War I draft registration card from June 1917 lists his office address as upstairs at 215 Jefferson Street, which was in the heart of the old downtown near the State Capitol along the banks of the Missouri River.[6] He and his wife Katherine lived at 609 Cherry Street.[7]

Military Service

In 1917 Dr. Moore volunteered for the army and was commissioned as a first lieutenant in the U.S. Army Medical Reserve Corps. He was sent to Fort Des Moines, Iowa, for military training, arriving there August 27, 1917. After completing 69 days of training, he was assigned to Camp Dodge, Iowa, as a medical officer with the 366th Infantry Regiment of the 92nd Division.[8] He served with that unit throughout his active combat operations in France.

The 366th engaged the Germans beginning in late August in the St. Dié Sector. It sustained its first casualties as it entered the trenches to relieve another American unit. It successfully repulsed a German attack to retake the town of Frapelle in this so-called "quiet sector." The 366th had moved there from a training area and before the relief was completed two men were killed and six severely wounded. The roads traveled by their supply trains were bombed—shelled with shrapnel, high explosives and gas shells—every night.

The 366th spent 28 days in that sector as the men gained experience and confidence. From there they moved to the Meuse-Argonne. They were ordered to build a road across "no-man's land" and amid gas, shrapnel, and high explosive shells they did their work, with few casualties. Then they were moved to the Marbache sector where they remained until the Armistice in November. Their biggest battle of the war was fought during the last few days of the war on November 9–11 in the attack near Metz. The 366th sustained 16 killed, 186 wounded with 63 gassed in that action alone.[9]

During his service in France Dr. Moore cared for many sick and wounded men.[10] He was also a victim of a gas shell, which troubled him in later years and probably shortened

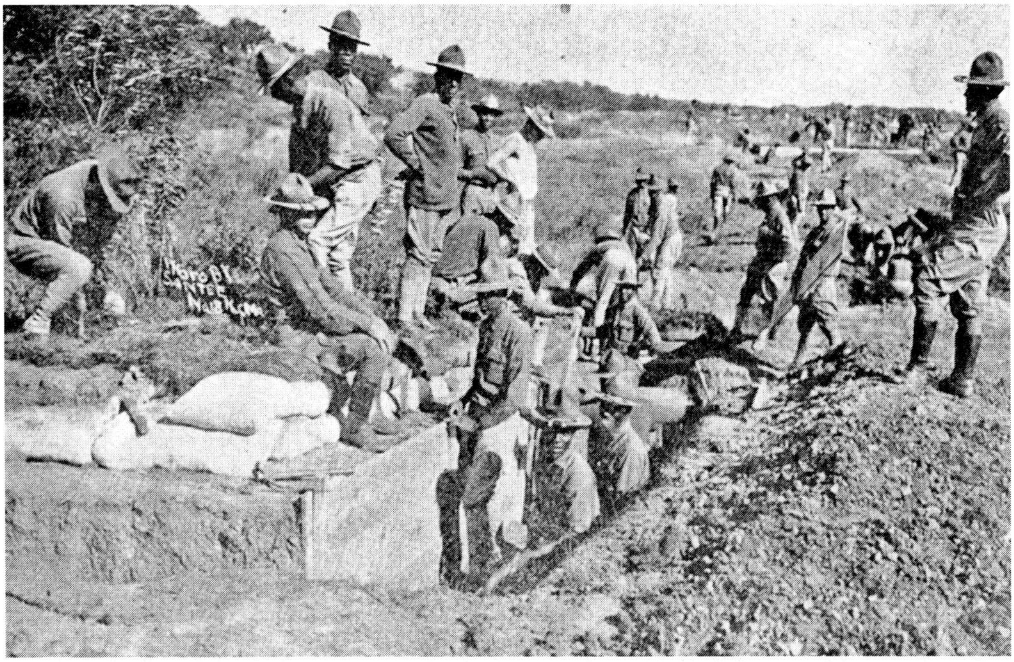

Officers in field training at Fort Des Moines (National Archives).

his life. After he returned to America in February 1919 he was ordered from Camp Upton, New York, to Camp Shelby, Mississippi, as the medical officer caring for 219 officers and men from various units of the 92nd Division. They were all being sent to Camp Shelby to be discharged. Lieutenant Moore was honorably discharged there on March 19.

Career

While Lieutenant Moore served overseas with the army, his wife Katherine Brown Moore lived in Jacksonville, Florida. She had been a schoolteacher from Athens, Georgia. Following his discharge they were reunited and moved back to Jefferson City, Missouri, where they lived at 609 Cherry Street, near Lincoln University, a historically black college.[11] The University had been started following the Civil War by returning U.S. Colored troops and is still an active institution today.

A published history of Jefferson City and Cole County lists Dr. Moore on the Cole County Honor Role for his service in the World War. Interestingly, his name is not listed among the Colored Soldiers, in all likelihood because he was an officer.

By 1920, Dr. Moore and his wife relocated to Colorado Springs, Colorado. There were more than 30,000 people living there, and 1,000 of them were African Americans. The city's only black physician Dr. R. S. Grant had left Colorado Springs in 1919. The Moores lived downtown at 317 West Monument Street, where he opened a practice. His younger brother William lived with them and was working as a hotel bellboy.[12] The dry Colorado climate and health facilities were likely good for Dr. Moore. His gassing in World War I made his lungs weak and ultimately led to pulmonary problems and then tuberculosis.

In 1922 he received a bonus of $190 (equivalent to $2,650 in 2013) from the State of Missouri for his military service in the First World War. The family's address was now 105½ Tejon Street. In October 1922, Dr. Moore announced the opening of the Lincoln Sanatorium (hospital) for Colored people. It was a two-and-a-half story brick house with four bedrooms, built in 1905, at 314 West Willamette Avenue. The sanatorium opened with space for 10 patients. Contributions were collected to provide care for patients unable to pay for proper care at other hospitals. Dr. Moore and his wife lived in rooms above the sanatorium. Their first son, Isaac Jr., was born in the sanatorium in 1924. In 1925 Dr. Moore closed the hospital for reasons that are unclear and moved into a new home at 738 North Spruce Street, just around the corner. According to a longtime resident, Eula V. Andrews, the neighborhood was interracial and white and black families lived alongside one another and interacted easily. In 1926 another son, Frederick, was born.[13]

Dr. Moore continued to practice from his home on North Spruce and was on the staff of St. Francis Hospital. St. Francis Hospital was the first hospital in Colorado Springs. Established in 1887, the hospital began as a treatment clinic for injured railroad workers who were involved in the construction of the Midland Railroad's Colorado Springs to Leadville Line. It was founded by Dr. B. P. Anderson, a physician and surgeon for the Midland Railroad Company, at a time when the railroad was the driving force behind the growth of Colorado Springs and the rest of the west. By 1925, St. Francis Hospital was more than 35 years old and served the entire Colorado Springs community.

Dr. Moore was a highly respected member of the community. By 1930, his son Isaac Jr., was six years old and Frederick was three-and-a-half.[14] "He belonged to the Episcopal Church and was a Mason and past exalted ruler of the local Colored lodge of Elks. He took an active interest in civic affairs affecting the Colored residents of the city, and was well-known" around town.[15]

Dr. Moore's life was cut short the following year in 1931. He passed away at the Fitzsimons Army Hospital in Denver from chronic pulmonary tuberculosis. The hospital, founded by the U.S. Army during World War I, arose from the need to treat the large number of casualties from the chemical (gas) weapons in Europe. Denver's reputation as a prime location for the treatment of tuberculosis led local citizens to lobby the army on behalf of Denver as the site for the new hospital. It was named the Fitzsimons Army Hospital after Lieutenant William T. Fitzsimons, the first American medical officer killed in World War I.[16]

Dr. Moore received a veteran's burial at Evergreen Cemetery in Colorado Springs. He was barely 40 years old and had been practicing medicine in Colorado for a little more than 10 years. His widow, a teacher, and their two boys remained in Colorado Springs until at least 1940; then they relocated to Los Angeles, California.

Moore's oldest son, Isaac Jr., graduated from Thomas Jefferson High School in Los Angeles and the University of Southern California (USC) before returning to Colorado, where he graduated from law school in 1949. He was only the second African American to graduate from the Colorado University Law School. In 1950 he married Dorothy Williams, a teacher-librarian. The couple settled in Denver. He became a member of the Colorado State Legislature and served in the House during the late 1950s and mid–1960s. He fought successfully for social justice and worked as a practicing attorney until his retirement in 1998.[17] His personal papers are held at the Denver Public Library's African American Research Library.

Notes

1. 1900 U.S. Federal Census.
2. 1910 U.S. Federal Census.
3. AMA Deceased Physician Card, National Library of Medicine, Bethesda, MD.
4. Todd L. Savitt, *Race & Medicine in Nineteenth- and Early- Twentieth-Century America*" (Kent, OH: Kent State University Press, 2007) 347.
5. James E. Ford, *A History of Jefferson City* (Jefferson City: New Day Press, 1938) 219–222, 231–244.
6. World War I Draft Registration Card, 1917–1918, ancestry.com.
7. *1917 R.E. Hackman's Jefferson City Directory*, 206.
8. Table of Medical Reserve Corps—Colored—Receiving Instruction, Medical Training Camp, Fort Des Moines, Iowa, RG-112, Records of the Army Surgeon General, National Archives, College Park, MD.
9. 92d Division, Summary of Operations in the World War, Prepared by the American Battle Monuments Commission, United States Government Printing Office, Washington, D.C., 1944, www.history.army.mil/topics/afam/92div.htm.
10. Emmett J. Scott, *The American Negro in the World War* (Homewood Press, 1919), Chapter XI.
11. Soldiers' Records: War of 1812—World War I, Moore, Isaac Edward, Missouri Digital Heritage Collection.
12. 1920 U.S. Federal Census.
13. John Stokes Holley, *The Invisible People of the Pikes Peak Region: An Afro-American Chronicle* (The Friends of the Colorado Springs Pioneers Museum, 1990) Chapter Ten, Special Collections, Pikes Peak Library District.
14. 1930 U.S. Federal Census.

15. "Dr. Isaac E. Moore Is Dead in Denver," *Colorado Springs Gazette*, March 17, 1931, 1.
16. Fitzsimons Hospital, en.wikipedia.org/wiki/Fitzsimons_Army_Medical_Center (accessed September 23, 2013).
17. *Isaac E. Moore, Jr. Papers*, Blair-Caldwell African American Research Library, Denver Public Library, aarl.denverlibrary.org/archives/imoore.html (accessed September 20, 2013).

Homer Erwin NASH

6 May 1887–19 March 1981
Meharry Medical College, 1910

Roots and Education

Homer Nash was born in White Plains (Greene County), located between Augusta and Atlanta, Georgia, to Elizabeth and William Nash. His mother was a maid and his father a laborer. White Plains was an agricultural area. Until the depression of the 1920s, the area experienced growth. This was an area where cotton was king. At one time before the Civil War, there were 7,000 slaves and 350 whites in Greene County. There were extensive businesses to serve the plantation economy. After the Civil War, many of the town's businesses were sold to the African American community. Andrew Carnegie funded the purchase of the building for the town's library and started its collection with 50 books.

The boll weevil hit the area around 1917 and changed White Plains forever. Businesses closed and families left; the railroad no longer stopped there.[1]

It is extraordinary that a physician such as Homer Nash had such roots. He received his earliest education in White Plains and went on to high school in Atlanta. From there he worked his way through Meharry Medical School in Nashville, Tennessee. He graduated in 1910 and opened his practice in Atlanta, Georgia. He cared for patients and was involved in the community there for 71 years.

Until the early part of the 20th century the only black medical men known to the black community were untrained voodoo priests and folk healers. "Real" doctors were white. When black doctors opened practices in the south, they were considered by prospective patients to be inadequate at best. Dr. Nash is reported saying, "The cooks and maids and poor people looked at me and said, 'Ain't no Negro Doctor gonna give me no medicine!'"[2]

Dr. Nash married Marie Antoinette Graves. Her father was a prominent real estate man in Atlanta.[3] The couple had five children, Catherine, Helen, Harriet, Dorothy and Homer Jr. Two children, Helen and Homer Jr., followed him into medicine.

Dr. Nash's Republican roots were quickly recognized in his Atlanta community. When President Theodore Roosevelt came to Atlanta in 1910, he addressed the African American community at the First Congregational Church. Dr. Nash led the discussion during this program at the Lincoln Lyceum. The president's remarks made favorable reference to the black soldiers among his Rough Riders troops. The following day, the president spoke to the white community at Atlanta's Auditorium-Armory.[4]

Military Service

At the age of 30, Dr. Nash registered for service in the U.S. Army Medical Reserve Corps. He left his family and practice in Atlanta and reported for basic training at the Fort Des Moines' Medical Officers Training Camp on September 12, 1917. After 53 days, First Lieutenant Nash was transferred to the 366th Field Hospital at Camp Funston, Kansas, prior to its departure for France in June 1918.

By November, he was a surgeon at the field hospital, as well as the hospital's evacuation officer. Part of his job was to write reports on in-coming and out-going patients. It was a mobile hospital with its location changing as the battles moved. On November 11 (Armistice Day), for example, the hospital was near Metz. He reported about 300 gas cases were brought into the hospital within one hour by its 41 ambulances. Lieutenant Nash reported 160 were not gassed at all, likely panicking when fellow soldiers were. The uninjured men were transferred to the casual camp for reassignment. His report included evidence of his frustration that the hospital's telephone contact with this casual camp was non-existent that final day of the war. The files of the 366th Field Hospital include an incredible number of daily reports from Lieutenant Nash on the movement of soldiers in and out of the hospital.

He was home in Atlanta when his honorable discharge came through on March 15, 1919. At the time Dr. and Mrs. Nash were living in three rooms at 116 Howell Street in Atlanta.

Career

Dr. Nash became involved in numerous community services including the Atlanta Tuberculosis Association and the Carrie Steele-Pitts Home. Mrs. Carrie Steele began finding babies and abandoned children while she was working at Atlanta's Union Railroad Station. She began to care for these children, placing them in an empty boxcar during the day and taking them home with her at night. In 1888 Mrs. Steele chartered the organization, selling her home to generate funds for her orphan's homes. Dr. Nash provided health care and helped with fundraising.[5]

For 33 years, Dr. Nash volunteered at the Fulton County Clinic, persuading mothers to immunize their children. He was called upon by a number of groups to address various aspects of health care. In 1934 the South Carolina state committee on tuberculosis in the African American community had him speak in Columbia on "The Family Doctor and the Tuberculosis Patient." The press coverage included the statement, "Negroes are dying seven times as fast as white people with this dreaded disease."[6]

In 1936 he was president of the Atlanta Medical Association and on the medical staff of the Atlanta Tuberculosis Association. In 1937, at one of the local medical meetings, he reported on a study he published about 48 cases being treated by the clinic. The *Atlanta Daily World* called him "an illustrious, honest, hardworking member" of the medical profession.[7] In 1938 his findings on "Tuberculosis Among Negroes" were published by the American College of Chest Physicians.[8]

Dr. Nash was an extremely popular Atlanta speaker. In 1937 he was hired by the Atlanta Federal Colored Forum to present a series of speeches on health issues. His first, on April 2, 1937, was "Social Diseases."[9] The next year, he was the main speaker during the 1938 National Negro Health Week. He drew a capacity audience.[10]

He became a nationally well-known expert on tuberculosis. When the U.S. federal government finally recognized the tuberculosis problem in 1939 it provided funds to build a 150-bed annex to Freedmen's Hospital in Washington, D.C. Howard University called a conference of those physicians well known for their work with the disease. Dr. Nash was included on the program. By that time he was a staff physician of the Atlanta Tuberculosis Association and had written numerous articles on the subject of community needs to combat the disease.[11]

By 1956, the Nash family moved to Washington, D.C. They purchased a home at 1983 Simpson Street, NW. His office was at 239 Auburn Avenue, NE. From his office, he saw his patients or offered his advice over the phone. He worked at Freedmen's Hospital for a number of years. He also gave speeches and continued his activities in local, state and national medical associations.

During the 1960s, the couple moved back to Atlanta. Medical organizations presented him with numerous citations including "Father of Medicine in Georgia" from Morehouse College. He was named 1963 General Practitioner of the Year by the National Medical Association. The Atlanta Medical Association named their outstanding physician award the Nash-Carter Award after Dr. Nash and his good friend, Dr. Raymond H. Carter. The two doctors served together in France during the First World War. When Dr. Nash reached into his eighties, he was Atlanta's oldest practicing physician.[12]

Dr. Nash had just attended a friend's funeral and returned to his office on the day he died in Atlanta at the age of 93. After a huge service at Atlanta's First Congregational Church, he was buried at South-View Cemetery in Atlanta.

There he joined a number of other prestigious African Americans including the Reverend Martin Luther King, Sr. (1899–1984), father of Martin Luther King, Jr., and an important civil rights leader in his own right.

NOTES

1. Whiteplainsga.com/about/history (accessed March 8, 2015).

2. Thomas J. Ward, Jr., *The Struggle for Patients, Black Physicians in the Jim Crow South* (Fayetteville: University of Arkansas Press, 2003) 124.
3. "Things You Ought to Know," *Atlanta Daily World*, September 27, 1936, 4.
4. "Escort for Roosevelt," *Atlanta Constitution*, October 4, 1910, 7.
5. csph.org/our-history (accessed September 4, 2014).
6. "News of Brewer Junior College," *The Index-Journal*, November 18, 1934, 4.
7. "Dr. H. E. Nash Re-Installed President of Local Med Association," *Atlanta Daily World*, January 27, 1937.
8. *Ibid.*, "Atlanta Physician Has Article...," March 25, 1938, 1.
9. *Ibid.*, "Dr. H. E. Nash to Lecture Tonight," Apt 1, 1937, 1.
10. *Ibid.*, "Health Week Mass Meet Tonight," April 4, 1938, 1.
11. "The Mason-Dixon Line," *Pittsburgh Courier*, June 10, 1939, 18.
12. Funeral Services Program for Dr. Homer E. Nash, Sr., First Congregational Church, Atlanta, Georgia.

Hosea Jefferson NICHOLS

12 August 1870–21 April 1936
Howard Medical College, 1899

Roots and Education

Hosea J. Nichols was born in 1870 in Sardis, Mississippi (about 50 miles due south of Memphis, Tennessee). His father, William Nichols, was a minister and served during the Civil War with the Tennessee U.S. Colored Infantry and the 59th U.S. Colored Infantry.[1] His mother, Lucy Spann Nichols, was from North Carolina. They had a large family with seven children, and Hosea was the second youngest. His father died when Hosea was quite young.[2]

Young Nichols attended public schools in Sardis, and from 1889 to 1893, he attended the Le Moyne Normal Institute in Memphis, Tennessee. LeMoyne was founded in 1871 by the American Missionary Association as a primary and normal school for training freedmen. It functioned primarily as a teacher training school until the 1930s when it became a four-year college. After graduation Nichols taught in the public schools of Shelby County, Tennessee, for two years before going to Howard University Medical College in Washington, D.C., in 1895, where he graduated in 1899.[3]

After medical school Dr. Nichols went to Quincy, Illinois, to practice medicine. Quincy is a Mississippi River city located in western Illinois on the border with Missouri. In 1900 his office was at 234½ 6th Avenue North. On October 9, 1901, Nichols married a Bedford County Tennessee woman named Annie M. Davis. His wife was a trained nurse who had been born in 1872. He and Annie lived at 819 N 8th Street, where he had his office. They lived there until 1920 and raised their three young daughters, Wanda, Hazel and Alice, in that house.

Dr. Nichols' activities went well beyond practicing medicine. When the Quincy Branch of the NAACP was organized in 1912, he was elected president and served in that role until 1917. In May 1914 he attended the 6th Annual Conference of the NAACP in Baltimore and Washington, D.C.[4] On July 23–24 of the same year he presided over the Interstate Racial Conference held in Quincy at the Bethany AME Church. Dr. W. E. B. Du Bois of New York gave a talk at the conference on "The World Problem of the Color Line."[5] In January 1915 Dr. Nichols was Toastmaster at a banquet given by the men of the Quincy NAACP for their wives at their hall in Sixth Street. Twenty-five members had been added in the last membership drive.[6]

By 1916 Dr. Nichols was one of three well-known African Americans prominent in local societies and affairs who were under consideration for the one Negro post on the Quincy Board of Education.[7] It was planned to place his or Mrs. Frances Monroe's name on the ballot for the Lincoln District.[8] While no record of the outcome can be found, his nomination is a testimonial to Dr. Nichols' standing in the community.

Military Service

He volunteered for service in 1917 and was commissioned as a first lieutenant in the U.S. Army Medical Reserve Corps.[9] At 47, Lieutenant Nichols was the oldest medical officer completing the Medical Officers Training Camp (MOTC) for Colored officers at Fort Des Moines, Iowa. After 43 days of military training, he was sent to Camp Funston at Fort Riley, Kansas. He was assigned to the 366th Field Hospital of the 92nd Division's 317th Sanitary (Medical) Train. In February 1918 he was granted leave to see his elderly mother who was dangerously ill in Sardis, Mississippi.[10] He returned to camp where he was assigned to work in the infirmary of the 317th Sanitary Train. His military service ended following six months of active duty in March 1918. He resigned his commission to return home to his family and practice.[11] His mother's poor health condition and his age undoubtedly were factors in his decision to leave the army three months before he would have deployed overseas.

Career

When Dr. Nichols returned to Quincy, he jumped back into his community and civic activities. He was in charge of an elaborate parade and farewell celebration in July 1918 for African American draftees being sent to Camp Dodge, Iowa. Plans included an African American band called the Chauffeur's Band, as well as music and speeches.[12]

In 1919 Nichols was named chairman of the Negro Workers' Advisory Committee for three neighboring counties. The committee was established under the Illinois State Labor Department, and it was to give close attention to the needs of African American soldiers returning from service.[13]

Later in 1919 Dr. Nichols, at 50, and his family decided to move from Quincy to Detroit, Michigan. The great migration of African Americans to the industrial north was in full swing, and Detroit was a very popular destination because of the industry there. By the mid–1920s Detroit was the fastest growing metropolitan area and the fourth largest city in the United States. Many of the early arrivals had been recruited by General Motors and Dupont. The health situation for the southern black migrants was poor and medical facilities were very limited. Many of the African American migrants knew nothing about immunization. During the 1920s, 50 percent of Detroit's smallpox victims lived in the crowded St. Antoine district. Tuberculosis was rampant. Pneumonia became their greatest cause of death. Health officials finally responded in a small way, opening a couple of small healthcare centers. Dunbar Memorial Hospital was opened in 1918. Five years later, it had cared for 3,000 patients. The white hospitals were not opened to them so access to healthcare would not be possible for Detroit's African American residents until later decades.

For many years Dr. Nichols brought health care to his community. During the 1920s, the Urban League began to distribute information about health care to the newcomers. National Negro Health Week actually took messages about hygiene and sanitation to the pulpit. Local physicians like Dr. Nichols would "preach" their sermons about staying healthy at the local churches.[14]

In 1920 the Nichols family had a house at 1016 Joseph Campau Street in Detroit, and his office was in their home. They were well located in an African American enclave only seven blocks north of the Detroit riverfront. In 1930, his three daughters, all in their early to mid–20s, were still living at home. Hazel had become a social worker in recreation, and the youngest, Alice, was a public school teacher.[15]

Dr. Nichols practiced medicine there for more than 15 years. He died of pneumonia at the age of 65. In 1937 his youngest daughter, Mrs. Alice E. Nichols-Dent, wrote to the American Medical Association reporting his death.[16] She wrote from her home at 1014 Joseph Campau Avenue, right next door to where her family lived in Detroit for so many years.

NOTES

1. "William Nichols," Civil War Pension Index 1861–1934, ancestry.com.
2. 1880 U.S. Federal Census.
3. Daniel Smith Lamb, Howard University Medical Department, Washington, D.C. *A Historical, Biographical and Statistical Souvenir* (Washington, D.C., 1900).
4. "Race Question Is Discussed," *The Quincy Whig*, May 20, 1914, 2, archive.quincylibrary.org.
5. "Dr. Du Bois Speaks at Mass Meeting of Colored People," *The Quincy Whig*, July 25, 1914, 8.
6. "Brevities," *The Quincy Daily Journal*, January 29, 1915, 7, archive.quincylibrary.org.
7. "Colored Folks to Have Candidate," *The Quincy Daily Journal*, March 24, 1916, 3.
8. "One School Petition Filed; Others Soon," *The Quincy Daily Journal*, March 30, 1916, 8.
9. "Quincy, ILL., Negro Doctor Passes," *The Kansas City Sun*, August 11, 1917, 2.
10. "Lieut. Nichols, M.R.C., Here," *The Quincy Daily Journal*, February 14, 1918, 10.
11. "Medical Mobilization," *JAMA: Journal of the American Medical Association*, Vol. 70, 1104.
12. "Park Program Planned for Colored Boys," *The Quincy Daily Journal*, July 23, 1918, 2.
13. "Name Dr. Nichols as Head Negro Committee," *The Quincy Daily Journal*, April 17, 1919, 2.
14. Elizabeth Anne Martin, *Detroit and the Great Mi-*

gration 1916–1929, bentley.umich.edu/research/publications/migration (accessed October 5, 2013).
15. 1930 U.S. Federal Census.
16. AMA Deceased Physician Card, National Library of Medicine, Bethesda, MD.

Hudson Jones OLIVER, Jr.

3 September 1889–20 September 1955
Howard Medical College, 1913

Roots and Education

Hudson J. Oliver, Jr., was born in New York. When he was quite young his parents, Cecelia (Washington) and Hudson Oliver moved to Jersey City, New Jersey. His father was employed by the well-known steel agent, Thomas Prosser & Son, for nearly 40 years. He had a brother, Clinton, and three sisters—Cecelia, Gladys and Ray. The Oliver children grew up at 35 Corbin Avenue in Jersey City and attended the city's public elementary schools. The family was Catholic so Hudson went to one of the Blessed Sacrament high schools.

After high school (where "Huddy" was a star football and basketball player), he enrolled in Howard University in 1909. He was a "stocky-built little lad ... a crack forward. He put Howard on the map in basketball ... one of the most colorful court-men of the East in his day."[1] "Huddy" went on to Howard's Medical College in Washington, D.C., and graduated in 1913. Following graduation he interned at Freedmen's Hospital in D.C. before establishing a practice in 1914 in Asbury Park, New Jersey. While there he met and married schoolteacher Orville M. Washington. The Olivers were living there in 1917 when he volunteered for the U.S. Army's Medical Reserve Corps.

Military Service

First Lieutenant Oliver reported for duty at the Medical Officers Training Camp, Fort Des Moines, on August 11, 1917. He trained there until the first graduates left on November 3, 1917. His assignment was the 92nd Division's 367th Infantry Regiment being organized at Camp Upton, New York. They sailed from Hoboken, New Jersey, on June 19. After an uneventful voyage, the 367th arrived in France on June 29, 1918.

Within the 367th medical detachment, Oliver worked with five fellow MOTC graduates—Edwin Lee from Kansas City, Kansas; Albert Punche from Cleburne, Texas; Walter Jackson from Baltimore, Maryland; Frank Raiford of Atlanta, Georgia; and, Rosco Wilson from Florence, South Carolina. At sea, they gave the men physicals and cared for those who were seasick. After they landed in Brest, France, they were kept at the old Pontanezen Barracks for several days.[2]

From there they went by train to Bourbonne-les-Bains, where the 92nd Division was first assembled. While the soldiers were trained in bayonet fighting, grenade throwing and the use of the machine gun, the medical corps had light duty (only a few cases of mumps). That was fortunate at the outset as they lacked medical supplies. They spent time training the men in sanitation and chlorination of water by adding water to the 36-gallon Lyster bag. Only repeated inspections got the point across that this was the only water pure enough for the men to drink.

They were next introduced to combat in the St. Dié sector of the rugged Vosges mountains. The 367th was assigned duty near Frapelle, where the Germans attacked them. "Despite being subjected to heavy artillery and gas shelling, the 367th withstood the attack and held the line until it was relieved on 20 September 1918."[3]

As fall came and the rains worsened, the doctors of the 367th spent more time treating those with illnesses like the flu, pneumonia, venereal diseases and tuberculosis. During October and through to the end of the war on November 11, the medical detachment of the 367th treated the wounded and gassed, victims of the final push against the Germans. His regiment sustained light casualties in the final days of the war when the regiment was deployed and attacked the Germans on the west side of the Moselle River near Metz. By the spring of 1919, most of these Americans would be home.

Career

After the war, Dr. Oliver returned to his practice in Asbury Park. In 1921 the Olivers moved into New York City, where they bought a house at 257 West 139th Street in Harlem.

Their children, Hudson and Orville Y., grew up there. His offices were in his home for the rest of his life. In the 1930s his aunt Maria and two boarders lived with them. In the 1940s his wife's father Charles lived with them.

In 1923 Dr. Oliver took time to reach out to the youth of Harlem at the St. Christopher Club of St. Philip's Parish. He talked to them about the importance of planning a career other than athletics.[4] Mrs. Oliver was involved with the youth of the city and taught school for many years.

Dr. Oliver was among the leadership of the Elks. He held the position of exalted ruler of Monarch Lodge, No. 3 several times. In 1927 he presided over the Convention Committee for the various lodges throughout the New York metro area.[5]

In 1928 he was appointed to New York's Mayor Hylan's Committee of 100 to plan the 300th anniversary of the purchase of Manhattan. He was the first African American to be so honored. The mayor said of him, "Your known interest in the city and your desire to promote its progress and prosperity prompt my extending to you a cordial invitation to serve as a member of the Mayor's Committee."[6]

Dr. Oliver specialized in "female surgery." He conducted clinics at Harlem Hospital until Dr. Louis T. Wright took its leadership in the 1930s and appointed Dr. Oliver a member of the staff. He was a member of the National Medical Association (NMA) as well as New York's state and local associations. He participated in the Harlem's Physicians Reading Club where new approaches to medicine were shared.

When the contentious amalgamation of the North Harlem and Manhattan medical societies was accomplished, the leaders of both organizations were relieved of their positions. Dr. Oliver was elected vice president of the new Central Harlem Medical Society[7] and helped shape the new organization.

When New York's International Hospital made its annual staff appointments in 1931, Dr. Hudson was among some of the leading physicians and surgeons of the community to accept places on the staff. This appointment recognized his expertise in anesthesiology.[8]

Life was not all work and no play for the Olivers. In 1936 they gave one of their "swanky parties" in their "beautifully appointed home." It included "music from the magic fingers of Bruce Wendell," Mrs. Murray's "uplifting voice," "delicacies fit for a king," and bridge. Forty-one guests from New York's African American society were feted.[9] Dr. Oliver was a dedicated bridge player. He was one of the "Killers' Team" and participated in the Eastern Bridge League.[10]

He was also active in the Catholic Church. In 1939 when he was president of the Catholic Inter-Racial Guild, his son Hudson Jr. was a senior and member of St. Peter's College track team. During a meet at Catholic University in Washington, D.C., young Hudson was barred from participation in track on account of his race. It seems the college had a rule "prohibiting Negro and white athletes from taking part in the same meets in Washington, D.C."[11] The headline on page one of the *New York Age* indicates the clamor that this raised in New York: "Catholic University Bars Dr. Oliver's Son from D.C. Track Meet." Racism in athletics was still prevalent in the nation's capital.

He was in his 60s when he was diagnosed with cancer. He died of it at the age of 66 at one of the Veterans Administration hospitals in New York.[12] Early in his life, Hudson Oliver began taking leadership roles in high school sports. He honed those skills in medical school, practiced them in France, and shared them with his community and his profession for the rest of his life.

Notes

1. "'Huddy' Oliver Started a Golden Age of Basketball," *Afro-American*, January 21, 1928, 13.
2. Historical Division, Office of the Surgeon General, 92nd Division, Box 314–2, National Archives, College Park, MD.
3. Timothy C. Dowling, *Personal Perspectives, World War I* (ABC-CLIO, 2006) 17.
4. "Name of Everard Daniels Received with Hearty Cheers," *New York Amsterdam News*, October 3, 1923, 4.
5. "With the Elks," *New York Amsterdam News*, January 26, 1927, 10.
6. "'Huddy' Oliver Started a Golden Age of Basketball," *Afro-American*, January 21, 1928, 13.
7. "Dr. Wright Called 'Little Czar' as Harlem Medics Seek to Oust Him," *Journal and Guide*, April 7, 1934, 14.
8. "International Hospital Appoints Yearly Staff," *The New York Age*, August 29, 1931, 5.
9. "Society Whirls with the Hudson Olivers," *New York Amsterdam News*, December 12, 1936, 8.
10. "Harlemites Battle in 2-Night Bridge Tourney," Afro-American, May 30, 1936, 20.

11. "Catholic University Bars Dr. Oliver's Son from DC Track Meet," *The New York Age*, March 18, 1939, 1.
12. AMA Deceased Physicians card, National Library of Medicine, Bethesda, MD.

James Alexander OWEN

6 September 1891–6 July 1955
Meharry Medical College, 1916

Roots and Education

James A. Owen was born in Natchez, Mississippi. His parents were both educators. His father, Samuel Henry Clay Owen, was a teacher and president of Natchez College. His mother, Sarah Josephine Mazique, was a teacher and matron at the same school. She was in charge of domestic and medical arrangements. The family was part of the small educated elite of the African American community. They lived in a nice residential area only a few blocks from the downtown commercial area and close to the city's best African American schools.[1]

James and his twin Henry were the eldest of five brothers. All five boys were educated in the segregated public school system in Natchez, and four of them became medical professionals. This was extraordinary considering that even the best of the black schools in Natchez were not equal to public schools located outside of the Jim Crow south.

James graduated with an A.B. from Natchez College in 1912 before attending Meharry Medical College in Nashville. He earned his M.D. from Meharry in 1916. Opportunities for internships were limited for African American physicians, but he secured one in Kansas City, Missouri, at the Old General Hospital No. 2. In 1917, as he was completing his internship, America entered the First World War. He volunteered for the U.S. Army Medical Reserve Corps and received a commission as a first lieutenant.[2]

Military Service

First Lieutenant Owen reported to the Medical Officers Training Camp (MOTC) for military training at Fort Des Moines on August 17, 1917. He was one of the youngest doctors in camp. He trained there for 79 days before leaving for Camp Funston at Fort Riley, Kansas, where he was assigned to the 317th Sanitary (Medical) Train of the 92nd Division.[3] While at Camp Funston he was detailed to study the *American Journal of Roentgenology* (radiology) to present at a meeting of medical officers in March 1918. He was then assigned to the 366th Field Hospital along with fellow MOTC graduates lieutenants Nash, Brannon, Wilson, and Whittaker. He went on to serve throughout the war with this unit.

In June 1918 the 92nd Division was sent to France. Some equipment was slow in coming, but his field hospital was equipped with a Mobile Field Laboratory in August 1918. On September 3, 1918, there were 119 patients in their field hospital, and just two days later on September 5, the number had jumped to 142, with the vast majority suffering from mustard gas inhalation. The hospital reported treating 258 cases of gas poisoning during just the last two weeks of October 1918. One of them died, 139 required extended hospitalization, and 135 required further evacuation to the base hospital.[4]

In addition to treating patients, Lieutenant Owen was also charged with the field hospital's administrative duties, including funds and property accountability and monthly reports to the division surgeon on topics like self-inflicted wounds or venereal disease cases.[5] A

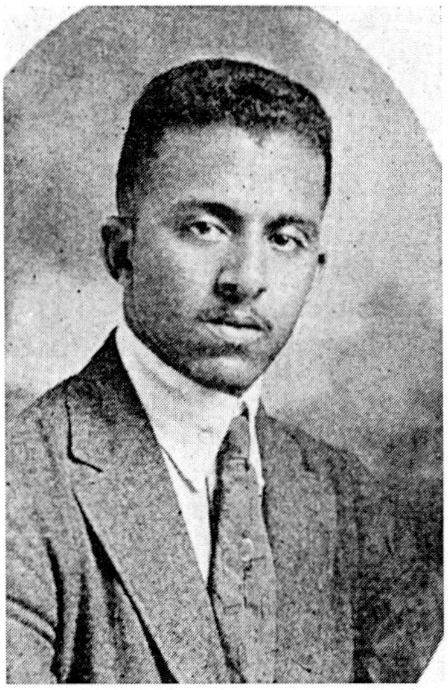

James A. Owen (National Pictorial, members of the National Medical Association, 1925, courtesy of Kansas City Public Library).

description of his service printed in the Meharry Annual in 1919 noted that he had been the Supply Officer for the division's triage hospital at Millery, France. That hospital received positive special mention in a letter from the Chief Surgeon. The article went on to say Owen was loved and respected by all who knew him and proved to be an officer of rare ability.[6] After the war ended he attained the rank of captain in the Medical Reserve.

Career

Dr. Owen returned home in 1919 and made his way to Sapulpa, a small town near Tulsa, Oklahoma. Oil had been discovered five miles from Sapulpa in 1905. It was quite a boomtown with its own railroad spur by the time Dr. Owen arrived. In 1920 he was single and working there in a hospital.[7]

While in Sapulpa he met Marie E. Thomas who was a teacher and originally from Tuskegee, Alabama. They were married on July 30, 1921, in Cleveland, Ohio.

James and Marie moved to Cleveland and lived for eight years at 2160 East 76th Street, before moving to nearby 2168 East 74th Street.[8] In the 1920s Cleveland was a fast growing northern industrial city and needed physicians. Dr. Owen opened his practice at 2437 East 46th Street, where he and his army associate Dr. Linell L. Rodgers shared a medical secretary. These two physicians and Dr. Charles H. Garvin had all been members of the 92nd Division, and all became important community leaders in Cleveland's African American community.

In November 1925 Dr. Owen was one of 10 African American physicians who founded the Cleveland Medical Reading Club to keep abreast of programs and advances in the medical field.[9] In 1926 he was listed as a prominent Ohioan, who along with his friend Dr. Charles H. Garvin and others backed the formation of a unique fraternal insurance society in Cleveland.[10] They later became two of its eight trustees.[11]

In the early 1930s Dr. Owen moved his practice to new quarters at 7818 Cedar Avenue. His years in Cleveland were dynamic. He was a member of the Cleveland Medical, Dental and Pharmaceutical Association (CMA) and was its president in 1929. He was also a member of the National Medical Association (NMA) and served as its second vice president.

Dr. Owen was also a leader in the local Democratic Party and served as Ohio state director of the Democratic National Campaign in 1928. He ran unsuccessfully for the Cleveland City Council in 1929 and 1933, running on a platform that included better sanitation and increased access to medical care.[12]

In 1932 he became a Democratic Committeeman for Cleveland's 18th Ward, and he was on the Democratic County Executive Committee for Cuyahoga County. He served in those capacities until 1940. As if that were not enough, he was also a member of the NAACP, the National Urban League and the YMCA. His community involvement extended to his membership in fraternal organizations like the Masons, Elks, Kappa Alpha Psi, the Woodmen and the local Baptist church.

In the 1930s the governor of Ohio appointed Dr. Owen a trustee of the Combined Normal and Industrial Departments at Wilberforce College. He became embroiled in the controversy surrounding Wilberforce President D. Ormonde Walker's attempt to bring the university under the domination of the AME Church. Dr. Owen released a statement: "Indignation throughout Ohio is running very high ... [it] threatens the very future of the institution." Despite this, Dr. Walker was not removed and continued as university president until 1941, and Dr. Owen remained a member of Wilberforce board of trustees for 16 years.[13]

Dr. Owen occasionally found life in Cleveland challenging. In February 1933 two men entered his office and ordered him to "put 'em up." Instead, Dr. Owen "drew a gun from the desk and fired, chasing the men into the hall. [One got away, the other] had one wound to the right leg, two in the right side, and two fingers shot off."[14] Dr. Owen said he carried a pistol since having been robbed in 1931.[15]

In 1940 Dr. and Mrs. Owen decided to leave Cleveland and move to Detroit. His twin brother, Dr. Henry Owen, M.D. (Samuel H. C. Owen, Jr., Meharry class of 1917), was a successful practicing physician there. He encouraged his twin brother to pursue the opportunity presented by the phenomenal wartime growth of the "Motor City." James made the move and opened a medical office, and was on the staff of two African American-owned and operated Detroit hospitals, Parkside and Wayne Diagnostic hospitals. Both hospitals were important to Detroit's large African American community.

Parkside was a 54-bed hospital and one of its eight founders was his brother, Henry Owen. His brother also served as the medical director of Parkside, chief of the Department of Surgery and a member of its board of trustees.

The Wayne Diagnostic Hospital had two locations, including a mental health facility, with a total of 96 beds in 1949. It was considered one of the "best" medical facilities with which African American physicians could affiliate. In 1952 it underwent a major expansion that included a second operating room, a second delivery room, an autopsy room, a pharmacy, an enlarged medical laboratory and numerous support departments.[16]

In Detroit, Dr. James Owen once again became involved with local and professional and civic organizations. He maintained his close affiliation with the National Medical Association (NMA) and became a member of its board of trustees.

In July 1954 Dr. Owen and his wife traveled to Europe where he attended the International Congress of Obstetrics and Gynecology at Geneva, Switzerland. After the conference they visited centers of medical interest in Paris and other parts of Europe.[17]

Dr. Owen died the following year on July 6, 1955, in Detroit. He was 54 years old. Marie, his wife of 34 years, survived him, as did one younger brother, Dr. Lee M. Owen, of Vicksburg, Mississippi.[18]

His was a life filled with achievement, caring and stewardship. His activities on behalf of his fellow man and his community were extraordinary, and his passing was a great loss to his community.

NOTES

1. 1900 and 1910 U.S. Federal Census.
2. Thomas Yenser, Editor & Publisher, *Who's Who in Colored America* (Fifth Edition) (New York, 1944), 395.
3. Table of Medical Reserve Corps—Colored—Receiving Instruction, Medical Training Camp, Fort Des Moines, Iowa, RG-112, Records of the Army Surgeon General, National Archives, College Park, MD.
4. *Ibid.*
5. Record Group 120, AEF Records of Combat Divisions, 92nd Division, 317th Sanitary Train, Field Hospital 366, National Archives, College Park, MD.
6. "*The Meharry Annual, Military Review 1919*," Harold D. West Collection, Meharry Archives, Nashville, TN, 43.
7. 1920 U.S. Federal Census.
8. 1930 U.S. Federal Census.
9. The Cleveland Medical Reading Club, trees.ancestry.com/tree/4236907.
10. "License Is Granted New Fraternal Society," *Pittsburgh Courier*, September 18, 1926, 8.
11. "Form Company Save Business of Aid Association," *The New York Age*, March 19, 1927, 3.
12. "The Encyclopedia of Cleveland History," ech.case.edu/cgi (accessed April 3, 2015).
13. "Names Trustees for Negro School," *Evening Independent*, Massillon, Ohio, September 7, 1939, 8.
14. "Two Shot in Attempt to Rob Doctor," *Pittsburgh Courier*, February 25, 1933, 4.
15. "Cleveland," *Sandusky Star Journal*, February 17, 1933, 11.
16. *Black-Owned and Operated Hospitals in the Detroit Metropolitan Area During the 20th Century*, www.med.umich.edu/haahc/hospitals/hospital1.htm.
17. "Professional News—Personal," *Journal of the National Medical Association (JNMA)*, March 1955, Vol. 47 No. 2, 136.
18. "Professional News—Deaths," *Journal of the National Medical Association (JNMA)*, January 1956, Vol. 48 No. 1, 73, 75.

Frank Adrian PEARL

2 September 1886–24 July 1948
Howard Medical College, 1912

Roots and Education

Frank Pearl was born in Atchison, Kansas. In the 1890s his family moved westward to Silver Bow in Butte, Montana. Butte was in booming mining country. He lived there with his stepfather, John F. Davis, mother Sarah J. Davis, and older brother, Milton Pearl. Young Frank attended the public schools of Butte and then Butte Business College. He went on to train at the Topeka Vocational Institute in Topeka, Kansas, an industrial and educational institute for African American students. It prepared them for agricultural or mechanical pursuits. From there, he went to Howard University in Washington, D.C., where he earned a medical degree with honors in 1912.

Dr. Pearl returned to Kansas and established a medical practice downtown at 614½ Commercial Street in Atchison. Atchison is located on the great Missouri River 50 miles Northwest of Kansas City, Missouri. It was a commercial center in the early 1900s and the eastern terminus of the famed Atchison, Topeka and Santa Fe Railroad.

Pearl quickly became involved with the professional and social life of the area. In January 1915 he was one of many out-of-town guests attending a major social event in Kansas City given by the "Ochya Girls, who were described as the leaders in Kansas City's social life among the younger set."[1] Later in 1915 Dr. Pearl participated in the Pan-Medical Association of Missouri meeting in Kansas City and opened a discussion on the "Relationship of Alcohol to Epilepsy and Degeneracy."[2] He was still listed as single when he registered for the World War I draft in Atchison in June 1917.

Military Service

In 1917 Pearl was one of 16 Howard University medical school graduates who volunteered for service in the army. He was commissioned a first lieutenant in the Medical Reserve

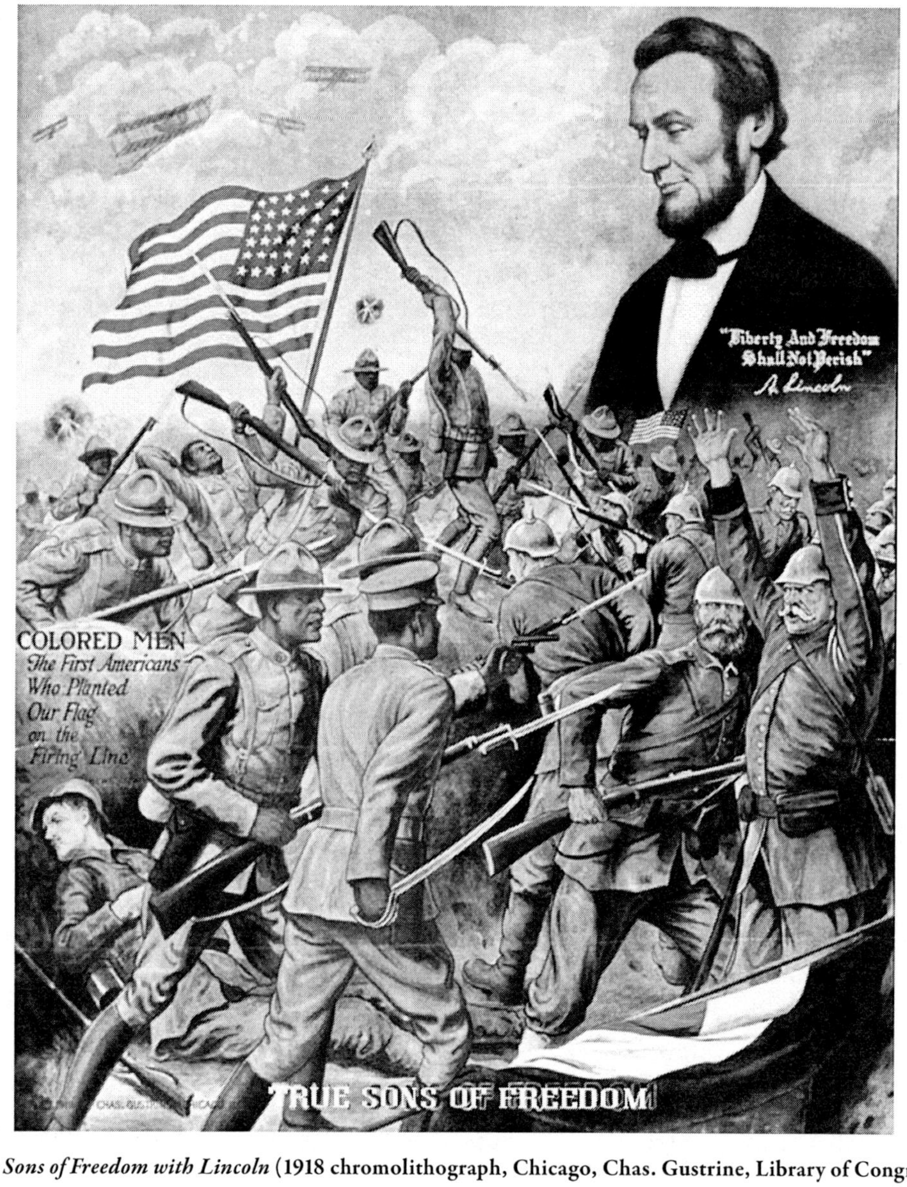
"Liberty And Freedom Shall Not Perish"
A. Lincoln
COLORED MEN
The First Americans Who Planted Our Flag on the Firing Line
TRUE SONS OF FREEDOM

True Sons of Freedom with Lincoln (1918 chromolithograph, Chicago, Chas. Gustrine, Library of Congress).

Corps. He was described as one of seven doctors from Atchison who had "given up a lucrative practice to join the colors."[3] He arrived at the Medical Officers Training Camp (MOTC) at Fort Des Moines on August 27. After 69 days of training, Lieutenant Pearl was ordered to the 317th Sanitary (Medical) Train of the 92nd Division at Camp Funston at Fort Riley, Kansas. There he was assigned to the division's 368th Ambulance Company under the command of Captain H. H. Walker, another African American physician who had trained at Fort Des Moines.

A March 1918 newspaper article regarding YMCA No. 11 (Colored Service) at Camp Funston commented twice about Pearl, saying he was one of a group of three officers from the 368th that gave a "swell" party, and at another time he was one of seven fellow officers who took an interest in the religious work of the Bible school.[4] In France, he continued to serve with the 368th Ambulance Company. Ambulance companies treated and evacuated soldiers from frontline aid stations to field hospitals, and transported the sick and wounded to specialized base hospitals. Some were animal drawn.

In September 1918 he was reassigned to the 367th Field Hospital. In general terms, the work of the field hospitals were triage and treating non-transportable wounded, slightly wounded, and gassed and sick. Usually simple records were made of each patient during triage. Cases were classified, dressings changed, shock treated and hot food provided. Emergency surgery might be conducted there, too.[5]

He rose to the rank of Captain, and after the war, he returned to the United States to Camp Zachary Taylor, Kentucky, where he was discharged in March 1919.

Career

After his service in World War I, Dr. Pearl headed west. He stopped briefly in Detroit, Michigan, before deciding at the end of 1919 to continue his studies and practice medicine in California. An avid researcher, Dr. Pearl continued graduate studies at the University of Southern California and Los Angeles General Hospital.

In February 1920 he was receiving patients at his office located at 1205½ Central Avenue, in the heart of the Los Angeles African American community.[6] During the 1920s he married Etta May Smith, a former Baltimore teacher who became a career social worker. Dr. Pearl was not only active medically, but also socially and politically. In October 1933 he was elected a vice president with the Civil Liberties organization in Los Angeles at its annual meeting.[7] By this time his medical office had moved to Suite 220 in the Blodgett Building at 2510 Central Avenue.

When a new Eastside Los Angeles citizens' political action committee was formed in 1934, Dr. Pearl authored a lengthy article for the *Los Angeles Sentinel* explaining its purpose and value.[8]

Another newspaper article speaks volumes about Dr. Pearl: "Fire Destroys Furniture of California Pastor."

> A fire that caused about $2500 worth of damage to the furniture of Rev. Guy J. Johnson almost claimed the lives of Dr. Frank Pearl, James Keys, and Clyde Davis who were clearing the house of the pastor's furniture.
>
> The blaze was first discovered over the living room, and these men started to help save the effects of the resident. They were successful in doing so except a divan which they could not get out the door. At this juncture, Dr. Pearl and his workers threw the rug over the furniture and stepped out of the door.
>
> The time between this act and the falling of the roof, which was a wall of fire, was almost indistinguishable. Davis and Keys thought the medical man had been covered with the falling flames and ran around the back of the house to see if he had stepped clear. Pearl was not injured.
>
> When interviewed by the reporter, Dr. Pearl stated that he and Davis were turning out of 25th Street when they saw smoke billowing in the vicinity of Adams and Hooper. They turned the car towards it, and when they arrived they saw the place crowded with people yelling "Fire! Fire!" but nobody had turned in an alarm.
>
> Pearl and Davis raced to turn in an alarm and started to clear the room of furniture. Soon afterward the roof fell.
>
> Dr. Pearl looked upon the matter rather philosophically while seated in his office about two hours after the fire. He asked himself why he, a man who had passed the medical examina-

tion of the state, would be fighting a fire? He answered his own question by stating that he could not bear to see the man's furniture burn while he was able to save it.[9]

In 1937 Dr. Pearl's reputation was tarnished when he was named as one of 13 persons indicted by a grand jury for participating in "fake accident insurance rings" that defrauded insurance companies by filing false damage claims. Interestingly, according to the *Chicago Defender*, 11 where white and their names were not mentioned in the early news accounts of the indictments.[10] He emphatically denied the charges. Pearl was later found guilty by a jury on two counts of conspiracy to commit theft. He was convicted of soliciting two women to make a false accident report.[11] In December 1937 he was sentenced to a year in the county jail, five years probation, a fine of $300 and restitution to an insurance company. He requested permission from the court to apply for probation.

How the Pearl matter was finally resolved is unclear from press reports; however, penalties and jail terms were reportedly imposed on 11 of the persons indicted. It appears Dr. Pearl may not have had to serve a year in the county jail because late the following year, in November 1938, he relocated his medical office from Suite 220 to Suite 303 in his same office building.[12] Fortunately for the African American community, he was able to continue his medical practice. In fact, in October 1940, Dr. Pearl announced a new location and practice hours for his medical office at 2403 South Central Avenue.[13] In August of the following year, he joined other doctors in the *California Eagle*, welcoming the members of the National Convention of Colored Graduate Nurses to Los Angeles for their 33rd annual convention.[14]

Dr. Pearl lived and practiced in an area of the city then known as South Central Los Angeles, the heart of the African American community. It was also the home of the University of Southern California. Six other African American physicians, also Army MOTC graduates who served in France, practiced in Los Angeles. Two were considered native Californians, Dr. Claudius Ballard and Dr. Leonard Stovall. Their medical practices were located in the same area of the city, and they were all active in the local African American medical society. The others veterans were Dr. Jack Smitherman, Dr. William A. Tarleton, Dr. Arthur J. Booker, and Dr. James T. Whittaker. Except for Dr. Whittaker, whose focus was in Pasadena, the other six doctors all concentrated their practices in downtown Los Angeles.

In 1942, during the Second World War, Dr. Pearl was named a member of a special committee formed to launch the first liberty ship to be named for an African American, the *Booker T. Washington*.[15] In 1944 he was named as a member of the executive committee of the California Colored Voters' League for Dewey and Bricker.[16] One of the objectives of the group was to promote the integration of the Negro into American life.

Throughout his life he maintained an interest in the military. He was a member of the American Legion, the Veterans of Foreign Wars, and the National Guard (where he was described as an excellent horseman and sharpshooter). During World War II, he headed the National Disaster Relief Committee of the Office of National Defense for the Los Angeles area. Politically active, he was a member of the Los Angeles Republican Central Committee.

At age 61, Dr. Pearl retired with a heart condition two years before his death in 1948. He used that time to continue his medical research. This time he was the subject. The *Los Angeles Sentinel* tells us for two years he studied the dietary problems of heart patients. He hoped that records he kept of his own condition, when released, would greatly enrich medical history.

His lengthy obituary in the *Los Angeles Sentinel* described him as a leading physician and surgeon in California. He was active in the National Medical Association and the American Medical Association, and became a Fellow of the American College of Physicians and Surgeons.

At his funeral seven local military and fraternal organizations officiated and a group of outstanding citizens served as pallbearers. Dr. Pearl was survived by his wife, Etta May Pearl, and his older brother, Milton, of Warm Springs, Montana. His wife continued to work as a social worker and supervisor of casework at the

Los Angeles County Department of Charities.[17] He is buried at the Angelus Rosedale Cemetery in Los Angeles with his wife, who died 36 years later, on Christmas Eve 1984.

NOTES

1. "Ochya Girls Party," *The Kansas City Sun*, January 16, 1915.
2. "General Program Fifth Annual Session of the Missouri Pan-Medical Association," *Journal of the National Medical Association*, July–September 1915, Vol. 7, No. 3, 233–235.
3. "Seven Atchison Doctors Are in Military Service," *The Topeka Daily Capital*, February 9, 1918, 3.
4. Russell S. Brown, *Y.M.C.A. No. 11 (Colored Service) March* 9, 1918, Jesse Moorland Papers, Box 126–72, Howard University Manuscript Archives, Washington, D.C.
5. U.S. Army Medical Department, Office of Medical History, Vol. VIII Field Operations, Chapter IV, Medical Service of the Division in Combat, GPO 1925, Washington, D.C., history.amedd.army.mil (accessed April 23, 2015).
6. "Space Ad Physician & Surgeon," *California Eagle*, February 20, 1920, 3.
7. "Dr. W.F. Watkins Again Chosen President of Civil Liberties," *California Eagle*, October 20, 1933.
8. "Citizens Committee Aims Explained by Dr. Pearl," *Los Angeles Sentinel*, August 23, 1934, 6.
9. "Fire Destroys Furniture of Calif. Pastor," *Atlanta Daily World*, June 16, 1934, 1.
10. "Leading Coast Physician Indicted in Recent Probe," *Chicago Defender*, October 2, 1937, 2.
11. "Doctor Convicted in Fraud Case," *Los Angeles Times*, November 4, 1937, 14.
12. "Space Ad Announcing Office Relocation," *California Eagle*, November 8, 1938, 8.
13. "Dr. Frank Pearl Tells Removal of Offices," *Los Angeles Sentinel*, October 24, 1940, 4.
14. "Nurses Gather in Los Angeles for Six-Day Convention," *California Eagle*, August 14, 1941, 1.
15. "Marian Anderson to Christen Ship Named After Booker T.," *Cleveland Call and Post*, September 26, 1942, 9.
16. "Dewey Backs Army Probe," *Pittsburgh Courier*, September 30, 1944, 1.
17. "Heart Attack Fatal to Dr. Frank Pearl," Obituary, *Los Angeles Sentinel*, July 29, 1948, 6.

James Maxie PONDER

22 February 1888–4 March 1958
Meharry Medical College, 1915

Roots and Education

Ponder was born to William and Addie (Williams) Ponder in Jacksonville, Florida. After graduating from Howard Academy in Ocala, young Ponder went on to Benedict College in Columbia, South Carolina, and then to Meharry Medical College in Nashville, Tennessee. He graduated from Meharry in 1915. He returned to Florida and began his medical practice in Ocala where he ran his practice out of his home.[1] Early in 1917 he married Fanny Ayer.

Military Service

First Lieutenant Ponder was called to service in the Army Medical Reserve Corps on August 7, 1917. He reported to Fort Des Moines for basic training and from there he went to Camp Meade, Maryland, with the 368th Infantry Regiment of the 92nd Division. In June he departed for France through Hoboken, New Jersey, for service with the 368th. The 92nd Division's first offensive action of the war was undertaken by his regiment in late September 1918 when the 368th took part in the Meuse-Argonne offensive. It was attached to a French unit and positioned between the French and New York's 77th regiment. "In front of this position vast stretches of enemy wire entanglement extended at intervals in all the intervening 'no-man's land.'" German machine-gun emplacements were beyond that area. Lieutenant Colonel T. A. Rothwell, Regular Army, was very proud of the enlisted men in his unit. He wrote they were "especially good soldiers during gas attacks." They could deal with it when the weather was wet and the gas would lie close to the ground, but "with the breaking out of the sun, it would rise in clouds suddenly and play havoc with the troops."[2]

The 368th experienced 450 men killed, wounded and gassed during two unsuccessful attempts to advance. Ultimately, they took the village of Binarville.[3] Ponder and the other medical team members had their hands full dealing with all the battle casualties, especially a large number who had been gassed. Many soldiers returned home following the war with lung damage from gas that would contribute to their premature deaths.

One of his fellow physicians, Dr. T. E. Jones, earned a Distinguished Service Cross for his actions in that campaign. Ponder's unit saw action in the Vosges Mountains, the Meuse-Argonne, and near Metz, before returning home through Camp Upton, New York, on February 15, 1919. He was honorably discharged on March 7, 1919.

As a young physician in World War I, James Ponder had put his new skills to work in the medical corps. At the end of the war, he was rewarded for his outstanding work during the influenza pandemic in France with a presidential citation for "meritorious service in the field of epidemic medicine." This prepared him for an almost single-handed fight against a smallpox epidemic in South St. Petersburg, Florida, during the late 1920s.

Career

After his military service, Dr. Ponder returned to his practice in Ocala. His son Ernest Ayer was young, but he remembered the family kitchen being used as an emergency operating room. He also remembered "the victims of accidents, fights, cuts and gunfight wounds all showed up at the family home late at night, and my father would go to work patching them up."[4] Payment for these medical services was often in the form of chickens, vegetables or hams.

In 1924 Dr. and Mrs. Ponder moved to St. Petersburg, in Pinellas County, Florida. Sometime in the 1920s they took in Florine as a foster daughter. She remained part of the family for the rest of their lives.

The family lived at 1209 5th Avenue, South. It is likely he was recruited by the city because that same year, he was appointed assistant city physician for the African American community.[5] He was without an office so he set up his medical practice in two rooms of the city's black-owned Royal Express Bus Line Building. While seemingly not the optimal location for a medical practice, the spot proved to be fortuitous for Dr. Ponder. His practice thrived among the thousands of African Americans who flooded into St. Petersburg—many by bus—during the late 1920s.[6] He became the city physician and administered medical care to the underprivileged until his retirement in 1951.[7]

Mercy Hospital was built in 1923. He was the first African American physician admitted to practice there. He would become one of the most influential leaders of St. Petersburg's African American community. He was recognized as spearheading the construction of Mercy's much-needed wing for prenatal care.

Among his community activities, Dr. Ponder was involved in the county schools. He was designated chairman of Trustees for Black Schools in Pinellas County. In this position, he was the voice of the black community and was able to improve the local black schools.[8] He was also the first African American physician to be elected as an active member of the Pinellas County Medical Society.

In 1929 Dr. Ponder became the first African American in the southern states to be extended membership in the National Council of World War Veterans. The organization chose him as state commander because he had served 20 months on active duty, with 8 months in France and 3 of those in combat areas. He was also the one person who was largely instrumental in bringing together African American veterans in Florida.[9]

He was a role model to those in the city's African American community who were interested in medical careers.[10] Dr. Ponder is said to have written the first prescription for Webb's Drug Store, opened for the city's African Americans. When he died in 1958, the flag at city hall was flown at half staff during his funeral.

Dr. Ponder died of a heart attack in the Veterans Administration Hospital[11] in Bay Pines, Florida. Mercy Hospital no longer exists, but a bronze plaque in his memory can be found at the Bayfront Medical Center. His obituary noted he was the "first Negro to practice medicine in St. Petersburg." He was survived by his widow, his son and daughter, and three grandchildren.[12]

NOTES

1. Thomas J. Ward, *Black Physicians in the Jim Crow South* (Fayetteville: University of Arkansas Press, 2003), 113.
2. W. Allison Sweeney, *History of the American Negro in the Great War* (New York: Negro Universities Press, 1919), 207.
3. Emmett J. Scott, *The American Negro in the World War* (Reprint, Arno Press and the New York Times, 1969), 141.
4. Sally P. Vihlen, *The Black Physician in Florida* (Gainesville: University of Florida, 1994), 60.
5. Thomas Yenser, Editor and Publisher, *Who's Who in Colored America, 1938–40* (New York, 1940), 419.
6. Sally P. Vihlen, "Dr. Noble Frisby, Interview," *The Black Physician in Florida*, 48.
7. faculty.usfsp.edu/jsokolov/mclin/res.4.1.html (accessed July 18, 2014).
8. Sally P. Vihlen, "Serving the Poorest, C. Calvin Smith," *The Black Physician in Florida*, 292.
9. "Florida Veterans Name Race Man State Commander," *Pittsburgh Courier*, December 7, 1929, 2.
10. www.stpete.org/historic_preservation/historic_landmarks/local_landmarks/docs/Mercy_Hospital.pdf (accessed July 18, 2014).
11. AMA Deceased Physician card, National Library of Medicine, Bethesda, MD.

12. "Dr. J. M. Ponder," *Pittsburgh Courier*, March 22, 1958, 6.

Albert Emerson PUNCHE

12 August 1874–2 July 1956
University of Illinois, 1914

Roots and Education

Albert E. Punche was born to Hampdon (Hamp) and Isabella Punche in Mount Enterprise, Rusk County, Texas. He had two sisters, Alice and Rachael and a brother, Sidney. The "Mount" in the town's name was actually no more than a hill, but it was rich in iron ore. It was the lumber industry, not mining, that contributed to the town's growth. By 1880, the town had three sawmills, a hotel, two cotton gins, a school, three churches, and a population of 150. Logging was a big industry in Mount Enterprise. So much so that when the Texas and New Orleans Railroad came to within 1½ miles of the town, the town moved to the railroad line in 1894. It became the new Mount Enterprise, and the old location was called the old Mount Enterprise. The major industry in the 1800s was Charles Vinson's manufacturing company. It made a variety of wood products from wagons to furniture to caskets.[1]

After school in Mount Enterprise, Albert enrolled in Prairie View State Normal School. Prairie View was the first state-supported college in Texas for African Americans. He graduated and began his teaching career in Cleburne, Texas. In the summer of 1902, he taught a summer school class at the University of Michigan. In 1903 The Dallas Morning News listed him as principal of the black high school in Cleburne.[2]

Ida Dubroca began teaching in the intermediate grades in Cleburne in 1899.[3] Professor Punche married her on March 22, 1903, in Johnson, Texas. They had two daughters, Chaldade L. Punche and Ossalee Veda Punche, and a son, Albert Dubroca. Chaldade does not appear in any records after the 1920 U.S. Census, which lists her then as 13. Ossalee graduated from Prairie View College and then Wilberforce University in Ohio. She was a member of

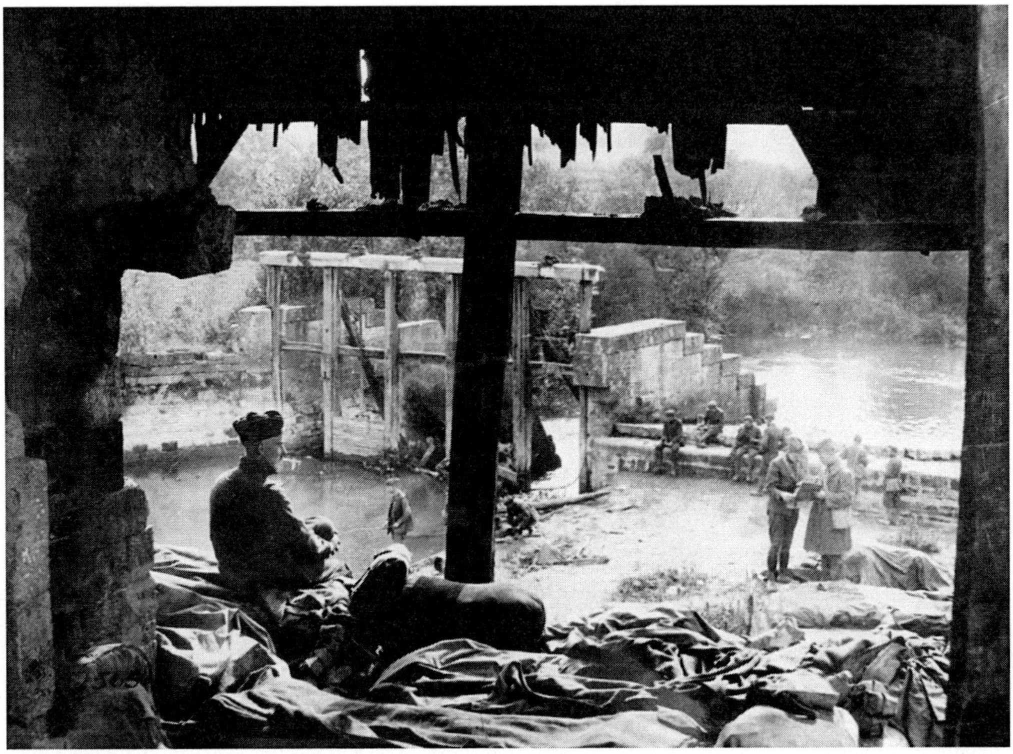

Temporary field hospital (National Archives).

Alpha Kappa Alpha and Gamma Rho sororities and was described as their brilliant daughter.[4]

In addition to his high school duties, Punche was involved in community activities that affected the school. On October 12, 1905, the *Dallas Morning News* reported on a meeting called by "the conservative element of the race." It requested "colored citizens of Cleburne and Johnson County to meet at the courthouse at 2 p.m. on Sunday, October 15, 1905." He was listed among the 34 signatories. During the previous 90 days, three assaults had been committed on white women within a radius of 100 miles of Cleburne. The purpose of the gathering was to "show to the world ... we are on the side of law and order ... and create a more friendly feeling with our white friends of the South by showing them we will do all in our power to see that their homes are safe."[5]

By 1911 Punche decided to leave education for medicine. He attended the Meharry Medical College of Walden University in Nashville for two years. He then transferred to the University of Illinois Medical School in Chicago where he received his M.D. in 1914. The alumni records at the University of Illinois show his address as 507 North Douglas Avenue and subsequently a business address 605 East Chambers Street in Cleburne.[6]

Military Service

Ida and Albert Punche were married with two children and a third on the way, when he volunteered to serve in the U.S. Army and reported to the Medical Officer Training Camp (MOTC) at Fort Des Moines on August 4, 1917. At 45, he was one of the oldest volunteer doctors. He said he was a Baptist.[7] Completing his MOTC training, First Lieutenant Punche was then assigned to the 366th Field Hospital of the 317th Sanitary Train and reported to Camp Funston, Kansas.

While stationed there on February 16, 1918, Ida gave birth to his son in Cleburne, Texas. He received the news and certainly would have been granted leave to visit with the family prior to his departure to France in June 1918.

While overseas, casualties were light in the 92nd Division until the late fall of 1918. While Dr. Punche and his fellow physicians spent much of their time preventing disease, they also treated soldiers for respiratory ailments, influenza, venereal diseases, injuries and assorted non-combat medical problems, including trench foot. Trench foot occurs when the feet are wet for long periods of time. It can be painful, but can also be cured if the foot is treated before the skin and tissue of the foot begins to die and fall off. The best treatment is air-drying and elevating the feet and getting them out of wet shoes and socks.[8] Unfortunately, this was trench warfare (and that meant walking in constant wetness). The best way to avoid trench foot was to have a shoe that protected the feet from the wet conditions. The 1917 trench boot was an improvement. It had two rows of stitching, a waterproofing solution on the inside, and an insole with reinforced canvas. In 1918 the Pershing boot or "Little Tank" was introduced. It had an extra third row of stitching with three full soles, thicker leather and a superior sole construction. This was the soldier's best defense against trench foot, but it was not delivered until late in the war so physicians were dealing with foot problems throughout their time in France.[9]

On September 2, the 92nd Division repulsed an enemy raid at La Fontenelle in the St. Dié sector. At the end of September, they were sent to the Meuse-Argonne where the 368th Infantry took part in the action. On October 10, they pushed into the Marbache sector where an African American observer commented the "aggressiveness of the patrols of the 92nd Division changed the complexion of things speedily. They [the 92nd] inflicted many casualties on the Germans and took many prisoners."[10]

The division's greatest drive was near Metz on November 9, two days before the war ended. "A sense of race pride seemed to stir and actuate every man. An opportunity to enact a mighty role was upon them, and they played it well."[11] Casualties were heavy. The war ended the next day, November 11, 1918, but he and the other physicians of the 92nd were busy tending to the wounded for many weeks after the war.

The *Dallas Express* reported Punche's return from France in its April 19, 1919, issue.[12] In May he spoke at the AME Church about his war experiences.[13] The *Texas State Journal of Medicine* reported his honorable discharge from the U.S. Army Medical Corps in June.[14]

Career

After the war Dr. Punche returned to his family, home and medical practice in Cleburne. He did not close the Cleburne office, but in 1922 he opened an office in nearby Fort Worth, Texas, at 900 Jones Street. By 1926, his home and office were at 307A East Ninth Street. According to the 1930 U.S. Census, he was 61 with dual addresses for his home and practice in Cleburne and Fort Worth (about 30 miles apart). His wife appears to have stayed in Cleburne, but he and his 14-year-old son lived in the house in Fort Worth.

Dr. Punche's daughter Ossalee was certainly the star of the next generation of the Punche family. In June 1935 she was awarded her Bachelor of Science degree from Wilberforce University.[15] On November 5, 1938, the *Pittsburgh Courier* carried a large photograph of "brilliant Fort Worth girl" Ossalee Veda Punche.

In 1939 Ossalee and Rogenia Anola Goldthwaite published the "Bibliography of George Washington Carver." In 1940 she published, "A Tentative Guidance Program for the Negro Junior High School Grade Levels of Texas."[16] It appears to have been written as a thesis for her master's degree from Prairie View State College.

Their son, Albert Dubroca Punche, did not attain greatness. At age 23 (on May 15, 1941), he was murdered at 606 East First Street in Fort Worth.[17] He was stabbed to death in the throat by a 20-year-old woman. It was Dr. Punche himself who signed his son's death certificate.[18]

In August of 1941 at the age of 67, Dr. Punche left Fort Worth for a visit to Chicago, where he participated in the annual meeting the National Medical Association (NMA), and likely enjoyed a reunion with a few veteran physicians he had known at Meharry and Fort Des Moines.

In the late 1940s, at about the age of 75, he retired and moved in with his daughter Ossalee Punche Lockett and her family at 8225 LaSalle Street, Detroit, Michigan. He was living with Ossalee when he died. She took care of his burial with a military headstone in Detroit Memorial Park Cemetery. His wife, Ida, died in Riverside, California, in August 1966.

NOTES

1. www.tshaonline.org/handbook/online/articles/hlm93 (accessed September 11, 2014).
2. fortworthafricanamericandoctors.wordpress.com/1920s/punche-albert-e/albert-e-punche-biography (accessed December 11, 2011).
3. Telephone Interview with Senior Librarian, Shirley Apley, MLS, Fort Worth Library, July 11, 2011.
4. *Pittsburgh Courier*, November 5, 1938, 24.
5. *Ibid.*
6. Reference Librarian Susan Glover: University of Illinois Special Collections, 1914 Yearbook, July 21, 2011.
7. John L. Thompson, *History and Views of Colored Officers Training Camp for 1917 at Fort Des Moines, Iowa* (Des Moines: *The Bystander*, 1917) 81.
8. emergency.cdc.gov (accessed March 29, 2015).
9. *The Pershing Boot*, worldwar1.com (accessed March 15, 2015).
10. W. Allison Sweeney, *The American Negro in the Great World War* (New York: Negro Universities Press, 1919) 200.
11. *Ibid.*, 201.
12. "Cleburne," *The Dallas Express*, April 19, 1919, 5.
13. *Ibid.*, May 3, 1919, 6.
14. *Texas State Journal of Medicine*, Vol. XV, June 1919, No. 2.
15. "Mitchell Speaks—Too Many Pass at Wilberforce Univ," *Afro-American*, June 22, 1935, 10.
16. Ossalee Veda Punche, *A Tentative Guidance Program for the Negro Junior High School Grade Levels of Texas* (Prairie View State College, Graduate Division, Publisher, 1940).
17. "Jailed in Stabbing," *Fort Worth Press*, May 16, 1941.
18. Texas Department of Health, Bureau of Vital Statistics, Certificate 24732, filed May 19, 1941.

Frank Perryn RAIFORD, Jr.

24 September 1890–12 March 1966
University of Michigan, 1917

Roots and Education

Frank Raiford, Jr., was born to Frank and Ella Pearl Raiford in Columbus, Georgia. His father was a Columbus native who moved his family to Atlanta where "he operated a hat check business in numerous Atlanta clubs and private homes for about 45 years. He and his checking concessions were most frequently seen in the

Municipal Auditorium." The family lived at 174 Howell Street. His father was a longtime member of the nearby First Congregational Church, where he acted as superintendent of the Sunday school. There were five children in the family: Frank Jr., Beatrice, Mamie, Rosa, and a younger brother, Johnnie. Beatrice would become a schoolteacher. His father, Frank Sr., lived a very long life, working into his mid–80s. He didn't retire until 1950 and then passed away in 1958 at the age of 92.[1]

Frank Jr. received an excellent education. He completed his college preparatory work at Atlanta University and later graduated with an A.B. from Lincoln University in Philadelphia in 1913. He went on to study at the University of Michigan Medical School from 1913 to 1917. He was 26 when he received his medical degree. America was preparing to enter the First World War, and Frank registered for the draft while he was still at the University of Michigan.

African American physicians were the last to be recruited. First, the army had to be sold on the idea of black combat troops, then black officers. Then it finally occurred to the military that physicians would be needed for those segregated combat divisions. By the time he volunteered for the Army Medical Reserve Corps, Raiford had returned home and was living in Atlanta.[2]

Military Service

First Lieutenant Raiford was called to active duty and reported to the Medical Officers Training Camp (MOTC) at Fort Des Moines. He arrived October 8 and completed his training November 3, 1917. He was then sent to the 317th Sanitary (Medical) Train of the 92nd Division at Camp Funston, Kansas, where he was assigned to the 368th Field Hospital. While on leave in Chicago, Lieutenant Raiford and Lula Alberta Watts were married just before Christmas on December 23, 1917.

Back at Camp Funston, Raiford suffered a fractured fibula (calf bone) in the "line of duty" and was out of action in May while it healed. He returned to duty in time to leave for France. After arriving in France he had a recurrent problem with his leg that required his hospitalization briefly in July at Camp Hospital No. 21 at the Bourbonne-les-Bains training area. He recovered and was sent with seven other doctors for a week of training at the Gas School at Dijon in early August, before the division was

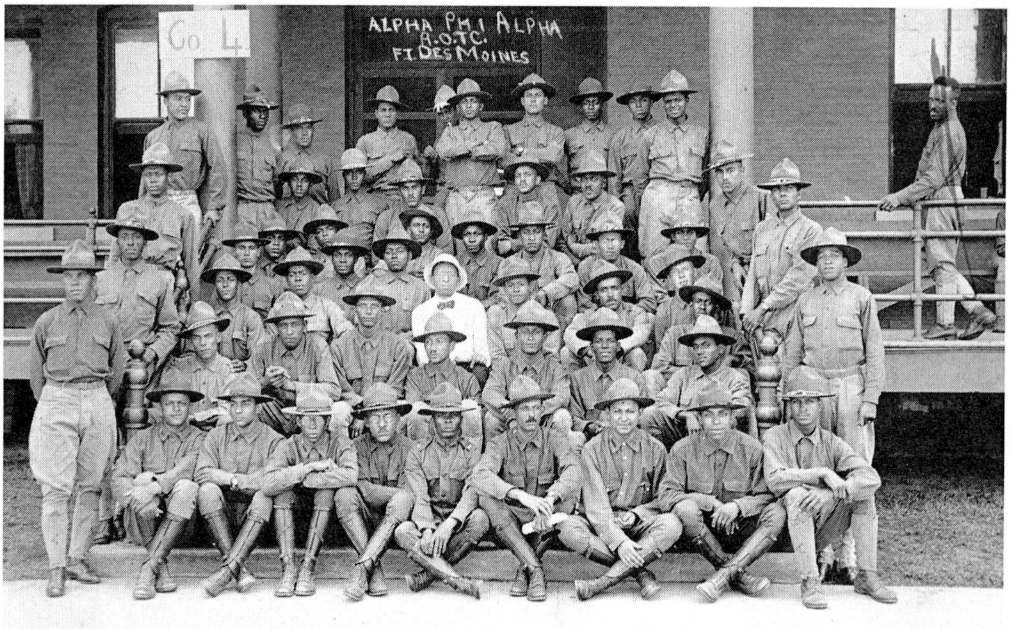

Alpha Phi Alpha, the first Black, intercollegiate Greek-lettered fraternity founded in 1906 at Cornell University (courtesy Rare and Manuscript Collections, Cornell University Library).

committed to battle. Infantrymen who were gassed were treated in specially equipped sections of a hospital. The section had a large shower bath, a large supply of blankets, pajamas, and bed sacks. Specialized equipment included oxygen-inhalation sets, sodium bicarbonate one percent solution, Novocain one percent solution, albolene, camphorated oil in ampules, caffeine citrate in ampules and quarter-grain solution of morphine in ampules. This equipment and the supplies were placed in each ward. Shower baths were provided, with a large supply of soap, towels, and sodium bicarbonate. Patients were those who suffered from surface contact with mustard gas, those who inhaled noxious gas, and those who were exposed to both. Many soldiers were in the last category, exposed to both types of gas. They were bathed frequently. Blisters on the skin were opened and the fluid caught on gauze to keep it from affecting the healthy skin. Eyes were washed frequently. Treatment was time consuming, but it improved the patient's chances of avoiding complications. On the wards patients were given stimulating drinks, such as coffee and cocoa. Morphine was administered as needed for the pain. Patients did recover, but only after a long convalescence.[3]

Lieutenant Raiford continued to serve with the 368th Field Hospital until October 1918. He was then reassigned to the medical detachment of the 367th Infantry Regiment, shortly before the division's final offensive of the war near Metz. The 367th fought well and suffered light casualties as the war drew to a close. After returning from France in February 1919, Lieutenant Raiford was discharged from the army.

Career

In 1919 Frank and Lula were reunited and moved to Detroit, a city of opportunity because of the "great migration" of southern African Americans during World War I. By 1920, they had two children: a daughter, Frances, and a new baby boy, Frank P. Raiford, III.[4] They lived at 2225 Maple Street downtown, only a half mile from his office at 1901 St. Antoine.

Raiford built a successful medical practice in Detroit. By 1930 the family, with young Frances, age 11, and Frank III, age 10, had moved to 1710 McDougall Street where they lived for many years.[5]

In 1934 Dr. Raiford was one of the three founders of the Trinity Hospital (1934–1962) at East Congress and DuBois Street. His hospital was known "for its postgraduate surgical training and residency program for African American physicians. At that time, there was a need not only for housing and treatment for the ill, but for the training and guidance of the African American medical community. Trinity was Detroit's first African American hospital to operate a cancer detection center. Among some of its pioneering procedures were deep x-ray therapy for treating cancer and physiotherapy. It grew as a training facility and as an institution of excellence until it outgrew its building. It reopened as Boulevard General Hospital on West Grand Boulevard."[6] In 1942, it was moved to 681 East Vernor Street and expanded to 140 beds.

Dr. Raiford was a member of the Alpha Phi Alpha fraternity, serving as president of the local Gamma Lambda chapter in 1924. The next years must have been very good for Dr. Raiford and his wife. In 1935 a social item appeared noting "the largest and one of the most fashionable parties of the season was that given by Dr. and Mrs. Frank Raiford for their daughter, Frances, at the Lucy Thurman Branch YWCA Thursday night. Balloons, and other decorations enlivened the surroundings as the group danced to the music of a fourteen piece orchestra." It was a 16th birthday party for Frances and was attended by more than 60 people.

During the 1940s and 1950s the Raifords were often reported in the society pages of the African American press. In March 1941, for example, they were guests at a festive reception for many friends and family in Atlanta.[7] Dr. Raiford and his wife made many trips to Atlanta to visit with his parents.

In 1946 Dr. Raiford's son, Frank III, began working at Trinity Hospital as a practitioner and part-time administrator. Like his father, he attended the University of Michigan, graduating from the medical school in 1943. He interned at Cleveland City Hospital and served in the army as a medic during World War II beforc joining his father back in Detroit.

In 1953 a newspaper reporting on a big Saturday wedding in Detroit said among the guests was Raiford's daughter Frances, "one of the best honey-brown girls we've met" and wife of Attorney William Polk.[8]

In 1958 Dr. Raiford's father, Frank Sr., was brought from Atlanta to Detroit and hospitalized in his son's Trinity Hospital. He passed away there at 92.

Dr. Frank Raiford, Jr., continued to practice medicine, working with his son, Frank III. He maintained his affiliation with Boulevard General Hospital for many years.

Dr. and Mrs. Raiford also continued to enjoy an active social life. They are mentioned in the society columns as the town's "socialites" participating in Detroit's "Fun Days."[9] They went to Chicago for a Kid Gavilan boxing match and then had a houseguest, Phoebe Birney, dean of women at Clark University, Atlanta.[10]

He lived a long and productive life helping the members of Detroit's African American community. He died at 75 years old in 1966 of a cerebral hemorrhage.[11] His son Frank III continued to practice medicine in Detroit for several more decades.[12]

Notes

1. "Raiford Rites at Congregational Church Today," *Atlanta Daily World*, June 28, 1958, 1.
2. World War I Draft Registration Card, ancestry.com.
3. U.S. Army Medical Department, Office of Medical History, Vol. VIII Field Operations, Chapter IV, Medical Service of the Division in Combat (Washington, D.C.: GPO, 1925) history.amedd.army.mil (accessed April 23, 2015).
4. 1920 U.S. Federal Census.
5. 1930 U.S. Federal Census.
6. *Kellogg African American Health Care Project*, www.med.umich.edu/haahc/Hospitals/hospital.htm (accessed September 9, 2014).
7. "BETTY NOTES: Dr. and Mrs. Raiford Are Honor Guests," *Atlanta Daily World*, March 5, 1941, 3.
8. "Toki Types," *Pittsburgh Courier*, June 27, 1953, 10.
9. *Ibid.*, June 1956, 15.
10. *Ibid.*, April 17, 1954, 8.
11. "AMA Deceased Physician Card, National Library of Medicine, Bethesda, MD.
12. "Obituary, Frank P. Raiford, III, MD," Wayne County Medical Society of Southeast Michigan.

Emory Wallace RICHIE

25 January 1887–21 July 1937
Howard Medical College, 1916

Roots and Education

Emory Richie was the son of Louis P. Richie, a blacksmith in Abbeville, South Carolina. His mother, Emma P. Richie, was a nurse. Emory's father died by the time he was a teen. In 1900 he was 13 and lived on Main Street in Abbeville with his mother and an older sister, Florence. His mother owned the house free and clear of a mortgage. His sister Florence died young May 13, 1902, and was buried in Lakeview Cemetery in Abbeville. In 1905 Emory earned a bachelor of science degree at the A & M College (now South Carolina State University) in Orangeburg, about 100 miles from his home.

By 1910 he had moved on to study at Howard University in Washington, D.C. He graduated in May from the Commercial (Business) Department at Howard University. There were eight other people in his class.[1] In 1912 he entered Howard's Medical College. He graduated with a medical degree in 1916. Dr. Richie then worked for a year as an intern at Freedmen's Hospital in Washington. Freedmen's Hospital was a federally owned hospital located at Howard University where many African American physicians trained and worked. His mother stayed in Abbeville on Harrisburg Street and worked as a "sick nurse" for a private family. She continued to work there in 1920 at age 65.[2]

Military Service

As America entered the First World War in 1917, Howard University urged its graduates to enlist. Richie volunteered and at age 30, he was commissioned as a first lieutenant and sent to Fort Des Moines for military training at the Medical Officers Training Camp (MOTC). He was one of 16 Howard graduates in camp.

Lieutenant Ritchie received only 38 days of training before he was sent to Camp Funston at Fort Riley, Kansas.[3] He was assigned to the 317th Sanitary (Medical) Train, 92nd Division, as a medical officer with the 349th Machine Gun Battalion.

On March 2, 1918, he submitted a report to the division surgeon from the "Office of Surgeon at the Infirmary" of the 349th M.G. Battalion noting there had been no discharges because of tuberculosis among Kansas soldiers.[4] On March 3, 1918, he was working in the 17th

Infirmary where he was assisted by Lieutenant Jonathan N. Rucker. By July 1918, the 92nd Division was en route to France without Richie. He had fallen ill at Camp Funston and was hospitalized at the Fort Riley Base Hospital.

After he recovered he was assigned to U.S. Army General Hospital No. 3 in Colonia, New Jersey, near the army's main embarkation terminals. Ritchie spent the entire war at this 2,000 bed medical and surgical "clearing house" hospital. It served the ports of entry in New York City and Hoboken, New Jersey, for the returning wounded doughboys.

Various cases could be quickly sorted out on the basis of their medical requirements and promptly sent to the proper military hospitals for care. There was also a need for an orthopedic hospital since large numbers of the returning wounded had suffered orthopedic injuries. In the 15 months the hospital existed (1918–1919), more than 6,000 wounded Yanks arrived at Colonia, with the majority able to return to active civilian life.[5]

After the war ended in 1918, he was honorably discharged on June 30, 1919.[6] The *Journal of the American Medical Association* (JAMA) lists Dr. Emory Wallace Richie in "The War Service of the Medical Profession" honor roll as reported by the South Carolina Medical Association, 1917–18.[7]

Career

Dr. Richie never returned to live in South Carolina. He stayed in New Jersey the rest of his life. Official State of New Jersey records show that he became licensed by the New Jersey State Board of Medical Examiners in 1919. His home at the time was given as Elizabeth, New Jersey, not far from the Colonia hospital.[8]

In 1920 the U.S. Census reported that Dr. Richie and his wife, Mabelle Richie, lived at 232 Clay Street in nearby Hackensack. Hackensack city directories from 1921 to 1931 list Dr. Richie as a physician at 172 James Street. Because his wife is listed at the same address, it seems sure he conducted his medical practice in his home, which was common in those years.[9]

He practiced at the Hackensack Hospital as early as the 1930s. It became a very important institution in northern New Jersey. The hospital had opened in 1888 with 35 beds, and with major donations was overhauled and improved significantly in the 1920s. It has become one of the largest, most modern community hospitals in New Jersey with 500 beds.[10] That Dr. Richie, an African American, was on staff in the 1930s was unusual. It was not common for African American doctors to be able to practice at white hospitals in New Jersey. The hospital did not even accept its first African American intern until 1950.[11] His service there is a testament to his professionalism and skill.

The State Department of Health at the State House in Trenton reported to the American Medical Association that Richie died on July 21, 1937, from an acute stroke and kidney disease complications. He was still on the staff of Hackensack Hospital when he died there.[12]

Dr. Richie served his community in New Jersey for nearly 20 years before his untimely death in 1937 at only 50 years of age. He rests in the Hackensack Cemetery under a U.S. military headstone honoring his service in the First World War.[13]

NOTES

1. "Diplomas to Graduates," *Washington Evening Star*, May 24, 1910, 18.
2. 1910 and 1920 U.S. Federal Census.
3. Table of Medical Reserve Corps—Colored—Receiving Instruction, Medical Training Camp, Fort Des Moines, Iowa, RG-112, Records of the Army Surgeon General, National Archives, College Park, MD.
4. Record Group 120, Records of the 92d Division, 317th Sanitary Train, Memoranda 1918, National Archives, College Park, MD.
5. Virginia Bergen Troeger, *Colonia's WWI Hospital*, GardenStateLegacy.com Issue 8, June 2010, gardenstatelegacy.com/files/Colonias_WWI_Hospital_Troeger_GSL8.pdf (accessed January 5, 2013).
6. The Official Roster of South Carolina Soldiers, Sailors and Marines in the World War, 1917–18, Vol. 2, 1610, South Carolina Department of Archives & History, Reference Library, Columbia, SC.
7. "The War Service of the Medical Profession," *Journal of the American Medical Association (JAMA)*, June 1, 1918, Vol. 76, No. 22, 1714.
8. *Licentiates of the State Board of Medical Examiners of New Jersey for the Year of 1919, Physicians*, Documents of the Legislature of the State of New Jersey 1918–1919, Legislative Documents, Vol. VI, Document Number 68.
9. *U.S. City Directories, 1821–1989 (Beta), Hackensack, New Jersey*, ancestry.com.
10. George Mercer Scudder, *Historic Facts About Hackensack*, September 1999, Hackensack Hospital, 7–8, www.hackensacknow.org/HistoryFactsb.pdf.
11. John Lathen, 1st African American Intern at Hack-

ensack Hospital, www.hackensacknow.org/index.php?topic=1867.0 (accessed October 11, 2013).
12. AMA Deceased Physician Card, National Library of Medicine, Bethesda, MD.
13. U.S Headstone Applications, Military Veterans, ancestry.com.

Linell Leonard RODGERS

9 May 1894–17 February 1971
Meharry Medical College, 1916

Roots and Education

Linell Rodgers was the younger of two sons born to O.C. and Pemphey Rodgers in Sandersville, Mississippi, a very small town in southeast Mississippi about 10 miles north of Laurel. It's now considered part of metropolitan Laurel, a lumbering town founded in 1882. By 1910 the family moved south to Hattiesburg where O.C. worked in real estate for a land company, and they lived downtown at 400 East Second Street.[1] Remarkably, both of the Rodgers boys went on to become physicians.

Linell succeeded in entering Meharry Medical School in Nashville and graduated with his M.D. in 1916. The previous year, in April 1915, he had married Miss Ina J. Shanks in Tennessee. After graduation they moved to Kansas City, Missouri, where he interned at General Hospital No. 2 under the tutelage of the renowned Superintendent there, Dr. Thomas C. Unthank. When the city built a new municipal hospital in 1911, Dr. Unthank urged the city fathers to designate the old facility for black patients. He succeeded. By 1913, four black physicians were appointed to the hospital's staff, quickly followed by interns.

In 1917 Dr. Rodgers, his wife and young son, Linell Jr., moved to Chicago where he pursued post-graduate work and began to practice medicine. His older brother, Dr. David Charles Rodgers, also a Meharry graduate (1915), was already a physician and surgeon in Chicago.[2] Once there, Linell took a job as a laborer with International Harvester to help cover his family's expenses while he pursued his post-graduate studies and began to establish his practice.[3]

Military Service

When the United States entered the Great War in 1917, Rodgers volunteered for the U.S. Army Medical Reserve Corps. The *Illinois Medical Journal* reported Dr. Linell L. Rodgers of 526 East Bowen Avenue, Chicago, had received his commission.[4]

When First Lieutenant Rodgers reported to the Medical Officers Training Camp (MOTC) at Fort Des Moines, he was 23 years old, the youngest physician at the training camp, and one of its earliest arrivals. He trained there for 90 days before moving on to Camp Funston as a member of the 317th Sanitary (Medical) Train of the 92nd Division.[5] There he was assigned to the Train's 367th Field Hospital unit.

The field hospital provided young Rodgers with a wealth of experience. In July 1918 Rodgers was sent to Gas School in Dijon, France, for training in the prevention and treatment of gas casualties.[6]

In 1919 the *Meharry Annual Military Review* described Rodgers as a man who "served throughout the war as a member of and supply officer for the 367th Field Hospital. He won the esteem and respect of all his superior officers and the enlisted loved and trusted him in all matters pertaining to their comfort and welfare. No officer or enlisted man attempted to put anything over on Lieut. Rogers. In battle he was as cool and composed as in his Chicago office. His promotion to captaincy was delayed owing to the [unwritten] policy of certain higher officials to 'Keep down promotions in the 92nd Division.'"[7]

Like many other war veterans, Rodgers required medical treatment and hospitalization after he returned from overseas. In 1920 he remained in the army and was paid while he was a patient at U.S. Army Hospital No. 21 in Aurora outside of Denver, Colorado. This hospital was used as a recuperation hospital for many soldiers and veterans, particularly those suffering from the effects of gas warfare and tuberculosis. It was very large and had a 1,600-bed capacity during the war. By the end of 1920, the number of beds was reduced by half to 800 beds. The institution was renamed Fitzsimons Army Hospital in July 1920 and continued to operate through most of the 20th century.

Rodgers was released from the Fitzsimons General Hospital and honorably discharged on August 15, 1920, and returned to Chicago to his family. He listed his four dependents as his mother, Temple Rodgers; his wife, Ina J. Rodgers; his son, Linell Jr. (born 1915); and his daughter, Ethelyn Lenora (born 1917). They lived in three rooms at 4357 Calumet Avenue in south Chicago.

Career

Soon after Dr. Rodgers returned to Chicago, the family moved to Cleveland, Ohio. Cleveland in the 1920s was an economic beneficiary of industrial demand. Declining immigration had created an opportunity for black labor. As black migrants came north as part of the Great Migration, Cleveland's African American population grew to 72,000 by 1930.[8] The need for physicians was great, and they were being recruited.

By November 1925, Dr. Rodgers was one of 10 African American physicians who founded the Cleveland Medical Reading Club. It was organized to keep physicians abreast of programs and advances in the medical field. At its conception, there were no hospitals in Cleveland where black physicians could get internship training. In addition to Dr. Rodgers, Medical Reading Club founding members included Drs. Luther O. Baumgardner, E. J. Gunn, Charles H. Garvin, Leon Evans, Armand Evans, George Ferguson, James A. Owen, Oliver A. Taylor, and John H. McMorris. Drs. Garvin and Owen were also First World War veterans who had trained and served with Rodgers in France in the 92nd Division. By 1995, it had become one of the oldest continually meeting medical clubs in the city. It met monthly to discuss presentations by members. Membership was limited to 20 elected physicians.[9]

Life during the early 1930s in the Great Depression was not easy. Dr. Rodgers worked as a city district physician in Cleveland's Twelfth Ward until, in a highly political move, the mayor suspended three Democratic leaders of the Twelfth District Democratic Club from their positions. Rodgers was one of the three. The others were the club president and secretary.[10]

By 1930, Dr. Rodgers remarried, Arnita, who was from Ohio. The couple lived at 2286 East 93rd Street, near the old University Hospital and Case Western Reserve University School of Medicine. He shared a medical office with Dr. James A. Owen, a fellow MOTC graduate who had served in France with the 366th Field Hospital. By 1940, Dr. Rodgers and his wife had moved closer to Lake Erie into an attractive residential neighborhood with detached homes. His son, Linell Jr., who had previously been living in Chicago, was now with them. His son was 25 and working as a driver (chauffeur).[11]

By the early 1940s, Dr. Rodgers had relocated his office to 2282 East 55th Street, where it remained for the rest of his life.

Dr. Rodgers was very devoted to the Salvation Army's Mary B. Talbert Hospital, almost from its inception. The hospital started in 1925 as a rescue home assisting unmarried, pregnant African American women and girls in Cleveland. Dr. Rodgers was an attending physician there. The all-black home with 12 beds was named for an anti-lynching activist and second president of the National Association of Colored Women. It became the Mary B. Talbert Home and Hospital and in 1930 moved to 5905 Kinsman Road, the site of the former Booth Memorial Hospital. It was administered by the Salvation Army at that location until it was closed in 1960.[12]

In January 1951 Dr. Rodgers spoke at the annual doctors' dinner of the Mary B. Talbert Hospital. He is quoted as saying, "The Negro doctors and the Salvation Army have made a unique combination of medical skill and philanthropic endeavor which have gone hand-in-hand to build this institution and its far-reaching programs."[13] The programs included pre-natal care, maternity services, and post-natal education programs. He spoke of the hospital's accomplishments as a tribute to African American enterprise.

Arnita Rodgers shared his interest in caring for these women and helping them get on with their lives. Mrs. Rodgers was introduced in 1954 at the annual doctors' dinner because she had interested a new group of women, known as the Junior Board, into helping. They wanted to serve unmarried mothers of the community by setting up a beauty salon where instruction and morale building would be provided by trained volunteer beauticians. It was directed especially at young women leaving the hospital to go out and take their place in society.[14]

Dr. Rodgers and Dr. Owen were also early members of the Cleveland Medical Association (CMA). The CMA was the Northeastern Ohio local chapter of the National Medical Association. It represented African American physicians and conducted regular monthly educational programs. Rodgers and Owens conducted medical classes about asthma for the CMA membership in January and February 1931.[15]

His interest in civic matters is reflected in his letters to the editor of the *Cleveland Call* and *Post*. One of Rodgers' letters, signed as president of the Civic and Cultural Society, protested streetcar fare increases that would affect the poorest citizens who lacked alternative transportation and would unfairly raise wages of the transit workers.[16] He also wrote as a member of the Hensley Defense Committee seeking freedom for Edward Hensley, a Negro boy who had been convicted. In 1966 Rodgers spoke on behalf of the Corey Methodist Church supporting a city sales tax rather than a city income tax to address the city's 1967 deficit.[17]

In his practice, Dr. Rodgers was open to trying innovative approaches to managing pain. In 1957 he and a "dentist collaborated over the telephone to maintain a hypnotic spell over a woman while she had a tooth extracted." In an amusing account, Dr. Rodgers related the dentist broke the spell with instructions relayed by phone. "I told him to count to three and snap his finger ... he forgot and counted to six but it worked anyway."[18]

In 1958 he demonstrated for the managing editor of the *Cleveland Call and Post* the use of hypnosis to help prepare a patient for pain-free childbirth. The experiment was the second in a series to help young women achieve anesthesia hypnotically. Dr. Rodgers explained that only one-fourth of the patients induced into a trance are capable of achieving a sufficiently deep hypnotic state to make such procedures possible. He said it was also possible to produce anesthesia for post-operative pain. Using these practices, there was an absence of the nausea that often occurred in chemical anesthesia.[19]

Dr. and Mrs. Rodgers made significant contributions to the African American community in Cleveland. When he passed away at the age of 76 in 1971, he had been serving the citizens of that city for half a century. He is buried in Cleveland's lovely Lake View Cemetery, Section 50, Lot 221-A.[20]

Notes

1. 1910 U.S. Federal Census.
2. "List of Those Who Passed State Boards, Class of 1915," *Meharry News*, January 1916, Vol. 14, No. 3, 5, Meharry Medical College Archives, Nashville, TN.
3. World War I Draft Registration Card, ancestry.com.
4. *Illinois Medical Journal*, November 1917, 378.
5. Table of Medical Reserve Corps—Colored—Receiving Instruction, Medical Training Camp, Fort Des Moines, Iowa, RG-112, Records of the U.S. Army Surgeon General, National Archives, College Park, MD.
6. Record Group 120, Records of the AEF (World War I), 92nd Division, 317th Sanitary Train, Daily Report—29 July 1918, National Archives, College Park, MD.
7. *The Meharry Annual, Military Review 1919*, Harold D. West Collection, Meharry Medical College Archives, Nashville, TN, 54.
8. *African Americans—The Encyclopedia of Cleveland History*, ech.case.edu/cgi/article.pl?id=AA (accessed October 9, 2013).
9. The Cleveland Medical Reading Club, ancestry.com.
10. "Cleveland Mayor Suspend Workers," *The Zanesville, Ohio, Times Recorder*, May 21, 1932, 7.
11. 1940 U.S. Federal Census.
12. "Mary B. Talbert Home and Hospital," *The Encyclopedia of Cleveland History*, ech.case.edu/cgi/article.pl?id=MBTHAH (accessed October 9, 2013).
13. "Staff Doctors Praised at Annual Mary B. Talbert Hospital Dinner," *Cleveland Call and Post*, February 3, 1951, 8B.
14. "Cites 30% Increase in Illegitimate Births," *Cleveland Call and Post*, March 6, 1954, 5A.
15. "Program-Cleveland Medical Association," *Journal of the National Medical Association (JNMA)*, January 1931, Vol. XXIII No. 1, 45.
16. "Letter Box," *Cleveland Call and Post*, August 27, 1949, 4B.
17. "Church Class Rejects Any but Sales Tax," *Cleveland Call and Post*, September 17, 1966, 6A.
18. "Phone Hypnosis Helped Extraction," *Panama City News-Herald*, November 20, 1957, 2.
19. "Introduction to Hypnosis," *Cleveland Call and Post*, October 18, 1958, 5 C.
20. Ohio Deaths (1971), Linell L. Rodgers, February 17, 1971, ancestry.com.

Jonathan Nathaniel RUCKER

3 September 1892–8 February 1970
Meharry Medical College, 1914

Roots and Education

Rucker was born on a plantation outside Natchez, Mississippi. He was the second of six children of Peter C. and Ardella Screws Rucker.

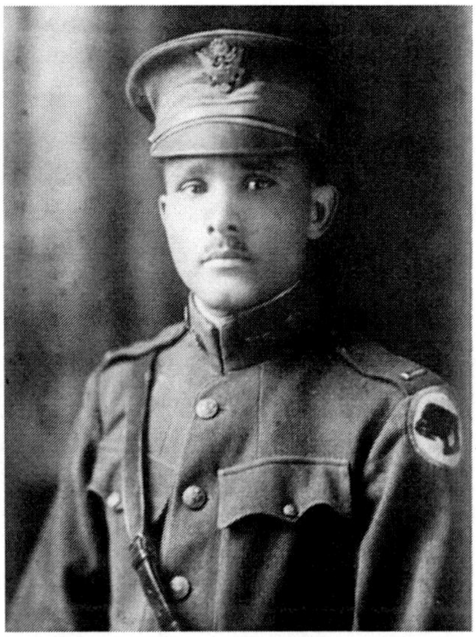

Lieutenant Jonathan N. Rucker, 317th Supply Train, 92nd Division (courtesy the Rucker family).

His grandfather and namesake, Jonathan Rucker (1809–1873) was the white plantation owner. He had two mulatto children, Peter and Sarah. Following their father's death in 1873, the two young children inherited the homestead. When Sarah died in 1875, Peter inherited the property. Peter was educated, received divinity training and became an active evangelical preacher in the African American community. He married Mary Ellen Ardella Screws in 1888. Ardella had trained at the Tuskegee Institute and was a home economics teacher. She taught at Natchez College and helped educate her local community as a Jeanes Teacher. The Jeanes program, created by a wealthy Quaker from Philadelphia named Anna T. Jeanes, distributed funding to maintain rural black schools in the South.

Their son, Jonathan, attended Adams County public schools in Natchez. He graduated from Natchez College (a high school-level institution) in 1911. His father died that same year.

Times were hard in Mississippi in the early 20th century. The boll weevil swept across the South, devastating its cotton crop and crippling the Southern economy. To continue his education, young Rucker worked his way up to Memphis, Tennessee, on a railway baggage car. Once there he worked long hours at a Memphis department store until he had enough money to make his way to Nashville. In Nashville, Rucker enrolled in Walden University to study theology and earned his D.D. He then entered Meharry Medical College.[1] Dr. Rucker ranked in the top four students of his 1914 medical school graduating class. Throughout his time in Nashville, Rucker excelled in the classroom and worked as a waiter at the Tulane Hotel.

After graduating, Rucker learned that a doctor was needed in Gallatin, a small city in Sumner County about 35 miles northeast of Nashville. He decided to open a practice there. It was a low-income rural area, where many times Rucker's patients paid him in farm products, such as potatoes and corn.[2]

Dr. Rucker was ordained as a Baptist minister in 1916, and he began his preaching career at Gallatin's First Baptist Church. He worked hard to build up the church. Through an innovative fund raising campaign, Rucker offered bricks "for sale" for five cents each and funded a new building and baptismal pool. Rucker was also the minister at nearby Durham's Chapel Baptist Church, where working alongside him as a teacher at Durham's Chapel school was his new wife, Fannie M. Ross Rucker. The couple had met years before while attending youth activities at church in Natchez. After they were married in June 1916, she joined him in Gallatin where they started a family.[3]

Military Service

Rucker's busy but relatively peaceful life in Gallatin changed dramatically when the United States officially entered the First World War on April 6, 1917. Soon after the declaration of war, the American government urged doctors to enlist and help with the war effort. Rucker was one of 43 Meharry-educated physicians and dentists who responded to this call. The army sent him to Fort Des Moines' Medical Officers Training Camp (MOTC).

After basic training, Lieutenant Rucker was assigned to the 92nd Division at Camp Funston, Kansas. He worked there in the 317th Sanitary (Medical) Train's infirmary before joining the division's 317th Motor Supply Train. By June 1918, his division set sail from New York to Brest, France. It traveled by military convoy on a large troopship, and there was constant fear of surprise attacks by German submarines. Rucker's convoy arrived safely in Brest in mid–July 1918. He was serving as the unit's only black officer under the command of Captain John N. Douglas. He was joined later by a black dentist and a chaplain. Lieutenant Rucker and his medical detachment cared for the 500 men of the motor supply train.

According to Captain Douglas' diary, "After arrival in Brest, the division marched up from the port several miles to a miserable 'rest camp' called Camp Pontanezen, an old and foul place with buildings dating from the time of Napoleon. They were cold, dank and fetid." They were soon moved eastward across France by railroad toward the battlefields of the Western Front in Lorraine. In mid–August, Rucker's 92nd Division suffered its first casualty in Epinal, when a truck driver fell victim to a German air raid. By the end of August, the division engaged in its first real combat in the trenches of the St. Dié sector of the Vosges Mountains in eastern France. Then, during September 1918, the soldiers were busy with massive divisional supply duties associated with the great Meuse-Argonne Offensive that was launched late in the month.

A month before the armistice on November 11, 1918, the 92nd "Buffalo" Division joined other units for a major attack on the city of Metz, a German stronghold. By the war's end, although the division had suffered more than 1,647 casualties in France, Rucker proudly wrote in an official report that there had been no deaths in his 317th Motor Supply Train. Despite many illnesses, injuries and hardships, Rucker had helped his men avoid any fatalities. He also provided another service. As a trained minister, Rucker took an interest in attending to his men's spiritual needs and often led and participated in Bible studies with his fellow soldiers.[4]

On February 15, 1919, Rucker and his medical detachment left France. After a year and a half in the army, Rucker was honorably discharged and returned to his family in Gallatin, Tennessee. For the rest of his life, he remained proud of his service with the Buffalo Division. For many years, every November 11 for Armistice Day, Rucker would don his army uniform and display it to the students in his school. It provided an opportunity to educate them about the Great War.[5]

Career

A new family member awaited his homecoming. His wife had given birth to their first child, Stella Adell Rucker, on December 20, 1918, while Rucker was still serving in France. The couple would have five more children: Jonathan N. Jr. (1920), John Ross (1921), and Joseph W. (1922), Benny Ferrell (1926) and Fannie Evelyn Mae (1930).

After his return from France, the Gallatin Board of Education asked him to become principal at the local Union High School.[6] He worked on the facility for many years. First, he expanded Union High academically, extending it from eight grades to twelve. Next, in order to accommodate the additional students, Rucker worked tirelessly and expanded the building itself. The cost of the new building was more than $17,000. Public funds provided $10,000 and the Rosenwald Fund contributed about $2,000.[7] The remaining $5,800 had to be raised by the African American community in Gallatin. Using the same method as he had for expanding the First Baptist Church, Rucker began a fund-raising campaign selling bricks. That technique raised the needed funds to complete the new school.

In addition to expanding the school building, Rucker secured funds to purchase a school bus. Because there was only enough money to buy the bus, Rucker personally paid for all of its servicing and repairs throughout the years. The bus carried students, and it transported the church choir, football team, basketball team, and many other community organizations.

Rucker changed the Union High School curriculum, adding new classes and programs. He also approached the president of Tennessee Agricultural and Industrial State College for two students to teach agricultural classes at Union High. The new courses taught students the science of cultivating crops and raising farm animals, incredibly important topics to the rural Gallatin community. An industrial teacher was also brought on staff at Union High. He taught masonry work, woodworking and automobile repair.[8]

Lastly, Rucker understood the importance of athletic activities. Although Union did not have a football field on campus, he managed to build up a successful football program. He negotiated with prominent African American members of the community who owned a large fairground and secured a space for the Union football team to practice and play. The fairground's bleachers, grandstand, and field were filled with football fans and the team when it was time for games. Rucker also built up a successful school basketball team. He approached the town's most prosperous tobacco producers and asked permission to use a local tobacco barn for a basketball court. The school only needed to provide the baskets.[9]

He later recalled with pride the many successful students who had graduated during his time as principal. Rucker noted in 1966 that the current principal was "one of my graduates," as well as nearly all the African American teachers in the Sumner County area. "I also baptized the principal."[10]

Dr. Rucker was a tireless community activist. In the Jim Crow South, Tennessee voters had to pay a poll tax in order to cast their ballot. Son John Ross recalled, "My dad fought the poll tax for years, knowing that many of the Negroes and minorities in the community could not afford it." Rucker also found ways to deal with local segregation laws. During the 1920s, whites in Gallatin decided to provide a place where African Americans could attend films at the neighborhood movie theater, but they were required to enter through the back door and view the movie from an upstairs balcony. To enable local African Americans to avoid it, Rucker purchased his own movie projector for the community's use. John Rucker recalled, "Each Friday and Saturday, [at] some place in the community there was going to be a movie."[11]

In 1930, Dr. Rucker's wife of 13 years died in childbirth. His mother, Mary Ardella Rucker, moved up from Natchez to help raise his children. The family needed more room so they moved to a farm just east of the city near the Durham Chapel Baptist Church where he pastored. The 14-room farmhouse was a busy place. In addition to the family, the Ruckers took in young men to work the farm and be educated.

The next year, Rucker remarried. His new wife, Elverlina Vertrees, was the daughter of Reverend Peter Vertrees, the former pastor at the First Baptist Church. She was a Gallatin native and a graduate of Union High School where Rucker was principal. She was also an accomplished music teacher. She gave birth to the last four of Rucker's ten children, Ellington (1933), Ina Claire (1935), Sandra Elaine (1946), and James Leach (1949).

Throughout the 1930s, Rucker continued his medical practice, ran the high school, preached, and became a very accomplished farmer. In the Gallatin community he pursued innovative methods and strongly believed in the cooperation of local farmers. He continuously experimented with crops, raising various kinds of corn and several types of fruit trees like pecan, pear, and peach that were usually only grown in more southern areas like Mississippi.

Rucker encouraged local farmers to form collaborative relationships in order to make sure Gallatin farms ran more easily and efficiently. He urged farmers to help each other during harvest season, reducing the need to hire extra help. Rucker was also instrumental in convincing farmers to grow sorghum, a type of crop similar to sugar came that could be used to feed livestock or as a food for families during the winter. After the farmers harvested the sorghum, the community would come together and work to prepare the sorghum and make it into molasses. They would then distribute this syrup among the farmers and their families. His son John Ross recalled, "Every year, around Thanksgiving ... a number of farmers would come to my dad's farm and they'd bring all the hogs they were going to kill. Sometimes there would be 15 or 16 hogs that the farmers would get together and kill, and dress out. Each farmer left that day with his meat supply for the winter."[12]

In 1938, Dr. Rucker almost died from a ruptured appendix. He was rushed 35 miles to the closest hospital in Nashville, and doctors at Meharry Medical were able to save his life by performing an appendectomy. This traumatic experience made Rucker aware of the dire need for an emergency care facility in Gallatin. Soon after, he opened a four-bed clinic there that could help people in need of immediate care. Shortly after that, in 1938–39, there was a fire at his office in Gallatin. Five years later, another incident shook the Rucker family. In 1943 a devastating fire destroyed their 14-room family farmhouse and almost all of their possessions, including the Bible that had been in the family since 1823.

The next year Rucker moved his family back to his hometown, Natchez, where his mother lived. She returned when he remarried.

He opened his medical practice in lively downtown Natchez. Mary Louise Mingee worked for him there for 15 years. She described Rucker as a respected community leader, known for his intelligence and shrewdness. She observed Rucker's kindness to the poor and his importance as a community leader, despite the racial discrimination he faced as an African American.[13] Rucker rented a building with his medical clinic located in the front and living quarters for his family in the rear. This location was good for his business because the nearby tavern and pool hall supplied Rucker with injured patients from evening altercations.

Rucker's practice remained constantly busy, and after a few years he relocated across the street to a larger facility. At the same time, the family moved into a larger house in a nearby residential neighborhood. With new space, Rucker established a four-bed clinic for patients who needed overnight care. The new office also contained a small pharmacy so Rucker could dispense his own medicine to his patients, saving them a substantial amount of money. Many of Rucker's patients were poor and paid for their visits and medicine in kind, either with farm produce or by providing labor. His clinic was very important because in those years African American physicians were not accorded privileges at the Natchez Hospital. If his patients required hospitalization, then they had to be attended by white physicians.

He became the pastor at three churches, Rose Hill Baptist Church, St. Mark Baptist Church, and St. Paul Baptist Church. Rose Hill Baptist Church was the largest of the three and the oldest black Baptist congregation in the state of Mississippi. His wife Elverlina led the church's choir and learned to play its pipe organ.

As a minister, Rucker promoted and organized church and community activities. He encouraged revivals, which he held usually two or three times a year at his churches. Rucker also created and became president of his local Black Ministers' Alliance, which met regularly to discuss ways to improve the welfare of the Natchez African American community.[14]

After the passing of his mother in Natchez in the early 1950s the Rucker family moved back to the Nashville area in 1959, where he became the minister of the First Baptist Church of East Nashville. Rucker continued his medical practice and became the resident physician at the Monterey Nursing Home, and a physician for students of the American Baptist Theological Seminary. He also maintained his medical office on the town's Main Street.

In 1964 fellow doctors from the Meharry Medical College presented Rucker with a 50-year "Service to Mankind" Award. Furthermore, a 1966 edition of the *Nashville Banner* newspaper underscored the achievements and uniqueness of Dr. Rucker, "he remains an almost extinct species—the physician who will respond to home calls."

Dr. Rucker continued his leadership roles

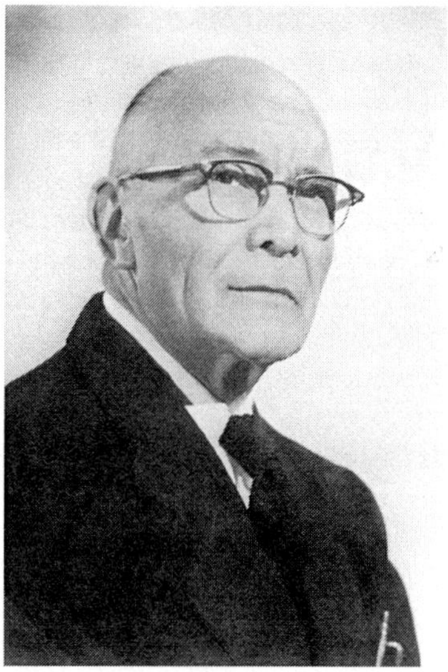

Dr. Jonathan N. Rucker, D.D., M.D. (courtesy the Rucker family).

in Nashville. Throughout the 1960s he was a chaplain of the Nashville City Council and frequently worked with the mayor, Clifton Beverly Briley. At the height of the Civil Rights Movement, Rucker remained a moderate and had many white friends and patients. Though his children did not heed his instructions, Rucker discouraged them from attending the sit-ins in Nashville because of his concern for their safety.[15]

In 1970 after a lifetime of achievements, Jonathan Rucker died of a stroke brought on by high blood pressure and diabetes. People from all over Nashville, Gallatin, and Natchez attended his funeral at the First Baptist Church. He is buried in Gallatin Cemetery alongside his wife of almost 40 years, Elverlina. The gravesite contains a marker from the U.S. government recognizing his military service in France during World War I. The granite headstone also bears the inscription "They shall mount up with wings as eagles" from the Bible verse Isaiah 40:31.

In addition to his accomplishments in farming, military service, church service, medicine, and community leadership, one of Rucker's most lasting legacies are his children. The proud and loving father of 10 children, he managed to send all of them to college, despite tight economic circumstances. His son John Ross recalled that the family "never had any money, but we had everything we needed." Owing in large part to their father's hard work, the children had the ability to enter a variety of important professions, including medicine, education, science, business, military service, community service, and law.

This distinguished African American man was a physician, minister, soldier, patriot, educator, farmer, father, and community activist. Living virtually his entire life in the South, Dr. Rucker touched the lives of thousands of people.

NOTES

1. www.mmc.edu/MeharryHistory.htm (accessed in 2001).
2. Velma Howell Brinkley and Mary Huddleston Malone, *Generations: A Pictorial Journey into the Lives of African Americans in Sumner County, Tennessee 1796–1996* (Nashville: Morgan Publications, 1996), 174.
3. "Marriages," *Meharry News*, July 1926, Vol. 14 No. 3.
4. Russell S. Brown, *YMCA No. 11 (Colored Service)*, March 9, 1918, Jesse Moorland Papers, Box 126–72, Howard University Manuscript Archives, Washington, D.C.
5. Personal interviews and correspondence in 2000 and 2001 with his son, John Ross Rucker, of Detroit, Michigan.
6. Velma Howell Binkley and Mary Huddleston Malone, *African American Life in Sumner County*, Images of America (Mount Pleasant, SC: Arcadia, 1998) 9–10, 13, 18–19, 33, 56, 124.
7. Julius Rosenwald (1862–1932) was an American merchant and philanthropist who became head of Sears, Roebuck & Co. and gave immense sums to philanthropic projects, especially for the education of African Americans. He founded the Rosenwald Fund in 1917 with the purpose of improving rural education, especially in the South, developing leadership among black and white Southerners through fellowships, and facilitating advanced education and health among African Americans.
8. Personal interviews conducted with John Ross Rucker in 2000–2001.
9. *Ibid.*
10. Churchwell, Robert, "*Highlights of Dr. Rucker's Active Career...*," *Nashville Banner*, September 2, 1966, Tennessee State Archives.
11. Personal interviews conducted with John Ross Rucker in 2000–2001.
12. *Ibid.*
13. Personal interviews conducted with Mary Louise Mingee, October 1–3, 2002 in Robbins, Illinois.
14. *Ibid.*
15. Personal interviews conducted with Dr. Joseph W. Rucker and James Leach Rucker in Nashville, Tennessee, November 2000.

George Lincoln SAMUELS

12 January 1884–14 January 1970
Meharry Medical College, 1909

Roots and Education

Samuels was born to Isaac and Jane Samuels in Bloomington, Illinois. His father, Isaac, was born on a farm in Nelson County, Kentucky, in about 1838 and had a most unusual history. Isaac was interested in more than farming. On August 27, 1864, at age 25, he enlisted in the U.S. Army and was assigned to the Union army's 5th U.S. Colored Cavalry (USCC). He participated in Burbridge's Raid from Kentucky into Southwestern Virginia between September 20–October 17, 1864.

The "Raid" included the first battle of Saltville, Virginia, as part of the Union forces under the command of General Stephen Gano Burbridge. Despite valiant attempts to break through Confederate lines, the cavalry was repeatedly repulsed. The battle became a defeat for the Union forces and, in the ensuing hours after its finish, a scene of criminal violence. Union injured, notably members of the 5th USCC, were murdered in their hospital beds by Confederate partisans.[1]

Private Samuels' army records show he and his unit saw more action at Lexington, Kentucky, on October 19 and Harrodsburg, Kentucky, on October 21.

In December 1864 Union general George Stoneman ordered the 5th USCC from western Kentucky to join in a raid from east Tennessee into southwestern Virginia. "Stoneman's Raid" involved moving the 5th USCC from Hopkinsville, Kentucky, on December 12 to Kingsport, Tennessee, on December 13. Then the Battle of Marion near Marion, Virginia, followed on December 17 and 18, and the second Battle of Saltville and destruction of the salt works on December 20 and 21. All were considered Union victories.[2]

Private Isaac Samuels' records indicate he continued service with the 5th USCC at Ghent, Paducah, LaGrange, Crab Orchard and Camp Nelson until August 1865, and then went into the army's Department of Arkansas until March 1866. He mustered out there on March 20, 1866.

Isaac returned north to Bloomington, Illinois, married Jane, and in 1884 their son George was born. Isaac still wasn't ready to settle for a small farm. He must have remembered the Arkansas land he saw while in the army—all that land near the Mississippi River and so few people. When the Oklahoma Land Rush was being organized, Isaac wanted in on it. His Civil War veteran status likely helped him qualify to register for it. No African Americans were included on the first day, but there was plenty of land for those who followed in the days afterward.

"The opening day was April 22, 1889, and it dawned bright and clear upon the hordes, an estimated fifty thousand strong, that surrounded the 'Unassigned Lands.' As noon approached, horsemen and wagons crowded forth to positions on the line, among them a few hardy women. Because of the social constraints of the day, few African Americans would be found at the front, though many came in immediately behind the initial rush and were rightfully 'Eighty-niners.'"[3]

Isaac Samuels ended up with 160 acres in the Deep Fork Township near the Deep Fork River close to what is today Dewey, Oklahoma. His wife Jane and son George joined him there. The 1900 U.S. Census lists the three of them on the farm. George was 16 at the time. His grandfather joined the family later and his parents adopted a daughter, Matilda Richardson Samuels. George was sent away to the east for a few years to be educated, but returned to Oklahoma.

In 1903 at the age of 19, George Samuels married. He and his wife Mary lived in Oklahoma until he entered Meharry Medical College in Nashville, Tennessee. The couple then lived in Nashville until he graduated in 1909. They returned to Oklahoma briefly where he established a practice in Luther, a small town about 25 miles from Oklahoma City. Future prospects there appeared limited. The next year they moved to Alton, Illinois.[4] Alton is a small city located on the banks of the Mississippi River about 20 miles north of St. Louis, Missouri. Its population was 30,000 people, of whom 25 percent were African American. During the early 20th century, the city's economy included heavy industry with a major steel company and glass bottle manufacturing. Dr. Samuels was Alton's first African American physician.

He and Mary boarded initially in 1912 they purchased a home at 1928 Marilla Street in Alton. By 1915 he was president of the NAACP branch in Alton. They joined the Union Baptist Church and in 1916 their only son, George Jr., was born.

Military Career

Dr. Samuels was 33 years old with a medical office at 405 Belle Street in Alton when he volunteered for service in the Medical Officers Reserve Corps. After 74 days of basic training at Fort Des Moines and 12 days of duty at Camp Funston, Kansas, Lieutenant Samuels was honorably discharged from the army November 13, 1917. The reason for his discharge is not reflected in military records. Several doctors were honorably discharged for medical reasons, for compassionate reasons relating to family or were judged unsuitable for overseas service. Whatever the reason, Dr. Samuels returned to Alton, his family, his practice and his community.

Career

In addition to his growing his practice, the good doctor must have also enjoyed writing because during the 1930s he wrote a column for the *Chicago Defender* about the social activities of Alton's African American community. The events he included in the column ranged from Miss Lois Manns surprising her mother with a birthday party, to a list of the delegates to the State Democratic Convention.[5]

In 1936 Samuels was one of the founders of the Booker Washington Center in Alton. This facility, with its large hall, kitchenette and a committee room, was a gathering place for the African American community. He served as the center's president for many years.[6]

Dr. Samuels took time from his practice in the early 1940s to pursue post-graduate work at Meharry and while involved in that program, he was elected president of the school's post-graduate department.[7]

The *Chicago Defender* reported on his activities in the Illinois State Medical Society and wrote about his travels. When he attended a state medical society meeting in 1943, the *Defender* described him as "a prominent physician and surgeon of Alton and who is known for his outstanding work in scientific medical and surgery work."[8] In 1945, the newspaper named him as one of the alumni aiding the building program at Meharry.[9]

The Negro Business Men's Association contributed to a host of African American community organizations in Alton—March of Dimes, the library fund, Girl Scout Camp fund, Boy Scout Trip No. 51 and books for the library. Dr. Samuels was involved in the leadership of the organization and served as its president for several years.[10]

His many civic activities included the George Washington Education Fund. The fund educated more than 200 students and supported seven schools. It was Dr. Samuels who led the 1950 memorial services for its founder.[11]

Samuels was justifiably proud of his son who graduated from Fisk University in Nashville and the Howard University College of Pharmacy in Washington, D.C. His son became a druggist and then a chemist for the largest African American solo-owned and operated manufacturing company in St. Louis, Missouri, Belva Manufacturing Co. The company made Hair-Rep oils, "the finest oils for Negroes' hair." Belva had a staff of black chemists "who know what it takes for Negroes' hair."[12]

Meharry recognized Dr. Samuels' contributions to his alma mater and medicine. In 1959 Samuels was presented with Meharry's "President Award" recognizing his 50 years of service.

Dr. Samuels died on January 14, 1970, at the Eunice Smith Nursing Home in Alton. He was 86 years old and succumbed to metastatic carcinoma of the prostate and multiple myeloma (cancer). He was buried in Alton Cemetery with a military headstone. Samuels had made a real difference to his adopted hometown. He not only reported on the activities of Alton's African American community, he was always involved in making changes to improve the lives of its citizens.

NOTES

1. en.wikipedia.org/wiki/5th_United_States_Colored_Cavalry (accessed September 21, 2013).
2. *Ibid.*
3. digital.library.okstate.edu/encyclopedia/entries/l/la014.html (accessed September 21, 2013).
4. "Obituary, Mrs. Mary Samuels," *Alton Evening Telegraph*, September 29, 1953.
5. "Alton, ILL.," *Chicago Defender*, August 24, 1935, 19.
6. "Booker Washington Center Anniversary," *Alton Evening Telegraph*, July 22, 1941, 2.
7. *Ibid.*, "Dr. Samuels Returns," June 13, 1942, 2.
8. "Attends Meet," *Chicago Defender*, November 14, 1943, 2.
9. "Alumni Who Aid Building Fund to Get Meharry Pins," *Chicago Defender*, April 14, 1945, 14.
10. "Negro Business Men Re-Elect All Officers for Year," *Alton Evening Telegraph*, February 5, 1947.
11. "Slave, Master Join in Rare Friendship," *Chicago Defender*, May 20, 1950, 14.
12. "Two of Leading Salesmen," *Atlanta Daily World*, August 12, 1941, 2.

Egbert Theophilus SCOTT

12 March 1884–4 December 1969
Leonard Medical School, 1913

Roots and Education

Scott came from a large, successful family in Wilmington, North Carolina. His father,

Benjamin Franklin Scott, was a grocer from Virginia. They lived at 519 Walnut Street only four blocks from Market Street, one of the city's main arteries.[1] His mother, Miriam Scott, taught at Williston, the local African American high school.[2] The school was the leading school in that part of North Carolina and a major social center for the local African American community.

The parents saw to it that all six children were well educated. Two brothers, Armond W. Scott and Thomas A. Scott, settled in Washington, D.C. Armond worked his way through Biddle University in Charlotte and Shaw University in Raleigh, where he earned his law degree. He opened a law practice briefly in Wilmington, but moved quickly to Washington, D.C., following the 1898 race riots in Wilmington. Armond practiced law in Washington for many years and in 1935 President Franklin Roosevelt appointed him to a judgeship in the District of Columbia. He served through the Truman and Eisenhower Administrations and became known as the dean of the D.C. Municipal Court. Brother Thomas worked for the railroad as a porter and waiter. Another brother, Arthur S. Scott, also a Biddle University graduate, operated a garage in Philadelphia. A fourth brother, Robert H. Scott, was an undertaker in Wilmington.[3] A fifth brother, Alfred Scott, became a national president of the prestigious Omega Psi Phi fraternity.[4]

Like several of his older brothers, Egbert Scott worked his way through Biddle University (now Johnson C. Smith University) in Charlotte, North Carolina. He graduated in 1909 with an arts and sciences degree. He was always an active alumnus and 50 years after his graduation he was presented with the Alumni Certificate of Merit at the annual alumni reception at the university's 1959 commencement exercises.[5]

After following his brother to Biddle, young Scott then went to Raleigh and Shaw University's Leonard Medical College. Leonard's white president, Charles F. Meserve, described the school's goal as training the "Consecrated, Skillful, Christian Physician.... Not *self*, but race must ever be his motto, and this requires not ability alone but the most rugged and strongest character."[6] There was no liquor or use of tobacco allowed on the grounds. During Scott's four years at Leonard, a new hospital was added and laboratories greatly improved. He was awarded his M.D. in 1913.

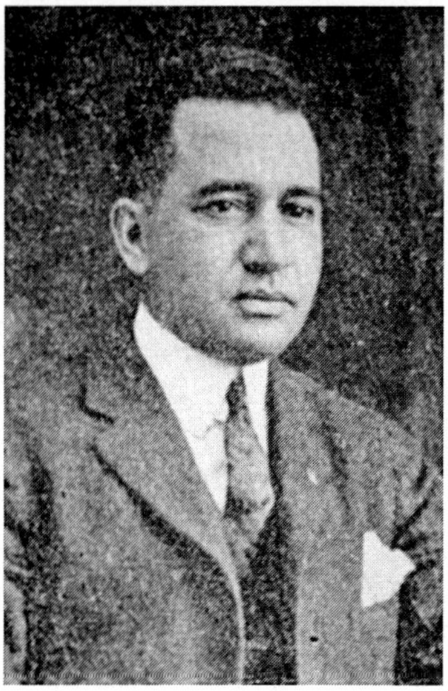

Dr. Egbert T. Scott (national pictorial, members of the National Medical Association, 1925, courtesy Kansas City Public Library).

After graduation, Dr. Scott interned in Washington, D.C., for a year at Freedmen's Hospital. It was very difficult for African American physicians to find hospitals for internships. Freedmen's had been established by the U.S. Government following the Civil War to provide care for freed, disabled and aged blacks. It was a teaching hospital and provided clinical education and training to future doctors.

In February 1914 Scott paid a visit to Philadelphia. The *Tribune*'s society page reported a young woman hosted an informal reception there in his honor before he returned to D.C.[7] Upon completing his internship in 1914, he moved to Philadelphia to establish a practice, and he worked at Mercy Hospital. Mercy had been established in 1905 for African Americans and was very important to that community in Philadelphia.

Military Service

Scott had only been in Philadelphia a short time when the United States entered the First World War. He volunteered for service in the Army Medical Reserve Corps in 1917 and received a commission as a first lieutenant. Lieutenant Scott was assigned to the Medical Officers Training Camp (MOTC) at Fort Des Moines, Iowa, where he received 70 days of training. He was then assigned to Camp Dix, New Jersey, with the 350th Field Artillery of the 92nd "Buffalo" Division.[8] At the same time, he was elected to membership in the Association of Military Surgeons in October 1917.[9]

In 1918 Dr. Scott saw active service with the 92nd Division in France. He served as medical doctor for the First Battalion of the 350th Field Artillery with fellow Fort Des Moines graduate, Dr. Arthur D. Browne. The care of the officers and men of the 1st Battalion was his primary responsibility. Although his unit arrived in June 1918, weeks of specialized training at the artillery school in La Courtine meant it was only able to support the infantry in combat during the closing months of the war, October and November. The combat casualties experienced by artillery units were far lighter than those of the infantry. Scott and his fellow doctors remained busy dealing primarily with sanitation issues, preventing disease, and treating disease and injuries rather than many wounds from air attacks, gas, machine guns or shrapnel. A field hospital report noted that only seven cases of gas poisonings in the last half of October 1918 happened in the artillery units, while the infantry suffered 210 cases during the same period.[10]

Influenza, pneumonia, lice, trench foot, trench fever and venereal disease were major problems. In fact, division troops suffered far more casualties from disease than from enemy action. The wide variety of organizational and health-related experiences Scott saw certainly made him a more effective physician when he returned home to America.

Captain Scott served in the U.S. Army Reserve in the 1920s and eventually was promoted to lieutenant colonel. He was proud of his service and maintained his military connections and interests long after he was discharged in New York on March 17, 1919.

He was a Charter Member of the American Legion "George T. Cornish Post" in Philadelphia, named for a Corporal Cornish who

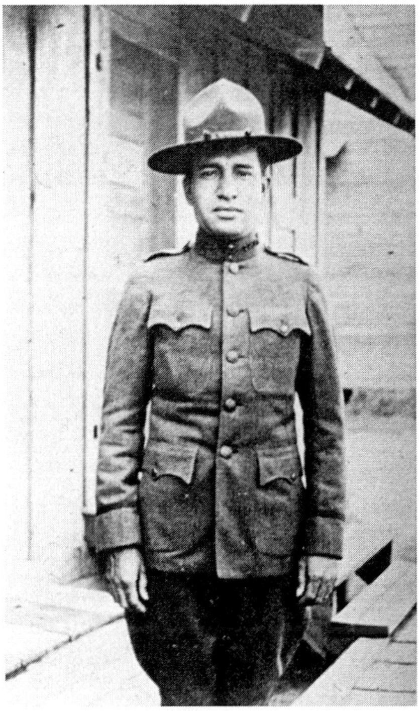

Lieutenant Egbert T. Scott (Betty Ann Davis Lawrence, *Philadelphia African Americans: Color, Class, and Style*, courtesy Hal S. Chase, Fort Des Moines Museum and Education Center).

lost his life in the Meuse-Argonne. The post was formed shortly after World War I, and Dr. Scott remained active with the Legion for many years. He served as the post's historian in the 1930s.

During the 1930s Dr. Scott was also an active member of the United War Veterans Organization of Philadelphia County. It was organized in 1933 to help local veterans with job opportunities, medical and dental care, and disability pensions.[11]

In 1933 the Scott family hosted a dinner party in honor of Benjamin Oliver Davis, Jr., a sophomore at West Point and the son of Colonel Benjamin O. Davis, Sr., of the Tuskegee Institute.[12] Cadet Davis would graduate from West point in 1936 and later command the famous Tuskegee airmen of the Second World War, and become the first African American four-star general in the U.S. Air Force.

In 1937 when enrollment applications were being solicited for 200 persons for a Citizens Military Training Camp (CMTC) at Fort

Howard, Maryland, Dr. Scott's name was one of five physicians, all commissioned officers of the Medical Reserve, who volunteered to conduct physical examinations and give inoculations free of charge to all candidates.[13] His devotion to his country and its veterans never waned.

Career

After the First World War, Dr. Scott resumed his general medical practice in Philadelphia and worked on the surgical staff at Mercy Hospital. He became an important leader at the hospital. In 1934 he attended the American Hospital Association (AHA) Convention in Philadelphia as a representative of Mercy Hospital. The AHA (white) and National Hospital Association (black) were cooperating on a survey with a view to standardizing hospitals.[14] In 1936 when Philadelphia's Mayor Wilson made an inspection tour of Mercy Hospital, Scott was called upon to explain the workings of his outpatient department. He made an excellent impression, and the mayor publically praised the hospital as equal to white hospitals.[15]

Dr. Scott was a pioneering surgeon at Mercy Hospital and worked closely with the superintendent. He also served as medical director and chief of Out-Patient Services at Mercy for 25 years. Mercy was only the second hospital formed to serve Philadelphia's African American community.[16] The Douglass Hospital had been formed 10 years earlier in 1895. Mercy eventually merged with its sister hospital to become Mercy-Douglass in 1948. It survived until 1973 when, after integration, it was no longer needed.

Scott played an active and important consulting role in the 1948 merger.[17] He continued as a senior surgeon and medical supervisor of the out-patient department at Mercy-Douglass Hospital for many more years. The merged hospital was vital to the African American community in Philadelphia and was described in 1951 as serving a huge community of 130,000 people, as well as being involved in medical research and the training of physicians and nurses.[18]

By 1921 he had joined the Philadelphia Medical Society. His professional memberships also included the American Medical Association (AMA), National Medical Association (NMA), Association of Military Surgeons of the United States, and the Society of Clinical Pathology.

Scott was also extremely involved in his community and maintained memberships in a number of fraternal organizations including the Masons, Odd Fellows, Elks, and Alpha Phi Alpha.[19] In the mid–1930s he worked in support of political activities of the local NAACP and the Democratic Party. He was a vestryman at the St. Thomas Episcopal Church at 52nd and Parrish streets.

He married Miss Ida Davis in the mid–1920s and by 1930 they had two children, Egbert Jr. and Jeanne. The family lived at 623 North 57th Street.[20] In 1935 Mrs. Scott was president of the Ladies Auxiliary of the Church of the Beloved Disciple at 57th and Vine, Philadelphia.[21] By 1940, with two teen-age children at home, she worked as a visiting social worker.[22] The couple was active in the city's African American community. Local newspapers from the 1930s to the 1960s frequently mention Dr. and Mrs. Scott as participants in variety of civic and social events.

In June 1944 he was one of 11 physicians honored by Mercy Hospital at a formal banquet at the Pyramid Club of Philadelphia with a Certificate of Merit for 25 years of service.[23]

By 1961, as he entered retirement, Dr. Scott was still listed as "Emeriti" by the Hospital. In 1963 he was honored by the Pennsylvania Medical Society for his 50 years of service as a physician.

When Dr. Scott passed away at the age of 85 in 1969, his obituary made the front page of the *Philadelphia Tribune*. It carried his photograph and the headline read: "Dr. Egbert Scott, Old Mercy Hospital Head, Dead at 85." The four-column article outlined his life of service. He died at Mercy-Douglass Hospital after a lengthy illness, and was interred at Eden Cemetery at Collingdale in Philadelphia. He was survived by his wife, Mrs. Ida Davis Scott, his son, Egbert Jr., his daughter, Jeanne, and four grandchildren.[24]

His death was also reported in Baltimore's *Afro-American* newspaper. The American Medical Association's report of his death said he died of congestive heart failure, uremia, and renal failure.[25] With Dr. Scott's passing, the city of Philadelphia and the nation lost an outstanding patriot, and a good and caring citizen.

NOTES

1. 1900 U.S. Federal Census.
2. "Mayor Moore to Welcome Mme. Jarboro," *Philadelphia Tribune*, November 23, 1933, 3.
3. "Arthur Scott Is a Victim of Heart Attack," *Philadelphia Tribune*, May 19, 1938, 1.
4. *Philadelphia Tribune*, November 23, 1933, 3.
5. "GE Chemist Honored at J.C. Smith," *Philadelphia Tribune*, June 13, 1959, 2.
6. Todd L. Savitt, *Race & Medicine in Nineteenth- and Early-Twentieth-Century America* (Kent, OH: Kent State University, 2007), 169.
7. "Flashes and Sparks," *Philadelphia Tribune*, March 7, 1914, 5.
8. Table of Medical Reserve Corps—Colored—Receiving Instruction, Medical Training Camp, Fort Des Moines, Iowa, RG-112 Records of the Army Surgeon General, National Archives, College Park, MD.
9. "Recently Elected Members," *The Military Surgeon*, November 1917, Vol. XLI, No. 5, Proceedings of the Twenty-Fifth Annual Meeting, 546.
10. RG 120, Records of Combat Divisions, 1918–1919, 92nd Division, Field Hospital 366, 317th Sanitary Train, November 1, 1918, National Archives, College Park, MD.
11. "Veterans, Join Now!!" Display Ad, *Philadelphia Tribune*, October 27, 1938, 2.
12. "Philly Society," *Afro-American*, December 9, 1933, 7.
13. "Medics Offer Aid to CMTC Enrollees," *Philadelphia Tribune*, March 18, 1937, 20.
14. "Hospital League Meets in Philly," *Afro-American*, October 6, 1934, 14.
15. "Mayor Wilson Praises Mercy Hospital as Being Equal to Others After Inspection," *Philadelphia Tribune*, May 7, 1936, 3.
16. Russell F. Minton, MD, "The History of Mercy-Douglass Hospital," *Journal of the National Medical Association (JNMA)*, May 1951, Vol. 43, No. 3, 153–159.
17. "Hospital Merger Closer," *Philadelphia Tribune*, December 23, 1947, 1.
18. Russell F. Minton, MD, "The History of Mercy-Douglass Hospital," *Journal of the National Medical Association (JNMA)*, May 1951, Vol. 43, No. 3, 153–159.
19. Joseph J. Boris, *Who's Who in Colored America* (New York: Who's Who in Colored America Corp., 1944), 455.
20. 1930 U.S. Federal Census.
21. "Mt. Zion M.E. Church," *Philadelphia Tribune*, January 24, 1935, 15.
22. 1940 U.S. Federal Census.
23. "Mercy Medics Honored at Pyramid Club," *Philadelphia Tribune*, June 17, 1944, 3.
24. "Dr. Egbert Scott, Old Mercy Hospital Head, Dead at 85," *Philadelphia Tribune*, December 9, 1969, 1.
25. AMA Deceased Physician Card, National Library of Medicine, Bethesda, MD.

William Henry SMITH

16 February 1872–5 August 1946
Louisville National Medical College, 1898

Roots and Education

William Henry Smith was born in Louisville, Kentucky, to Henry and Mary (Davis) Smith. His parents were both born nearby in Nelson County, Kentucky. He was educated in the Louisville Public School system and graduated from Central High School and State University in Louisville. He married Ann Weathers in 1891 when he was only 19 years old. He later graduated from Louisville National Medical College (LNMC) in 1898.

LNMC was the best of the unaffiliated (not connected to a church or college) African American medical schools at this time in history. It grew out of three physicians—William Henry Fitzbutler, Rufus Conrad and William Burney—training medical students in their offices.[1] The three physician-trustees secured other nearby physicians (including Louisville graduates) as instructors. Every year new facilities were added to continually conform to nationally accepted standards—an auxiliary hospital, a lengthened course of study, tougher graduation requirements, increased lab and clinical exposure for students. The school graduated about five students a year.

National medical standards continued to be strengthened. Toward the end of its life, Louisville graduates had a high failure rate on state exams. Finally, a poor Flexner report and lack of funds brought about the demise of the institution. In 1912 Louisville National Medical College closed.[2] Over its 24-year life, it graduated 175 doctors.

African American doctors had a difficult time finding internships. Dr. Smith managed to find work as an intern at the Central Kentucky State Hospital for the Insane between 1900 and 1906. Not all its patients had mental disorders—some suffered from brain damage, mental retardation or were simply poor or elderly. Following his internship Dr. Smith practiced medicine in Louisville. His wife, Ann, died some time before the 1910 Census, which lists him as a widower living at 66 West Eleventh Street in Louisville.

Military Service

When America entered the war in 1917, Smith volunteered to serve in the U.S. Army

Medical Reserve Corps. He received a commission as a first lieutenant and was sent to Fort Des Moines for military training. He arrived there October 4, 1917, and finished 39 days of training on November 11, 1917, when he was sent to Camp Funston. He was assigned to the 317th Sanitary (Medical) Train of the 92nd Division and was attached to its 368th Field Hospital where he worked in the camp infirmary. At age 45 he was one of the two oldest African American physicians at Camp Funston. The other was Dr. Hosea J. Nichols (47). It is likely that their physical condition and age precluded them from overseas field service with the division. Both left the army in April 1918 shortly before their unit deployed to France. Smith's military service was brief (less than seven months) when he was declared "surplus" and honorably discharged in the spring of 1918.[3]

Career

After his discharge, Dr. Smith returned to Louisville and resumed his practice. He would practice medicine there for the rest of his life.[4] He appears in the American Medical Directory in 1923 and 1927 with his office in the grand Kentucky Pythian Temple building. The Temple in Louisville, also known as Chestnut Street Branch-YMCA, was designed by Henry Wolters and built in 1914. It was listed on the National Register of Historic Places in 1978. The ideals of loyalty, honor and friendship are the centerpiece of the Pythian order.

Dr. Smith was personally involved in a number of professional medical organizations. He was a member of the National Medical Association (NMA), the Kentucky State Medical, Dental and Pharmaceutical Association, and the local Louisville Fall City Medical Society. He also became medical examiner for a large number of fraternal organizations, including the Knights of Pythias, the Atlanta Life Insurance Co. and the Court of Calanthe. His other fraternal organizations included the Masons, Elks, Odd Fellows and American Woodmen. He identified himself as a Baptist. Politically, he was a Republican as were most members of his community at that time. He was a member of the NAACP.

As early as the 1870s, Louisville had an established African American community of 15,000 and segregation in Louisville was entrenched there until well after the Second World War. It existed throughout Smith's entire lifetime. African Americans who required hospitalization received treatment in a segregated hospital known as the Red Cross Hospital (Colored). It was established in 1900 and by 1929 it had 30 beds, 4 bassinets and a school of nursing.

On February 19, 1924, Dr. Smith married Belle Wilson. They had one son, Haywood Smith. Their residence was at 2420 W. Madison Street, and his office was then at 555 South 10th Street. Subsequent residences and office addresses are listed in a number of Louisville city directories and American Medical Directories from 1918 to 1942. In 1935 the *Chicago Defender* reported his wife was quite ill and had been confined at home for some time. She apparently passed away that year. In late 1936, the *Defender* reported Dr. Smith, a "well-known physician," married Miss Thelma J. Samuels.[5]

When he died 10 years later at the age of 74, Dr. Smith had served his Louisville community as a physician for more than 40 years. He died of prostate cancer at the Nichols V.A. General Hospital in Louisville. Nichols was located at Conn and Manslick roads in southern Jefferson County, where it was operated by the U.S. Army Medical Department from November 1942 until March 31, 1946. On April 1, 1946, the army hospital turned the facility over to the Veterans Administration where it was designated "Nichols V.A. Hospital," and operated until April 2, 1952.

Dr. Smith is buried at the Zachary Taylor National Cemetery in Louisville where his tombstone reads, "1 LT U.S. ARMY WORLD WAR I."[6] His Kentucky death certificate lists his widow as Thelma Smith, age 43.

NOTES

1. Todd L. Savitt, *Race and Medicine in Nineteenth- and Early-Twentieth-Century America* (Kent, OH: Kent State University Press, 2007), 191.
2. *Ibid.*, 199.
3. RG 120, Records of the 92nd Division, 317th Sanitary Train, National Archives, College Park, MD.
4. Thomas Yenser, Editor, *Who's Who in Colored America*, Sixth Edition (New York, 1941), 475.

5. "Kentucky State News: Louisville News," *Chicago Defender*, September 7, 1935, 19 and September 19, 1936, 17.
6. U.S. Veterans Gravesites, ca. 1775–2006, ancestry.com.

Jackson (Jack) SMITHERMAN

29 July 1889–23 Apr 1949
Meharry Medical College, 1915

Roots and Education

Jack Smitherman was born in Birmingham, Alabama. His mother's maiden name was Mollie Coker. His father is not noted in any census records. Smitherman was educated in local Birmingham African American schools and went on to graduate from Selma University's Normal (Teachers) School. In 1912 he enrolled in Meharry Medical College, Nashville, Tennessee, and received his medical degree in 1915.

Oklahoma became a state in 1907. The newly created, Democrat-dominated state legislature passed racial segregation laws, commonly known as Jim Crow laws. Its 1907 constitution and laws had voter registration rules that disfranchised most blacks. This also barred them from serving on juries or in local office, a situation that lasted until Tulsa passed its own restrictions. On August 16, 1916, a city ordinance was enacted that forbade blacks or whites from residing on any block where three-fourths or more of the residents were of the other race. This made residential segregation mandatory in the city.[1]

In spite of the city's racial divide, Dr. Smitherman saw potential in a career there so in 1916 he relocated and worked to establish a medical practice there. Records show he was married to Laura Allen, had a small child, and his mother (Mollie) living with him at a rental property at 609 North Elgin Street. When the United States entered the First World War, he volunteered for the army's Medical Reserve Corps.

Military Service

First Lieutenant Smitherman reported for duty at the Medical Officers Training Camp in Des Moines on October 8, 1917. He was in training for 35 days before his transfer to Camp Funston, Kansas. There he was assigned to the 368th Field Hospital, 92nd Division. On May 1, 1918, Smitherman became ill and was judged "not fit for duty with the Field Hospital, on account of a diseased condition of the testicle, which makes attention to duty impossible." He was a patient in the infirmary two days later. After being treated, he recovered, returned to duty and was soon sent to France.

On September 6, 1918, as the military was preparing for the Meuse-Argonne offensive, Lieutenant Smitherman was transferred to the 368th Ambulance Company. Its ambulances were initially horse drawn and were responsible for transporting all sick and wounded within the divisional area from triage sites near the front line back to the field or gas hospitals.[2] Motorized ambulances were received just before the offensive, but the muddy bombed-out roads made all transport of soldiers and supplies difficult.

The offensive started on September 25, 1918, and the 368th Infantry was deeply involved in the early action and engaged on the left flank of the attack with the French army. They fought the Germans for several days near Binarville. In addition to working extraordinary hours with patients, the men of the 368th Ambulance Company had terrible living conditions. Those who could not be billeted with residents were housed in barns or whatever buildings were standing. The buildings were described as being dirty with human fecal matter on the floors and with no facilities for heat or light.[3] Smitherman saw the horrors of war first hand as he continued to serve with the 92nd Division until the end of the war. He returned with his unit to America in 1919 and was discharged.

Career

As cities absorbed returning veterans into the labor market following World War I, there was social tension and anti-black sentiment. At the same time, black veterans pushed to have their civil rights enforced, believing they had earned full citizenship by military service. The Ku Klux Klan was growing in urban areas. The economic slump after the war contributed to the KKK's popularity among whites. Dr. Smitherman experienced this white reaction after he returned to Tulsa while he worked to grow his practice until 1921.

On May 31 and June 1, 1921, more than 1,000 homes and businesses of African American residents of Tulsa were destroyed. The Greenwood District was known in Tulsa as "Black Wall Street." His office was upstairs at 122 North Greenwood Street. It likely did not survive the fires. At least 100 were killed during the Tulsa Race Riot. The city was placed under martial law.[4] Laura and Jackson Smitherman relocated to Los Angeles.

During the 1920s the Smithermans were doing well financially and socially in Los Angeles. In 1927 the *California Eagle* reported, "Dr. and Mrs. Smitherman are seen daily on the boulevard in their beautiful new Nash Victoria Coupe."[5] That same year, she entered the College of Music at the University of Southern California. He became active in the Southern California Medical, Dental and Pharmaceutical Association.

She took time to join with wives of other medical professionals to form the association's auxiliary. Its purpose was to bring the families of those in medicine together and assist in the production of any programs the association determined to develop. Mrs. Smitherman served as the auxiliary's first president.[6] Many of the programs were social. In 1932, for example, she hosted the auxiliary members for an evening of dancing and cards at the Appomattox Club.[7] The Los Angeles club was touted as the "finest Colored recreational club resort in the world."[8]

During the later 1930s, Dr. and Mrs. Smitherman continued with very active social lives. He was club physician and then an honorary member of the Ma-Po-Fi Social Club, a prestigious African American social club. The club's events usually included bridge and dancing. She was active on the Committee of Management of the Woodlawn Branch of the YWCA.

In August 1933 the couple was living at 215 East 45th Street in Los Angeles when Dr. Smitherman was entangled in a case of duplicity when a woman used him to "deliver" her baby. It was actually one of a set of twins delivered by Dr. Smitherman to another woman at the Los Angeles General Hospital. The woman's husband sued the wife, her accomplice friend, and the doctor for $25,000 in damages. The judgment was an award to the father for the humiliation he had suffered for a total of $1,500 from the three involved.[9]

In 1936 the doctor was involved in another controversy. The headlines ran "Society Doctor Hit by Charges." Smitherman was arrested and charged with an abortion on a 22-year-old white girl that resulted in her death.[10] In subsequent news of the arrest, he was described as "popular and debonair" and public opinion judged him innocent.[11] At the preliminary trial on December 26, the prosecution failed to attack a motion that charges be dismissed. The doctor was vindicated.[12]

The last seven years of his life during the 1940s proved to be very difficult. On February 12, 1943, Dr. Smitherman was remanded to San Quentin, California state prison, on a charge of second-degree murder (presumably following an abortion). His medical license was revoked on March 9, 1943.[13] He was eligible for release on parole on August 12, 1946. He died three years after his release while still on parole.

The Smithermans led a very active social life and certainly liked to show off their wealth. Unfortunately, he appears to have been involved in abortions and scams to pay for their lifestyle and eventually was caught and, in the end, lost everything.

NOTES

1. en.wikipedia.org/wiki/Tulsa_race_riot (accessed September 14, 1014).
2. RG 120, Records of the 92nd Division, Notes by Lieut. Col. J. S. White, MC, Division Surgeon, National Archives, College Park, MD.
3. RG 120, Records of the 92nd Division, "Condition of Billets," Field Hospital 368 memo to commanding officer by R. S. Kneeshaw, Capt MC, December 23, 1918, National Archives, College Park, MD.
4. Rudolph M. Lapp, *Afro-Americans in California* (New York, Boyd & Fraser, 1987) 43.
5. "Social Intelligence," *California Eagle*, September 16, 1927, 3.
6. Commodore Wynn, *Negro Who's Who in California* (California Publishing Co., 1948), 105.
7. "Los Angeles," *Chicago Defender*, June 4, 1932, 12.
8. content.cdlib/ark/1303/hb2870081f/?order=1 (accessed Sept 9, 2014).
9. "Fake Baby Story Costs Him $1500," *Afro-American*, March 3, 1934, 16.
10. "Society Doctor Hit by Charges," *Pittsburgh Courier*, December 19, 1936, 1.
11. "Sensational Case Stirs Coast," *Atlanta Daily World*, December 18, 1936, 1.
12. "Los Angeles Medic Freed," *Chicago Defender*, December 26, 1936.
13. AMA Deceased Physician Card, National Library of Medicine, Bethesda, MD.

Frederick Alexander STOKES

10 September 1873–25 August 1929
Indiana University, 1898

Roots and Education

Community service was at the core of the Stokes family. Frederick, born in Spartansburg, Indiana, next to the Ohio border, was the youngest son of the Reverend Lemuel Stokes, a well-known and popular minister of the AME Church of Indiana.[1] In 1907 at the AME annual conference, the Reverend Lemuel Stokes, 74, after 50 years of church work, asked to be relieved from further active duty.[2] Five years after his retirement, Rev. and Mrs. Lemuel Stokes celebrated their 50th wedding anniversary.[3]

In his early years Reverend Stokes was a clergyman in the Greenville Settlement in Randolph County in eastern Indiana near Ohio. It was a progressive community, home to a large number of members of the Society of Friends (Quakers).[4] Education and abolitionism were important movements within the community. Before the Civil War, it had three settlements of free African Americans (Cabin Creek, Greenville, and Snow Hill). The best known was the Greenville Settlement of 900 people in Greensfork Township. It was the site of the Union Literary Institute, one of the first racially integrated schools in the United States. Quakers and African Americans established the school in 1845, and it was chartered by the Indiana state legislature in 1847.[5]

That area is where Frederick Stokes was born. He received his earliest education at the old Quaker academy near his home. The family later moved to the town of Rockville, in the western part of the state, before finally settling in Indianapolis by the early 1890s. The family valued education. Frederick was close to his older brother, Edwin F. Stokes, who was an educator for more than 32 years in the Indianapolis public schools. In 1907 Edwin was Superintendent of the Flanner Guild Neighborhood House for the Industrial Training of Colored Boy and Girls.[6] Edwin Stokes' 1931 obituary described him as a pioneer in the manual training department. He was also a former trustee of the Bethel AME Church in Indianapolis. Edwin's wife, Eva McCullom Stokes, was a graduate of Wilberforce University and a teacher for many years.[7]

In 1880 at the age of 17, Fred Stokes followed his brother into teaching for two years. He then entered the pharmaceutical department of Purdue University in Lafayette and graduated in 1894. In 1894 the Atheneum Social and Literary Club was organized with "promising young physician" Fred A. Stokes as Secretary.[8] In 1895 he studied chemistry at the same university. In 1896 the erudite Stokes was a member of the board of directors of a group called "Indianapolis Literary."[9] After his postgraduate work in chemistry, he went to the Indiana Medical College in Indianapolis and graduated in 1898.[10]

Dr. Stokes' first medical appointment was as house physician at the Allen National Surgical Institute for eight months. The Institute, which had once been prominent, was then in receivership and had been taken over by the Indiana Medical College. From there he went to Terre Haute in early 1889 to establish a medical practice.[11] It could not have been very successful because he returned to Indianapolis the next year and took a government job in South Dakota on the Cheyenne River Indian Reservation.[12] The reservation was established by the U.S. government in the late 1800s to house a number of relocated Indian tribes.

In 1901 he returned to Indianapolis and opened a medical office at Senate Avenue and North Street.[13] He was entrepreneurial and that same year, before he had even turned 28, he opened a new drug store at 519 Indiana Avenue. It was described in a local newspaper as the only one in town owned by an African American.[14] He was later appointed house physician at the Indiana Home Hospital, and subsequently placed in charge of the Beech Grove Hospital branch of the Indiana Home Hospital. By 1907 the Indianapolis city directory lists him as a physician living at 1222 North Capitol Avenue with his elderly father and mother.

The city's African American newspaper *The Freeman* reported in May 1907 that Dr. Stokes had secured first place in a competitive U.S. Civil Service examination. He returned to the Cheyenne River Indian Reservation as its government physician.[15]

His wife, Zoe Jackson Stokes, was a teacher. She was born on April 23, 1877, in Washington, Ohio, near her husband's birthplace. She was the oldest child in a large family. They were married in Washington Court House in January 1907 at the AME Church and by spring were in South Dakota. While there, Frederick A. Stokes, Jr., was born in 1908.

Dr. Stokes served as a physician on Indian reservations for eight years from 1907 to 1915. In 1908 tuberculosis expert, Joseph A. Murphy, was hired to organize medical services for American Indians. In addition to tuberculosis, trachoma, an eye disease that led to blindness was also prevalent among the tribes. By 1909 trachoma had reached a crisis stage and the U.S. surgeon general told the commissioner of Indian Affairs that the disease was a distinct menace to the public health.

In 1912 President Wilson Howard Taft delivered a special address to Congress stressing that health conditions on Indian Reservations were very unsatisfactory. The president sought to increase the wages for Indian Service physicians, noting, "While there were efficient and self-sacrificing physicians in the Indian Department, 'the smallness of the salaries' which averaged about $1,186 per year (or less than half that of other government agencies) affected the qualifications and ability of the physicians employed by the Department."[16] Congress virtually ignored his request for a special appropriation of $253,350, granting the president only $90,000. This sad state of affairs was the environment of Stokes' medical job.

Stokes' expense reports to the Department of the Interior included basics like the cords of cottonwood and ash used to heat his home and clinic, or the various charges for care and feeding of his wagon team as he traveled in all weather to clinics or to schools to vaccinate Indian children. There is evidence of his frustration with his superintendent Thomas J. King for not understanding the need for meals or lodging when he occasionally was snowed in. One letter from Superintendent King, dated May 21, 1913, says, "There is enclosed herewith Treasury Warrant No 468 for $18.02, to reimburse you for traveling expenses—Apr. 21 to Apr. 25, as evidenced by the accompanying voucher, which you will please sign, have attested and returned to this office at your early convenience. I am also enclosing the signed voucher covering traveling expenses in February, to which you will please have the Notary Public affix his official seal."

Later in 1913 Stokes wrote to King again, still trying to collect for wood he bought in April of the previous year! His list of supplies needed for the "hospital" (really a clinic) he set up in Cherry Creek, South Dakota, included basic necessities such as a single bed, dish pan, frying pan, pot, spoons, broom, plates and other kitchen items. By December he has "practically nothing in my Dispensary" and wrote King again for basic medical supplies.

In early 1914 acting superintendent King was replaced. The medical supplies had not yet been received so Dr. Stokes requested permission to purchase some supplies on the open market: basic things like hydrogen peroxide, iodine, syringes, thermometers, ointment and soap. He heard from his new superintendent F. C. Campbell that he had checked on his predecessor King and in reply received a personally written letter of apology from an ex-senator from South Dakota saying, "I met Mr. King in Washington. He is utterly worthless, is incompetent and inefficient and has not a single qualification for the office."

Stokes response regarding the senator's assessment of King is worth sharing:

> Beyond a doubt there is some misunderstanding or misinformation in the mind of this person [King] concerning this expense account that, apparently has caused him so freely, candidly to vent the pent up spleen of his morbid mind on me and I fail to see wherein the garbled, inane and wholly irrelevant explanation could be construed as other than the venting of a personal animosity and having absolutely nothing to do with the validity of this expense account.[17]

Dr. and Mrs. Stokes returned home to Indiana periodically to visit relatives and family.[18] By 1914 Dr. Stokes was concerned about the poor quality of education available for his son.

The next year the family decided to return to Indianapolis, and he started a private practice. City directories in 1915 and 1916 list him then as an oculist, suggesting he had begun to specialize as an eye doctor, perhaps because of his experience treating trachoma. His business address was 158 East Market Street and his residence was 132 South Arlington Avenue. That residence would be the family home into the 1940s.

Military Service

Although Stokes was already 44 years old in 1917, he volunteered for service in the U.S. Army. In August 1917 he was one of the oldest physicians to arrive at the Fort Des Moines Medical Officers Training Camp. He described his varied career up to that point as "Physician U.S. Indian Service 8 years; pharmacist 5 years; hospital and private practice 4 years; specialist, diseases of the eye, 2½ years."[19]

Completing his training in November, he was then assigned to the 92nd Division, 317th Sanitary (Medical) Train at Camp Funston. In addition to treating soldiers, the doctors continued their medical education at Camp Funston. He was one of five physicians selected to review medical journals and report at medical meetings to the other physicians. For example, in March 1918, he was assigned to review the "Archives of Internal Medicine" for his report.[20]

The 92nd Division was sent to France in June 1918 where Stokes first served with the 367th Ambulance Company. Each ambulance company was to provide 12 ambulances to evacuate casualties from the battalion aid stations. The wounded were taken from the front to dressing stations 3,000 to 6,000 yards from the front where they were stabilized and then moved farther back to field hospitals. The length of time required to transport wounded soldiers from the front lines to the field hospitals was affected by road conditions, visibility, and traffic.[21]

Lieutenant Stokes was also detailed as the battalion gas officer for all four of the field hospitals in July 1918. In September 1918 he was transferred to the 365th Infantry Regiment's medical detachment where he worked more closely with the troops. He was dealing firsthand with the results of exposure to mustard and phosgene gases. The Germans introduced mustard gas in July 1918. "More casualties were caused by this gas than by all the rest of the gases in the war." The burns were said to take from three to five weeks to heal and made a man "practically useless for that length of time." Its effect on the eyes was loss of vision for anywhere from three days to three weeks.[22]

His regiment saw its most significant combat action during the attack by the AEF Second Army near Metz in early November 1918, shortly before the war ended. By the end of 1918, Stokes was serving again with the 367th Ambulance Company. He returned from France in the spring of 1919 and was discharged from the army as a captain in the Medical Reserve Corps on July 8, 1919.[23]

Career

Dr. Stokes returned to Indianapolis to his family, practice, and the Stokes-Bond pharmacy he had founded. Many African American physicians had drug stores, hospitals or other medical-related businesses to help support themselves and service their patients.

He was well acquainted with Dr. Joseph H. Ward of Indianapolis. They were the same age, graduated from the same medical school, trained together at Fort Des Moines, and served in the 92nd Division in France during World War I.

After the war, Major Ward was appointed medical officer in charge at the newly-built U.S. Veterans Hospital No. 91 for African American veterans in Tuskegee, Alabama. He recruited his friend Dr. Stokes to work with him in Tuskegee. In 1924 Stokes was named Executive Officer at the Veterans Hospital. He succeeded white physician Dr. George L. Johnson. When Major Ward came under fire in 1925, Stokes was mentioned along with Ward as being one of seven people being investigated.[24] That investigation went nowhere and is an example of the racial difficulties they faced.

Sadly, Stokes died in Tuskegee four years later from kidney failure. He was only 56. At the time of his death he held the rank of major in the Army Medical Reserve Corps.[25]

Dr. Stokes was adventurous, intelligent, articulate, curious, and caring. His life story is a testament to his belief that medicine, government service and education are paramount.

He is buried with other Stokes family members at beautiful Crown Hill Cemetery in Indianapolis with a military headstone.

NOTES

1. "Paragraphic News," *Washington Bee*, January 16, 1909, 8, 1.
2. "A.M.E. Meeting, 69th Annual Conference in Session This Week," *The Recorder*, September 14, 1907, 1.
3. "Terre Haute, IND," *The Indianapolis Recorder*, February 3, 1912, 1.
4. *Randolph County*, en.wikipedia.org/wiki/Randolph_County,_Indiana (accessed Sept 21, 2012).
5. *Union Literary Institute Recording Secretary's Book, 1845–1890*, Processed by Wilma L. Moore, March 27, 2010, Manuscript and Visual Collections Department, William Henry Smith Memorial Library, Indiana Historical Society.
6. "Directory of Charities," *The Indiana Bulletin*, December 1907, 37.
7. "Edwin Stokes Public School Teacher Dies," *The Indianapolis Recorder*, March 14, 1931, 1.
8. *Ibid.*, "City Happening—Personal," June 30, 1894, 10.
9. *Ibid.*, "Indianapolis Literary a Success," June 30, 1894, 8.
10. "Physician at Indian Reservation in Montana," *Indianapolis Freeman*, May 18, 1907, 3.
11. "Terra Haute Items," *The Indianapolis Recorder*, January 20, 1900, 1.
12. AMA Deceased Physician Card, National Library of Medicine, Bethesda, MD.
13. "Very Promising—Dr. Fred Stokes, Practicing Young Physician Returned to the City," *The Indianapolis Recorder*, February 9, 1901, 1.
14. *Ibid.*, "A New Drug Store—Dr. Fred Stokes Opens a New Place of Business," May 25, 1901, 1.
15. *Ibid.*, "Physician at Indian Reservation in Montana," May 18, 1907, 3.
16. *Ibid.*, 23–29.
17. "RG 75-Cheyenne River File for Dr. Frederick A. Stokes," National Archives and Records Administration, Central Plains Region, Kansas City, Missouri.
18. "Dr. Stokes in the City," *Indianapolis Freeman*, March 2, 1912, 8 and March 16, 1912, 8.
19. John L. Thompson, *History and Views of Colored Officers Training Camp for 1917 at Fort Des Moines, Iowa* (Des Moines: *The Bystander*, 1917) 88.
20. Record Group 120, Records of the 92d Division, 317th Sanitary Train, Memo March 3, 1918, National Archives, College Park, MD.
21. "The United States Army Medical Service Corps," Chapter 2, World War 1—The Ambulance Service, 43–44, history.amedd.army.mil/booksdocs/HistoryofUSArmyMSC/chapter2.html (accessed Sept 21, 2012).
22. www.armyhistory.mil (accessed March 30, 2015).
23. War Department, Q.M.C. Form No. 14, September 27, 1929.
24. "Major Ward Under Fire at Tuskegee Hospital," *Afro-American*, June 20, 1925, 1.
25. "Stokes in the City," *Indianapolis Freeman*, March 2, 1912, 8 and March 16, 1912, 8.

Leonard STOVALL

16 December 1887–18 February 1956
University of Southern California, 1912

Roots and Education

Leonard Stovall was born in Atlanta, Georgia, and came to Los Angeles as a very young child with his parents, Jerry and Mary Scott Stovall. Stovall was the fifth of seven children, four boys and three girls. Educated in Los Angeles public schools, in 1906 he became the first African American to graduate from Hollywood High School.

He worked his way through two years of pre-med undergraduate study at the University of Southern California doing truck farming: raising produce and selling it from a truck. Then he went on to the University of California Medical College in 1908, and graduated in 1912.[1] He was described at the time as "one of the most conscientious and able students of his class."[2]

Dr. Stovall immediately immersed himself in practicing medicine in Los Angeles and was active in numerous medical and fraternal organizations, and became a member of the NAACP.[3]

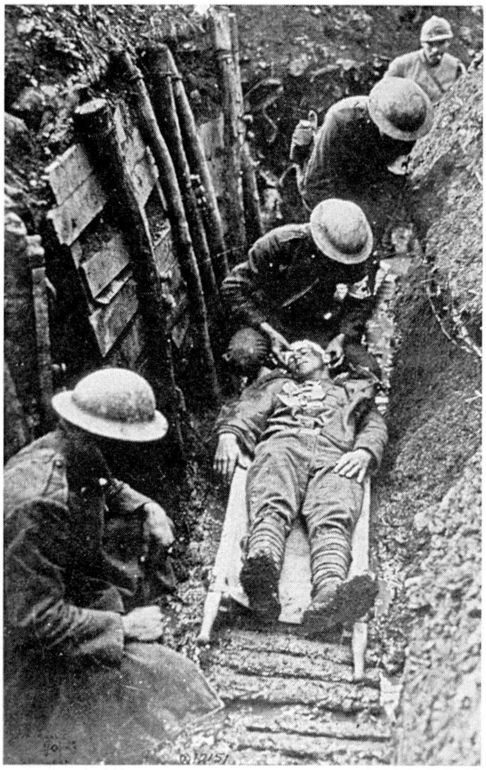

Caring for the wounded in trenches (courtesy U.S. National Library of Medicine).

In 1914, he was instrumental in forming the Southern California Physicians, Dentists and Pharmacists Association.[4] In 1914 Stovall presented a paper to the group on "Intestinal Disease in Children" and led a discussion regarding a paper on "Serum Therapy."[5] He shared his medical office upstairs at 1201 Central Avenue in downtown Los Angeles with his colleague and good friend Dr. Claudius Ballard. In 1917 when the government called on doctors to volunteer for the First World War, Dr. Stovall, still single and living at 1300 Fleming Street in Los Angeles, was commissioned as a first lieutenant in the Medical Reserve Corps and closed his office. His friend and associate Dr. Ballard followed his lead. At the time, he reported he was a member of the Wesley ME Church, and the Knights of Pythias, Foresters and AOF fraternal societies.[6]

Military Service

First Lieutenant Stovall arrived at the Medical Officers Training Camp at Fort Des Moines on August 2, 1917. After 94 days of training, he was ordered to Camp Funston, Kansas, and finally to the division's 365th Infantry Regiment at Camp Grant, Illinois, where he was a surgeon at the camp's infirmary.

He went to France as a medical officer with the First Battalion of the 365th. His regiment arrived overseas in June 1918 where it joined other elements of the 92nd Division. The French were there to help train our troops at Bourbonne-les-Bains before they were deployed to trenches in the Vosges mountain region near St. Dié. When the American troops arrived, this area became more active. Skirmishes between raiding parties were frequent. In an attempt to retake Frapelle, the enemy employed intensive artillery bombardment, mustard gas and flame projectors. It was a baptism by fire for the medical detachment as they treated the 34 wounded and gassed.[7]

From there the battalion was sent to the Meuse-Argonne and finally to the Marbache Sector. Here they saw the most significant combat action during the attack on Metz by the AEF Second Army in early November 1918.

After the war ended Stovall, was discharged in 1919 and returned to Los Angeles. During the one and a half years he spent in the army he cared for hundreds of sick, injured and wounded soldiers.

Career

Dr. Stovall's impact on the health of the African American community in Southern California is quite remarkable. In addition to maintaining a regular medical practice, he became a specialist in tuberculosis. A biographical sketch of Dr. Stovall was published in 1919 when he was only 31 years old. It summarized his amazing range of activities to that date as "visiting surgeon, Selwyn Emmett Graves Dispensary, University of Southern California; attending physician, Municipal Child Welfare Station, 1914; grand medical examiner, U.B.F. of California; physician for Foresters, Odd Fellows, Knights of Pythias; president, Georgia State Society; corresponding secretary, State Societies of Southern California; Republican; Methodist; member American Medical Association; California State Medical Association; Los Angeles County Medical Association; Southern California Physicians, Dentists, and Pharmacists Association."[8] He later became active with the National Tuberculosis Association.

As early as 1921, he was a member of an anti-tuberculosis committee that was planning to buy eight acres of land northeast of downtown Los Angeles for a tubercular sanitarium.[9]

He married Yolande McCullough in the early 1920s. She was born in Colorado, and moved to Los Angeles with her family where she became a schoolteacher. The Stovalls had two children, Gerald in 1925 and Yolande in 1929. Both of their children became distinguished physicians. His daughter joined him in his practice in 1955; a few years later his son joined them. Stovall's hobby was gardening, and he won several First Prizes for his carnations grown from seeds and a giant hybrid amaryllis.[10]

His concern for the community was reflected in many ways and in numerous activities. In 1928 he became an investor and director of a major African American business project to construct and operate the "Magnificent" Hotel Somerville in downtown Los Angeles at 41st and South Central Avenue.[11] "It was erected in June of 1928 in reaction not only to the complete lack of first rate accommodations in Los Angeles for blacks who were denied service at white-owned hotels, but also by a need for employment in the community.... It was the first hotel built by black people. Usually African Americans bought and refurbished old hotel buildings vacated by whites. The Somerville Hotel [renamed the Dunbar Hotel] took its place as the heart of African American culture in Los Angeles."[12]

In 1930, Dr. Stovall was the first African American appointed to the tuberculosis section of the staff of the Los Angeles City General Hospital. He had been specializing in the prevention and cure of tuberculosis for 12 years.[13]

In 1931 in an effort to improve the health of the African American community, he sponsored or gave health lectures at the YMCA every Monday evening.[14] In 1933 he gave health lectures during National Health Week events sponsored by the YMCA, YWCA, the City Health Department and other civic organizations.[15] He stayed involved in the YMCA for years. As late as 1950 he was still involved in the youth programs, giving free physical exams to the boys who participated in summer camp. The camp offered the boys eight days of high adventure in the San Bernardino mountains.[16]

By 1934 Stovall had laid the groundwork for a new institution. He established the Twenty-Eighth Street Health Center to treat the poor. It was established as an inter-racial, non-profit, non-sectarian clinic. Local physicians donated their time. Goals included facilitating early diagnosis of all diseases, especially tuberculosis. Six hundred and sixty patients were registered by 1934.[17]

Tuberculosis patients of the day were treated in long-term sanitariums. The disease claimed four times as many victims among the African American community as whites yet none of the sanitariums would treat them.[18] He gathered a group of his friends and formed the Outdoor Life and Health Association (OLHA).[19]

OLHA operated a 50-bed sanitarium in nearby Duarte, California, for patients of all races.[20] In 1937 he had help from local churches like the People's Independent Church of Christ, whose minister Rev. Russell set aside a Sunday evening benefit service.[21] A local ladies' bridge club also donated to the cause. It was said that more than 500 cases of tuberculosis were arrested as a result of Dr. Stovall's work. In 1938 he received a community service medal for erecting the Demonstration Rest Home in Monrovia. It was made possible by his Outdoor Life and Health Association.[22]

In 1941 Dr. Stovall became the medical director of the East Area Health Program. It was formed to improve health conditions in East Los Angeles. It was financed by the Los Angeles Tuberculosis and Health Association with Christmas Seal funds.[23]

In 1950 Dr. Stovall, still pioneering, was the first African American doctor to be seated in the House of Delegates of the State Medical Association.[24] His credentials for the appointment included his memberships in the American Medical Association and the American Trudeau Society. The latter was an organization that specialized in tuberculosis research.[25]

Twenty years later in 1954 the dread disease had been largely abated, and OLHA's strategic direction shifted to care for the elderly and disabled. The Duarte property was traded for two lots in East Los Angeles where two buildings named Fairmont Terrace were constructed for seniors. Sadly, Dr. Stovall passed away in 1956 at Good Samaritan Hospital three weeks before Fairmont Terrace opened.

After his death, the OLHA was renamed the Stovall Foundation in his honor, and Fairmont Terrace was renamed the Leonard Stovall Home for the Aged. It has since expanded and still operates providing housing and support for 300 low-income and disabled seniors.[26] He is buried with his wife in Evergreen Cemetery.

Tuberculosis was a scourge that was particularly prevalent among poor city dwellers during the late 1800s and early 1900s. It affected African Americans disproportionately. Dr. Stovall spent his life working to eradicate the disease. He also put tremendous effort into educating the black urban community on the benefit of a healthy life-style. Near the end of his life, he invested his money and time in helping the elderly with what we now call assisted living. He was truly a guiding spirit in the City of Angels.

NOTES
1. Delilah L. Beasley, *The Negro Trail Blazers of California* (Los Angeles, 1919), 248.
2. *Ibid.*
3. Commodore Wynn, "Dr. Leonard Stovall," *Negro Who's Who in California* (California Publishing Co., 1948), 51.
4. "Dentists and Pharmacists Unite with Physicians to Form State Society," *Journal of the National Medical Association (JNMA)*, July–September 1914, Vol. 6, No. 3, 212.
5. "Program of the Doctor, Dentist and Druggist Association of California," *Journal of the National Medical Association JNMA)*, July–Sep, 1915, Vol. 7, No. 3, 238.
6. John L. Thompson, *History and Views of Colored Officers Training Camp for 1917 at Fort Des Moines, Iowa* (Des Moines: *The Bystander*, 1917) 87.
7. Emmett J. Scott, "The Baptism of Fire and Gas," *The American Negro in the World War*, Chapter XI, net. lib.byu.edu/WWI (accessed April 2, 2015).
8. Delilah L. Beasley, *The Negro Trail Blazers of California*, 248.
9. "California, Los Angeles," *Chicago Defender*, April 2, 1921 13.
10. Wynn, *Negro Who's Who in California*, 51.
11. "Paid Advertisement, Hotel Somerville—Four Column," *California Eagle*, October 12, 1928.
12. "*Dunbar Hotel*," BlackPast.org, www.blackpast.org/aaw/dunbar-hotel-1928 (accessed August 23, 2014).
13. "The Inter-Racial Committee of Montclair, N.J., Precedents for the Service of Negro Doctors, Internes and Nurses in Public Hospitals," *Journal of National Medical Association (JNMA)*, July-Sep, 1931, 105.
14. "YMCA News," *California Eagle*, January 30, 1931, 31.
15. "California News, Los Angeles," *Chicago Defender*, April 22, 1933, 18.
16. "Summer Fun at 28th St. Y," *California Eagle*, June 14, 1950, 25.
17. "Health Center Boon to L.A. Poor, Prominent Physicians Head Los Angeles Inter-Racial Clinic—Brainchild of Dr. Stovall," *Pittsburgh Courier*, August 18, 1934, A9.
18. "Dr. Leonard Stovall, Founder of Duarte Rent Homes, Honored," *California Eagle*, February 15, 1951, 1.
19. *Ibid.*, "Spreading Joy by John Fowler," July 22, 1943, 8-A.
20. "Army 'Non Coms' Hold Meeting," *Pittsburgh Courier*, March 25, 1939, 3.
21. "Plan 'T.B.' Benefit Independent Service," *California Eagle*, October 28, 1937.
22. *Ibid.*, "S. C. Alumni Association Ends Year's Work," Sept 22, 1938, 9-A.
23. "To Plan East Area Health Program," *California Eagle*, April 17, 1941, 2-A.
24. "Voted Post with Coast Medic Group," *Chicago Defender*, May 13, 1950, 11.
25. "AMA to Seat Race Delegate," *Pittsburgh Courier*, June 24, 1950, 3.
26. "The Stovall Foundation and the Stovall Housing Corporation, Our History," www.stovallfoundation.org/our-history.html (accessed June 28, 2014).

Estil Young STRAWN

25 May 1887–5 October 1951
Howard Medical College, 1913

Roots and Education

Strawn was born in Columbia, Missouri, to Arthur Strawn, Sr., and Mary Bell Graves. Estil was the third son in large family of seven children, five sons and two daughters. He received his elementary education in Columbia, the home of the University of Missouri. He finished his high school years in nearby Jefferson City, the state capital, at the Lincoln Institute, now known as Lincoln University.

Estil graduated from Lincoln in 1905. He went on to study in Washington, D.C., at Howard University's Medical School from 1909 until he graduated in 1913. He stayed in D.C. for another year where he interned at Freedmen's Hospital. After taking post-graduate courses, he returned to St. Joseph in 1915 and established his medical practice.[1]

In February 1916 Dr. Strawn married Ruth L. Endicott, daughter of Mr. and Mrs. Joseph A. Endicott of St. Joseph. Her father had been a teacher in St. Joseph public schools since 1879, and taught at the Bartlett School for African Americans.

Estil and Ruth were wed at a small ceremony in Columbia in the Strawn family home on North Third Street. Ruth had been teaching school in Marshall, Missouri. After the early morning wedding, they attended church at the AME church and left that afternoon for St. Joseph to set up housekeeping in a home Dr. Strawn had just purchased.[2]

The following year, when America entered the First World War in 1917, Strawn volunteered to serve in the Army Medical Reserve Corps. His application notes the couple's address as 1908 Messanie Street in St. Joseph. He was accepted and was commissioned a first lieutenant.

Military Service

Lieutenant Strawn was ordered to active duty at Fort Des Moines, Iowa, in September 1917. He received 49 days of training at the Medical Officer Training Camp (MOTC) until November 3, 1917. He was then assigned to the

92nd Division at Camp Dodge, Iowa, where the 366th Infantry Regiment was being formed. He was one of six MOTC graduate physicians serving with the regiment's medical detachment.

His unit arrived in France in June 1918. The 366th Infantry was engaged in particularly heavy action toward the end of the war near Metz and suffered numerous casualties.

In a memorandum to the 366th Infantry battalion commander on November 17, 1918, just days after the armistice, Major A. E. Sawkins wrote of his men: "I cannot say too much in praise of the manner in which these officers handled their men. The men responded as though at a maneuver, although without food or sleep for 48 hours at time of the attack on morning of the 11th November, the men went into action in such a manner that I feel proud to command such fine, soldierly troops."[3]

While serving in France during World War I, Strawn rose to the rank of captain. After the war, he arrived in New York in February 1919, was discharged, and returned home to St. Joseph. He continued to serve in the Army Medical Reserve Corps after the war and had risen to the rank of major by his retirement. In 1922 he was branch chairman for the Citizens Military Training Camps (CMTC) program. He also was a member of the Association of Military Surgeons of the United States and the Reserve Officers Association.

Career

During the 1920s the Strawn home was at 2220 Sylvania Street in St. Joseph, Missouri, and his office remained at 1908 Messanie Street. The house on Sylvania was the family home for the rest of his long and productive life.[4] The Strawns had nine children, four daughters and five sons. All survived him. The family remained very close and had regularly scheduled family reunions every two years in places like Los Angeles and Kansas City. The four daughters all married and three lived in the midwest in Missouri, Kansas, and Nebraska. One moved to Orangeburg, South Carolina.

Dr. Strawn never went far from his Missouri roots. He was active professionally as a member of the National Medical Association (NMA), the State Medical Society and the Social Hygiene Association, which fought venereal disease. The African American community in St. Joseph was modest in size and very close. The Strawn family was active with the Ebenezer AME Church. In 1920 he served as toastmaster there for a reception and banquet for the visiting bishop of the 5th Episcopal District.[5] He practiced medicine in St. Joseph for 37 years.

The good doctor died at age 64 of cardiac failure due to hypertension. He was buried in Columbia.[6] His service to the community was long and dedicated. His and Ruth's legacy, through their very accomplished children, has extended his influence to many succeeding generations.

Clearly, his family was focused heavily on education. It is worth noting that in 1993 one son, Dr. Estil Y. Strawn, Jr., was the first black physician in Atlanta to perform in vitro fertilization (IVF). Another son, Alexander E. Strawn, had a distinguished teaching career and became dean of Student Affairs at Hampton University in Virginia. The other three sons were successful as well, one becoming a photogrammetric cartographer in Milwaukee, one a dentist in Los Angeles, and one a realtor in Kansas City.

NOTES

1. Thomas Yenser, Editor, Who's Who in Colored America, Seventh Edition (New York, 1950), 401.
2. Ada Byram, "St. Joseph, Missouri," *The Kansas City Sun*, February 19, 1916, 4.
3. Emmett J. Scott, *The American Negro in the World War*, Chapter XI, The Negro Combat Division, net.lib.byu.edu (accessed April 2, 2015).
4. "Physician Dies; Rites at Columbia for Dr. E. Y. Strawn," *St Joseph News-Press*, October 6, 1951, 2–3.
5. Ada Byram, "St. Joseph, Missouri," *The Kansas City Sun*, August 7, 1920, 2.
6. Missouri Death Certificate, Estil Young Strawn, State File No. 32691, Filed October 15, 1951.

William Albert TARLETON

10 June 1882–1920
Meharry Medical College, 1912

Roots and Education

Tarleton was born in Wilmington, North Carolina, and educated in the local black public schools. Throughout the south these were inferior to the white public schools. He went on to gain admission to a two-year program at Georgia State College, an African American school in Savannah. This land grant college issued its first degree in 1898. Today it is Savannah State University, a historically black university.

Obviously bright and ambitious, he left Savannah and attended Meharry Medical College in Nashville, Tennessee, where he graduated in 1912. He interned at the George H. Hubbard Hospital in Nashville and went on to assist the renowned Dr. Daniel Williams in Chicago, Illinois. Dr. Williams was an early heart surgeon who founded Provident Hospital, the first non-segregated hospital in the United States.

In 1914 Dr. Tarleton moved to Los Angeles, California, where he opened a private practice in the Germain building. In 1915 and 1916 he was active in the newly formed Southern California Medical Society for African American doctors. As early as March 1915, he was one of three local physicians (all of whom later served in the Army Medical Corps in the First World War) who presented at a Sunday Health Day Forum on the importance of maintaining good health. Tarleton spoke on "Disease and Inefficiency."[1] In September 1915 he led the discussion of a medical paper entitled "Specific Urethritis" written by George Taylor, M.D. At this time in Los Angeles history the growing economy had attracted immigrants from Asia and Mexico. The areas where they lived reported high rates of infant mortality and infectious disease. As fears of disease grew, Los Angeles County appointed its first public health officer, established free clinics for the poor and began an education program to combat disease.[2] The Sunday Health Day Forum was likely part of that program.

In 1915 he installed a newly popular French D'Arsonval Violet Ray Treatment and X-Ray Machine in his office.[3] These ultraviolet x-ray machines were supposed to oxygenate tissue to kill bacteria and infection while massaging the skin to resolve skin problems and slow the appearance of aging.[4] In January 1916 he presented a paper to the local medical group entitled "The D'Arsonval Current in High Blood Pressure." In April 1916 he led the discussion of a paper, "The X-Ray as an Aid to Diagnosis."[5] The devices were popular until the depression of 1929 put the manufacturers out of business.

Tarleton opened a combined medical office with dentist, Dr. B. A. Johnson, and they shared three suites (409–410–411) in the Germain Building at 224 South Spring Street. Los Angeles city directories for 1915 through 1917 list his office there in South Central Los Angeles. His residence in 1915 was 1339 East 23rd Street.

A June 30, 1917, Los Angeles newspaper report is an example of the humanitarian side of the good doctor. Dr. Tarleton was passing by when a woman was thrown from a streetcar. He picked her up, checked her for injuries and took her to her home.

His business and community activities continued apace; in mid–1917 listed his organizations as "Mason, Elk, Odd Fellow, Sir Knight, Knights of Pythias, Sons and Daughters of Africa."[6]

Military Service

In 1917 Dr. Tarleton, still single, volunteered for service in the army's Medical Reserve Corps and was commissioned a First Lieutenant. He reported to Fort Des Moines in August. He received 94 days of military training there at the Medical Officers Training Camp (MOTC). An August article in the *California Eagle* read, "A line from the doctor himself shows that he is full of enthusiasm and enjoying his work to the utmost. The doctor is sorely missed by his patients and a host of friends, as he was wide awake and abreast of the times and thoroughly progressive."[7] During his absence, Tarleton's friend, Dr. Frank A. Gordon, took over his offices in the Germain Building.

Upon completing his training Dr. Tarleton was sent to Camp Funston, Kansas, to the 92nd Division's 317th Sanitary (Medical) Train. He and six other MOTC graduates were assigned to the unit's 367th Field Hospital.

Unfortunately, he contracted spinal meningitis there in March 1918, was hospitalized until he recovered and was granted a leave of absence beginning March 31, 1918, pending discharge. On May 11, 1918, he received his orders to return home to Los Angeles until a final discharge from service. He received the orders before his unit deployed overseas in June 1918.[8] He was most probably found not physically fit for overseas service following his meningitis attack. In any case, Tarleton served honorably for eight months and returned to Los Angeles to resume his practice. In June 1918 he and his new wife, Hattie, traveled to Santa Barbara, where they visited with old friends from Topeka, Kansas. He was described as "the first Colored army officer in uniform that Santa Barbara has had the honor to entertain."[9]

Career

When he registered for the draft in 1918, he and Hattie were living at 1637 West 35th Place in Los Angeles and his office was back in the Germain Building. Between December 1918 and February 1920 Tarleton ran a series of advertisements in the *California Eagle* announcing he had "resumed his practice in the city and can be found at his former quarters."[10]

Evidently, he had regained his health by spring as evidenced by his activities. Dr. and Mrs. Tarleton were active in the tennis world and were founders of the Omega Tennis Club. In April 1919 he became president of the newly organized club. His name was mentioned in numerous social and tennis columns throughout the year in the *California Eagle*. He was also one-time head of the Western Federation of Tennis Clubs.[11] That group had been formed in 1916 to establish an alliance among the African American tennis clubs founded in Los Angeles. By 1921, 10 Los Angeles–area African American tennis clubs were affiliated with the federation.

He also joined the city's Progressive Business League, which had been formed to represent and promote business and professional interests in Los Angeles.[12]

In 1919 Dr. W. A. Tarleton added another sidelight to his already interesting life. He was a cast member in a feature film production entitled "*INJUSTICE*," an African American World War I drama that was released in July 1919. A review of the film describes the plot thusly: "Wealthy society girl Irene Waterloo is courted by a designing nobleman, Count Bertrade Delande, who had previously pledged himself to Gwendolyne Vanderbilt. Gwendolyne and her socially ambitious mother uncover evidence that Irene is really black, and Irene, shocked by the revelation, goes to Europe. Eventually she finds happiness with George Preston, who was formerly her porter." The film also treats the racism endured by blacks in Europe during World War I.[13]

According to the 1920 Census, his medical office was still located in the Germain Building, but he and Hattie had moved to 1657 West 37th Place.

In February 1920 Tarleton fell ill again. He and his wife moved 250 miles east to Needles, California, on the Arizona border, to live with Mrs. Tarleton's brother "for some time" while he recuperated.[14] They hoped the warm dry dessert air would help heal his lungs. Unfortunately, he died soon afterward from tuberculosis in Albuquerque, New Mexico, at the age of 39.[15] His body was returned to Los Angeles.[16] The African American medical community in Los Angeles was small at that time and Tarleton was missed. The community had been deprived prematurely of his skill, knowledge, energy, experience and commitment.

NOTES

1. "Sunday Was Health Day at the Forum. Drs. Stovall, Tarleton and Ballard Deliver Timely Addresses," *California Eagle*, March 25, 1915, 1.
2. www.ncbi.nim.nih.gov (accessed March 25, 2015).
3. F. L. Mather, Editor, *Who's Who of the Colored Race*, Chicago: Vol. One—1915, 259.
4. Gary J. Lockhart (1942–2001), *Electrical Healing and Violet Ray*, copyright 2000, unpublished.
5. "Society and Personal," *Journal of the National Medical Association (JNMA)*, April–June 1916, Vol. 8, No. 2, 124–125.
6. John L. Thompson, *History and Views of Colored Officers Training Camp for 1917 at Fort Des Moines, Iowa* (Des Moines: *The Bystander*, 1917) 89.
7. "First Lieutenant in U.S. Army Is Dr. William A. Tarleton," *California Eagle*, August 25, 1917, 1.
8. U.S. Army Finance Records—Tarleton, William Albert, 1st Lieut, M.R.C., National Archives, National Personnel Records Center, St. Louis, MO.
9. "Santa Barbara News," *California Eagle*, June 1, 1918, 5.
10. *California Eagle* advertisements, January–September 1919, 633.
11. *Ibid.*, Volume 36, 131.
12. "Progressive Business League Members," *California Eagle*, August 23, 1919, 8.
13. Alan Gevinson, *Within Our Gates: Ethnicity in American Feature Films, 1911–1960*, American Film Institute Catalog.
14. "Social Intelligence," *California Eagle*, February 14 & 21, 1920, 5.

15. AMA Deceased Physician Card, National Library of Medicine, Bethesda, MD.
16. Dr. William Albert Tarleton, Findagrave.com (accessed January 5, 2015).

John Quill TAYLOR

21 July 1884–23 September 1931
Meharry Medical College, 1911

Roots and Education

John Taylor was born to Edward V. Taylor and Amanda Taylor in Clifton, Texas. Clifton is a small rural town in central Texas located 35 miles northwest of Waco on the Bosque River. It was the site of a mill that provided flour and meal to Waco in the late 1800s. In the early 1880s the Santa Fe Railroad came through Clifton, making it easily accessible. In December 1906 a large portion of the downtown district was destroyed by fire.[1] That was also the year Taylor left Texas for Tennessee.

Taylor graduated from Meharry Medical College in Nashville in 1911 and settled in Memphis. In June 1915 the *Chicago Defender* reported, "Dr. J. Q. Taylor, physician and surgeon of Memphis, Tennessee, will be in the city this summer. He was here two summers ago [1913]."[2] A 1916 Memphis news item reported Dr. Taylor was caring for Sallie Jackson who was slowly recovering from an illness.[3] In 1917

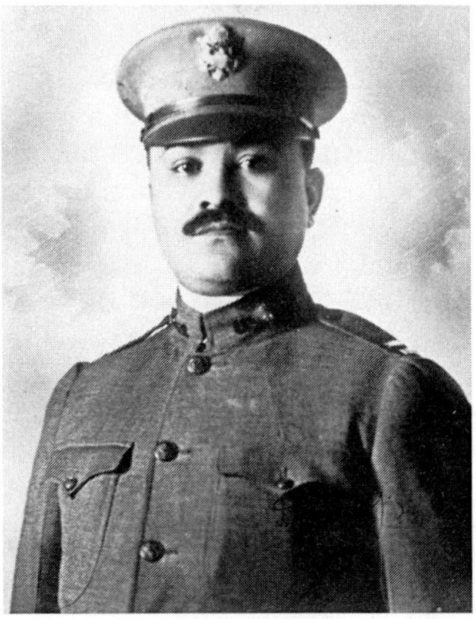

Captain John Q. Taylor, surgeon, First Battalion, 366th Infantry (courtesy University of Texas at San Antonio (UTSA) Libraries Special Collections).

it was reported he held a degree in ophthalmology, was a member of the Protestant Episcopal Church and the GUOOF (Grand United Order of Odd Fellows).[4]

He married Alice Clinton Woodson, a Memphis elementary school teacher. She was a direct descendent of Thomas Woodson, son of slave Sally Hemmings and her owner, Thomas Jefferson. Dr. Taylor and his wife lived at 692 Alston Avenue. They had a daughter, Edwina, and then a son, John Quill Taylor, Jr., was born September 25, 1921. That son later became extremely prominent in the African American community in Austin, Texas, where he became a college president and three star general in the Texas National Guard.[5]

Military Service

In early 1917 Dr. Taylor volunteered for service in the Army Medical Reserve Corps. He reported for duty at the Medical Officers Training Camp (MOTC) at Fort Des Moines on August 24. On November 3, 1917, he was transferred to nearby Camp Dodge, Iowa, the home of the 366th Infantry Regiment of the 92nd Division.[6] He was shipped to France with them in mid–1918.

In August 1918 the 366th was sent to what had been a quiet sector in the Vosges Mountains. Six days before their arrival, the U.S. 5th Infantry Division had captured the village of Frapelle. The 92nd Division replaced the 5th Division. Just as Taylor's 366th moved into the front-line trenches the enemy responded. They were greeted by artillery shelling with shrapnel and mustard gas.[7]

Lieutenant Taylor was among the doctors who were sickened by the toxic gas while caring for the 34 soldiers who were wounded and gassed. He was gravely ill. Most patients with mustard-gas burns had a complicating conjunctivitis. Slight conjunctivitis was relieved by irrigating the eyes with sodium-bicarbonate solution, followed by a few drops of albolene. Severe conjunctivitis was treated with a one percent solution of Novocain as often as required to relieve pain. Gauze wetted with one percent solution of sodium bicarbonate was placed over the eyes. Patients were given sponge baths as soon as their condition permitted. Patients were also given oxygen.[8] Later in life the effects of the gas likely contributed to Dr. Taylor's premature death.[9]

Taylor worked for Dr. Louis T. Wright in the 92nd Division's triage hospital at Millery during the last months of the war. Wright liked and admired Taylor and wrote that he worked on a division of the shock team with him and described him as "black-haired, brown faced, black eyed, handsome as a king." Wright described a racial incident in which he and Taylor were awaiting orders and taking a walk in the mountains when they encountered eight white privates from the South Carolina Wildcats division. "These privates began to follow us. It was near sundown. I then said to Taylor, 'This doesn't look good. Let's face it.' The wildcats then divided into two files, one behind each of us and I told Taylor, 'This is a showdown. Get your gun ready.' We suddenly turned and I said, 'About face,' with drawn guns, 'and we'll shoot any s.o.b. in the crowd.' That stopped them cold. We had our guns drawn. They did an about face and marched away."[10]

Taylor's heroism and leadership were recognized with several citations for bravery. He was promoted to captain and became its ear, eye, nose and throat specialist for the 317th Sanitary (Medical) Train for the remainder of the war.[11] After returning to America following the end of the war, he was discharged from the Army on April 8, 1919.

Career

Dr. Taylor returned to Memphis following the war. He had connections in Minnesota and in June 1919, soon after arriving home, Dr. Taylor and his wife spent time with friends at a cottage on Lake Pokegama. After his summer rest, they returned to Memphis, and he sought out other African American veterans.

On August 8, 1919, Captain Taylor became the first commander of a newly organized American Legion Post. It would serve the interests of "Memphis Negro World War Veterans, looking after their claims for service disabilities, compensation and hospitalization."[12] It was named the Austress Russell Post in honor of the first African American soldier killed overseas in the battle of the Argonne.[13] Many of its members served in the 92nd and 93rd combat divisions in France.

In the fall of 1919 Dr. Taylor registered for post-graduate work at the University of Minnesota in preparation for resuming his medical practice in Memphis.[14]

In 1920 he and his wife moved in with his wife's mother's family at 676 Pontotoc Avenue in Memphis. Unfortunately Dr. Taylor was still suffering after-effects from his First World War gassing. He suffered a hemorrhage in 1921. By 1930 he was separated from Alice and lived alone at 692 Alston Avenue, located less than two miles from today's National Civil Rights Museum.[15] He died there a year later.

His death certificate was signed by Dr. Dorsey B. Granberry, a friend and fellow MOTC graduate. Granberry wrote he had been caring for Dr. Taylor for five weeks before he died from a secondary cerebral hemorrhage in 1931. An October newspaper report from Memphis reported on rites for Dr. Taylor as follows: "Post No. 27 of the American Legion ... held mid-rites Wednesday night for the Dr. J. Q. Taylor, disabled ex-service comrade. He was the first post commander of the Austress Russell American Legion Post and contributed largely to the association."[16] Taylor is buried in the Memphis National Cemetery.[17] Because they were African Americans, members of the Austress Russell Post were not allowed to participate in the ceremony.

On November 21, 1940, "the biggest marching contingent of colored World War Veterans that has ever taken part in an Armistice Day program in this city," participated in a parade. All of the members of the post Dr. Taylor helped found marched to "perpetuate the memory of 6,500 men from Beale Street and its environs who served in the World War."[18] Dr. Taylor would have been proud and certainly enjoyed the spectacle.

NOTES

1. Live in Clifton, Texas, History Page, www.livein clifton.org/page/history.aspx (accessed April 4, 2015).
2. "Around and About Chicago," *Chicago Defender*, June 12, 1915, 5.
3. "Fred H. Lester," *Chicago Defender*, June 24, 1916, 8.
4. John L. Thompson, *History and Views of Colored Officers Training Camp for 1917 at Fort Des Moines, Iowa* (Des Moines: *The Bystander*, 1917) 89.

5. Memorial Obituaries, Lieutenant General John Quill Taylor King, Sr. PhD, obit.king-tears mortuary.com (accessed June 16, 2012).
6. Table of Medical Reserve Corps—Colored—Receiving Instruction, Medical Training Camp, Fort Des Moines, Iowa, RG-112, Records of the Army Surgeon General, National Archives, College Park, MD.
7. Emmett J. Scott, *The American Negro in the World War*, Chapter XI, net.lib.byu.edu/WWI (accessed April 3, 2015).
8. U.S. Army Medical Department, Office of Medical History, Vol. VIII Field Operations, Chapter IV, Medical Service of the Division in Combat (Washington, D.C.: GPO, 1925) history.amedd.army.mil (accessed April 23, 2015).
9. Robert V. Morris, *Tradition and Valor* (Manhattan, KS: Sunflower University Press, 1999) 53.
10. Louis T. Wright, "I Remember," (unpublished) Moorland Spingarn Research Center, Howard University, Washington, D.C., undated, 86, 89.
11. *Meharry Annual, Military Review 1919,* Harold D. West Collection, Meharry Medical College Archives, Nashville, Tennessee, 66.
12. "He Fell Facing Enemy," *Pittsburgh Courier*, November 23, 1940, 12.
13. *Ibid.*
14. "Minnesota," *Chicago Defender*, June 7, 1919, 17.
15. 1930 U.S. Federal Census.
16. "Tennessee, MEMPHIS," *Baltimore Afro-American*, October 3, 1931, 15.
17. Certificate of Death, Dr. John Q. Taylor, Tennessee Death Records, 1908–1951, ancestry.com.
18. "He Fell Facing Enemy," *Pittsburgh Courier*, 12.

Howard Randall THOMPSON

9 July 1887–10 August 1929
Indiana University, 1913

Roots and Education

Howard Thompson was born and raised in Nashville, Tennessee. His father William S. Thompson was a born a free man in February 1858 in Michigan. His mother Ella Cartwright Thompson was born December 1860 in Alabama. His older sister John (Johnnie) D. was born September 1885 and followed in their father's footsteps and became a teacher.

Thompson received his early education in Nashville's public school system. He finished his B.A. degree at Knoxville College in 1909. Knoxville College, an Historically Black College (HBCU), was founded in 1875 as part of the missionary effort of the United Presbyterian Church of North America to promote religious, moral, and educational leadership among the freed men and women. It is now a liberal arts college.[1]

Thompson enjoyed singing and must have had a wonderful voice. In 1912 he was one of a trio performing in the Presbyterian Church's annual spring musicale. The following year, he was a soloist with the orchestra at a concert at the Crown Garden Theater.[2]

Upon graduation he entered the Indiana University School of Medicine in Indianapolis. The 1913 Arbutus, his Indiana University year-

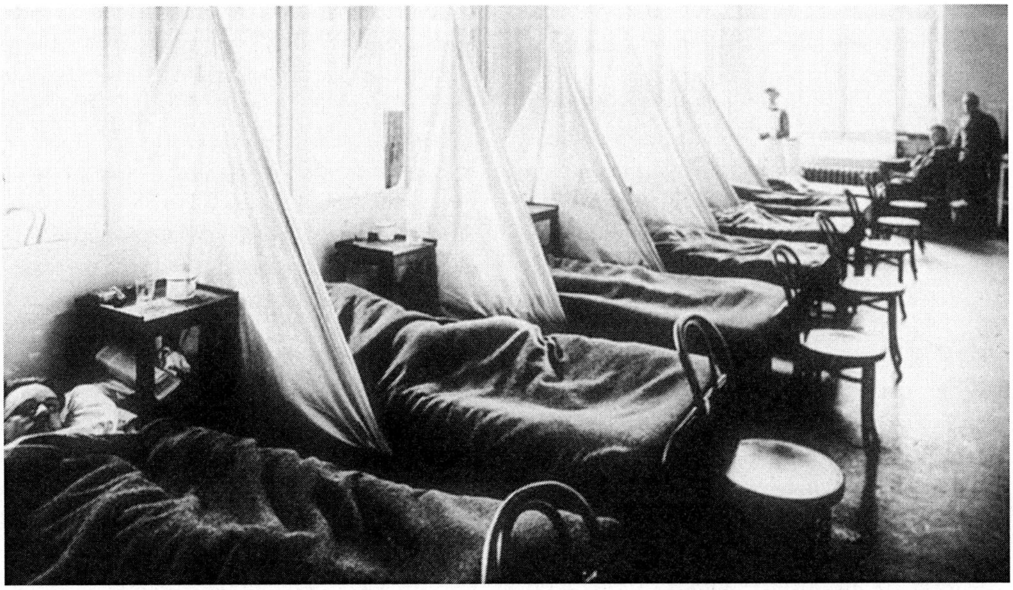

U.S. Army Camp No. 45, Aix-les-Bains, France, Influenza Ward No. 1, ca. 1918 (Reeve 14552, OHA 80: Reeve Photograph Collection, Otis Historical Archives, National Museum of Health and Medicine).

book, says of him, "Booker T. Washington Thompson, as he familiarly known, is noted for his deep bass voice and serious recurrent attack of spring fever after Washington Park season opens."[3] He graduated in 1913. He won, by competitive examination, an internship in the city hospital at Indianapolis, where he served for one year.

Dr. Thompson pursued an Allopath practice. This is the term given to a modern science-based practice. Records indicate he practiced medicine in Indianapolis for nearly two years before moving to Evansville, Indiana, on December 13, 1915, where he established his residence and a private practice.[4]

Military Service

According to his World War I draft registration card, Dr. Thompson registered in June 1917. He was living at 420 Chestnut Street in Evansville. Rather than waiting for his number to be called, he volunteered. He was 29 years old when he was commissioned a first lieutenant in the Army Medical Reserve Corps on July 20.[5]

Thompson arrived at Fort Des Moines for the Medical Officers Training Camp (MOTC) for Colored officers on August 17, 1917. After completing training, he was sent to Camp Grant, in Rockford, Illinois, with the 365th Infantry Regiment, 92nd Division. The regiment prepared there for overseas service.

He moved with the regiment to France in June 1918. Lieutenant Thompson joined the 317th Sanitary Train's 365th Field Hospital in September. Daily reports of casualties indicate he was sick in the hospital from September 14 to September 18, 1918 (likely with influenza), and returned to duty at the 365th Field Hospital. On November 5, he was transferred to the 365th Ambulance Company. This was just prior to the 365th Infantry's greatest battle in the attack on Metz, November 9–11. He would certainly have treated many battle casualties during the attack, which preceded the Armistice by only two days.

Captain Walter R. Sanders was the African American commander of Company E, 365th Infantry Regiment. His record of the attack is now available at the National Archives.[6]

In it he says, "How anyone survived under that fire is still a mystery to me. Enemy artillery had gotten word that we were in the wood and decided to end us right there. Stone, dirt, shrapnel, limbs and whole trees filled the air. The noise and concussion alone where enough to kill one. Talk about shell shock! The earth swayed, shook, and fairly bounced with the awful impact, flashes of fire, the metallic crack of high explosives, the awful explosives that dug holes 15 to 20 feet in diameter, the utter and complete pandemonium, the stench of hell, your friends blown to bits, their pieces dropping near, even striking you."

Lieutenant Thompson and his medics, while under fire, picked up the men who could possibly be saved and brought them out of the carnage. They then stabilized the patients and moved them to the rear where the more severely wounded were sent back to a field hospital.

Career

After the war, he returned to his practice in Evansville. His 1927 ledger of patients and billing information can be found at the Evansville African American Museum.

Dr. Thompson was active in his community. He became a member of the organizing committee that ultimately established the Welborn Walker Annex as a place to treat injured African American coal miners and the community at large.[7] He married Pauline Maxwell, a schoolteacher and worker for the United Service Organization (USO). She was also a member of the NAACP and a Girl Scout advisor. The couple lived at 404 Lincoln Avenue in the African American Baptisttown area of Evansville. They had three daughters—Jacques, Gloria and Patricia.

In the end, when Thompson became ill, he was taken to that same Welborn Walker Hospital Annex for surgery. Dr. James Welborn operated. Dr. Thompson died at the hospital on August 10, 1929. He was only 42. The cause of death was given as complications from appendicitis surgery, acute peritonitis.[8] To honor her brother, Dr. Thompson's sister John (Johnny D.) named her daughter Marie Howard Ferguson.

His widow Pauline survived him by 58 years and continued the family's tradition of service to Evansville African Americans. She was a member of the AME Church, the National Association of Colored Women and the College Women's Club. She also served on the Interracial Commission at Carver Community Center. She died in 1987 at the age of 89.[9]

Dr. Thompson, his wife and daughters are all buried at Evansville's Oak Hill Cemetery.[10] It is the city's oldest and largest public cemetery and holds the city's most influential citizens.

NOTES

1. "A Brief History of Knoxville College," www.knoxvillecollege.edu/about/brief-history (accessed October 10, 2012).
2. "Annual Spring Musicale," *Indianapolis News*, March 16, 1912, 17.
3. "Howard R. Thompson," *Indiana University 1913 Arbutus Yearbook*, U.S. School Yearbooks, ancestry.com.
4. *Directory of Deceased American Physicians, 1804–1929*, ancestry.com.
5. Dr. Thompson's Military Commission, World War I uniform, and medical bag are displayed in the collection of the Evansville (Indiana) African American Museum.
6. RG-120 Records of the American Expeditionary Forces (World War I). Records of Combat Divisions, 1918–1919, 92nd Division, Historical Decimal File—1.4 to 22.9 Box 1.
7. Darrel E. Bingham, *We Ask Only a Fair Trial* (Bloomington: Indiana University Press, 1987) 139.
8. "Death Claims Dr. Thompson." *Evansville Courier and Journal*, August 11, 1929, Clippings File, Willard Library, Evansville, Indiana.
9. Browning Genealogy Database, Evansville, Vanderburgh Public Library, browning.evpl.org (accessed November 6, 2012).
10. *Ibid.*

Silas Stewart THOMPSON

19 December 1881–24 July 1926
Howard Medical College, 1904

Roots and Education

Silas Thompson was born in South Carolina to Sumner and Mary Thompson. His father was a preacher. He had several younger siblings. By 1900 his family lived in Jacksonville, Florida, at 334 Bay Street and Silas, then 19, was living with them. He was single and already working as a schoolteacher.[1]

In the early 1900s he left for Washington, D.C., to study medicine at Howard University. He was one of 60 students who received his M.D. on May 10, 1904.[2] He was granted his medical license in D.C. in 1905, as an Allopath doctor. Thompson was employed as a physician at Freedmen's Hospital.

Dr. Thompson quickly became involved in Washington, D.C's social life. In 1907 he joined in the entertainment offered by Howard University's Florida Club.[3] The club is still active today, bringing students from that state together for several social events throughout the school year. It is also involved in community service projects.[4]

In 1908 the D.C. city directory lists his office at 1102 R Street, NW. In 1909, he was appointed president of the Eastern Star Home Association Trustees at an annual meeting at the Masonic Temple in Southeast Washington, D.C.[5] It was part of the Grand Chapter, Order of the Eastern Star of the District of Columbia. By 1910 he was married to Elizabeth Douglas Thompson, and they lived near the center of the city at 952 R Street, NW. His sister, Mamie Thompson, lived with them, as well as several lodgers.[6]

Dr. Thompson was an active member of the National Medical Association (NMA). In 1913 he was appointed as state vice-president for Washington, D.C. In 1914 the city directory carried a large and very bold listing for Dr. Thompson describing him as a "Physician and Surgeon with Office Hours until 10 a.m., 2 to 4 and 6 to 8 p.m. at 952 R St, NW." The ad included a telephone number. The same bold ad appeared in 1917, but the office address was now 937 R Street NW just across the street from his original home and office address. The original house was now only their residence. He practiced primarily in Washington, D.C., although he became licensed in Virginia in 1915.

Military Career

In 1917 as America entered the First World War, Dr. Thompson, at age 35, volunteered for the U.S. Army Medical Reserve Corps. He was awarded a commission as a first lieutenant. After completing his training, First Lieutenant Thompson was sent to Camp Dix, Wrightstown, New Jersey. He was assigned as a medical officer for the 92nd Division's Field Artillery Regiments (349th and 350th) and its 317th Trench Mortar Battery, which was training there prior to going overseas.

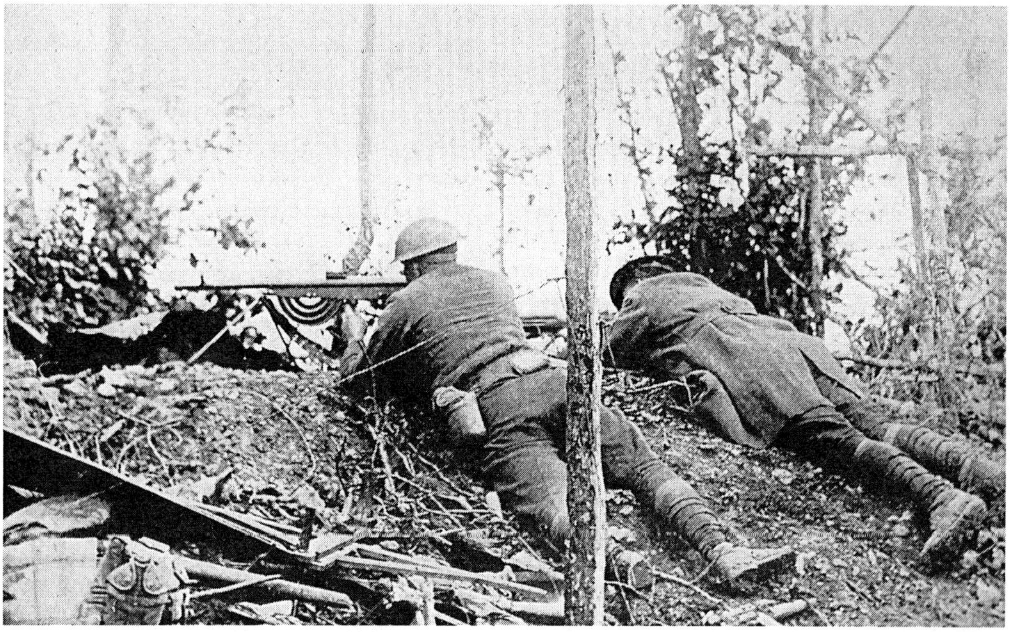

Machine gunners (National Archives).

In June 1918 the 92nd Division was deployed to France. He served with the artillery units during the war. By mid–August 1918 the units were sent for training to Camp La Courtine, one of the largest artillery camps in France. At the end of September and in early October the doctors and medics were extremely busy dealing with the Spanish Influenza epidemic. Many soldiers were being hospitalized while others were being moved into separate barracks and quarantined until the epidemic could be checked.[7]

In mid–October the artillery units began to move to the front to join the infantry units for the fight. The weather was cold and frosty. The artillery units entered the action only several weeks before the Armistice ended the war. The next several winter months were harsh and difficult. The doctors were quite busy attending to the soldiers' health as the division slowly made its way to the French coast to Brest for the trip home.

Career

After returning from overseas in 1919, Dr. Thompson travelled west to California and Nevada. His wife Elizabeth stayed behind. He acquired medical licenses in both states.[8] His sister was living at his home in Washington, D.C., at 937 R Street, NW. She had two young women lodgers. In late 1921 his wife Elizabeth sued Dr. Thompson in the Supreme Court of the District of Columbia seeking "a decree for maintenance and support."[9] The proceedings were contentious and covered in the *Nevada State Journal.* Although his wife was correct in her assertions that his move to Reno was only temporary, he was correct that she had deserted him when she refused to accompany him to California.[10] The jury was out only 15 minutes before granting the divorce on Dr. Thompson's terms. The divorce was finalized in Reno, Nevada, on October 31, 1922. He soon married a woman named Violet.[11]

For some years Howard alumni and members of the District of Columbia medical community had talked about the possibility of a National Capitol Country Club. In 1924 the group organized a board of directors and found volunteers willing to contribute to the effort. Dr. Thompson was quickly added to the group.[12] The club was chartered in Laurel, Maryland. It was only a nine-hole course, but it did provide a place for the African American establishment of Washington to practice the sport during the Jim Crow era.[13]

Dr. Thompson maintained his relationship with the Freedmen's Hospital and Howard University long after he graduated. His home and office were conveniently located less than a mile away from those institutions. In 1926 he was involved in Howard's Conclusion Campaign to raise $149,000 in order to secure a conditional gift of $250,000 from D. C.'s General Education Board.

Dr. Thompson was still married to Violet when he succumbed to cardio-renal disease at the age of 46. His military service in World War I entitled him to burial at the beautiful Arlington National Cemetery in Washington, D.C., where he rests in Section 4-E, Site 2721.[14]

Notes

1. 1900 U.S. Federal Census.
2. "News Items," *New York Medical Journal and Philadelphia Medical Journal Consolidated, Weekly Review of Medicine*, Vol. LXXIX, June 18, 1904, 1197.
3. "Florida Club Entertains," *Washington Bee*, October 12, 1907, 5.
4. www.facebook.com/.../Howard-University-Florida-Club (accessed April 3, 2015).
5. "Annie V. Moore Elected," *Washington Bee*, February 6, 1909, 1.
6. 1910 U.S. Federal Census.
7. "With the 351st in France," *a Diary Compiled by Sergeant William O. Ross and Corporal Duke L. Slaughter*, Baltimore, MD, Afro-American Company, Pennsylvania State Archives, Harrisburg, 22.
8. *Directory of Deceased American Physicians, 1804–1929*, American Medical Association, ancestry.com.
9. "Legal Notices," *The Washington Law Reporter*, Vol. XLIX, 699.
10. "Colored Physician Wins Divorce Suit," *Nevada State Journal*, October 31, 1922, 8.
11. "Wife Gets Estate of Dr. Silas Thompson," *Pittsburgh Courier*, August 14, 1926 1.
12. "Officers of the Board," *Pittsburgh Courier*, May 17, 1924, 7.
13. Marvin P. Dawkins and Graham Kinloch, *African American Golfers During the Jim Crow Era* (Westport, CT: Praeger, 2000) 24.
14. U.S. Veterans Gravesites, ca. 1775–2006, National Cemetery Administration, ancestry.com.

Thomas Clinton TINSLEY

15 November 1887–12 August 1954
University of West Tennessee, 1910

Roots and Education

Thomas Tinsley came from Henderson, North Carolina, in Vance County. He was the youngest of three brothers born there to Albert and Mollie Tinsley. In 1900 he was 12 years old and lived with his family on Hillard Street. His father was a painter and his mother worked as a laundress.[1] He was educated in the local black schools and entered the University of West Tennessee College of Medicine and Surgery in Memphis, graduating in 1910. He then passed the North Carolina State Board Examination and was granted a license to practice medicine in June 1910.

By 1912 he was established in Asheville and practicing medicine. In July he delivered an address entitled "Combined Efforts" at Asheville's Young Men's Institute (YMI), an African American cultural center.[2] The 1913 city directory records him living in Asheville and working as a physician from his home at 22 Eagle Street.[3] Another black physician in Asheville, Dr. William G. Torrance, opened the first black clinic in Asheville at 16 Eagle Street, before moving his family and clinic to 95 Hill Street in 1911.[4] The black medical community in Asheville was tiny in those years, so they must have known one another.

Military Service

Tinsley had returned to Henderson by the time America entered the First World War in 1917 where he lived at 720 Hillside Avenue. He was 29 years old and his draft registration card says he was self-employed as a physician there, with a wife and child. His wife was Lois Hoffman Tinsley of Knoxville, a schoolteacher.[5] His activities included membership in the United Presbyterian Church, and he was a Mason and Pythian.[6]

In 1917 he volunteered, was commissioned in the Army Medical Reserve Corps as a first lieutenant, and left his practice to serve. He was trained at Fort Des Moines, Iowa, for 79 days and then assigned to the 350th Machine Gun Battalion's Medical Detachment, 92nd Division, at Camp Grant in Rockford, Illinois. He commanded that medical detachment of more than a dozen men throughout the war.

His entire division went to France in the summer of 1918, and he arrived in Brest on June 19. After training at the village of Belmont, the battalion entered the trenches in September at the St. Dié sector near Frapelle (described as a hot sector), where it engaged in several battles and experienced its first artillery and gas attacks. The battalion used heavy Vickers machine guns that were transported on carts. His detachment's medical personnel were called on to attend to wounded and injured infantrymen of the 366th Regiment, who were being supported by the 350th Machine Gun battalion. From St. Dié, the division was sent to the Argonne Forest at the outset of the Meuse-Argonne campaign in late September.

Seleste L. Chandler, a former medical student and unit clerk described the combat: "Our [92nd] division lost quite a large number of men. I consider myself lucky not to be called during that awful slaughter. The ambulances were rushed both day and night with the injured. It was necessary to employ a number of trucks due to the shortage of ambulances. The sights were pitiful."[7]

From there the division transferred to the Marbache Sector, arriving October 8, where it fought until the war ended with the Armistice on November 11. Chandler wrote, "We were in very hot battles, losing many men. The weather was cold and they had to sleep on the ground, where many caught cold." On November 22 they were ordered to pull out and relocate to Pont-à-Mousson where an infirmary was established. According to Chandler, "Every morning they attended sick men from 7:00 am until 10:30 p.m. Finally, the division made its long, cold and slow way toward the embarkation port of Brest and returned home in February 1919."

Dr. Tinsley was awarded a "Croix de Guerre" medal by the French for his service.[8] He was honorably discharged from the army at Camp Lee, Virginia, on April 7, 1919, and returned home.

Career

In 1920 at the age of 32, he was issued a U.S. Passport and accepted a position as a physician in Mexico with Atlantic Refining Company of Philadelphia at its oil properties there.[9] After his tour in Mexico, he returned to the United States and from 1921 through 1924, Dr. Tinsley was in Durham, North Carolina, with an office at 203½ East Chapel Hill and a home at 802 Dowd. A few years later he had a home on Umstead near Pine Street.[10]

In 1921 he had the sad duty of signing the death certificate of a friend and fellow army doctor and Fort Des Moines MOTC graduate, Lieutenant William John Henry Booker, who died unexpectedly in April in Oxford, North Carolina.

Later that year he became a charter member of the Durham Alumni chapter of the Kappa Alpha Psi fraternity and served as its "The Keeper of Records" from 1921 to 1924.[11] Tinsley was an "out-of-town invited guest" at a Grand Ball to honor visitors from Monrovia, Liberia, in Raleigh in October 1922. It was described as the most significant and major social event in Raleigh for several years.[12]

The following year, in late summer 1923, he and his brother, Dr. J. A. Tinsley, and wife paid a visit to Philadelphia en route to the New Jersey shore.[13] In August 1924 he and his wife were described in a newspaper as "out-of-town" visitors attending a funeral for Mrs. Marian White in Raleigh.[14] In 1925 Tinsley attended the North State Dental Association meeting in Winston-Salem where he made a presentation entitled "Sinuses and Fecal Infection as Effecting Dentists and Physicians."[15] A brief social news report in May said Dr. Thomas Tinsley of Wilson, North Carolina, spent a few hours in Rocky Mount, North Carolina.[16] In 1928 an official roster of former World War I officers listed him and gave his address as 525 East Nash Street in Wilson.[17] In June 1930 he was listed in the U.S. Census as a patient at the U.S. Veterans Hospital #91 in Tuskegee, Alabama.

No information was forthcoming on the doctor's activities for the next 24 years until his death was reported in 1954. The request for a U.S. military headstone was signed by his wife, Mrs. Lois H. Tinsley of Knoxville, Tennessee. The headstone still stands over his grave at his birthplace in Henderson, North Carolina, in the Blacknall Cemetery.

NOTES

1. 1900 U.S. Federal Census.
2. "Y.M.I. Notes," *Asheville Gazette-News*, July 20, 1912, 2.
3. *1913 Asheville Directory*, U.S. City Directories, 1821–1989 (Beta) ancestry.com.
4. Annye S. Holt, "*The Black Physician's Presence in Asheville, North Carolina,*" Self-published, Annye S. Holt, 37 Erskine Ave, Asheville, NC.
5. World War I Draft Registration, ancestry.com.

6. John L. Thompson, *History and Views of Colored Officers Training Camp for 1917 at Fort Des Moines, Iowa* (Des Moines: *The Bystander*, 1917) 90.
7. *Diary of Seleste L. Chandler, Medical Detachment, 350th Machine Gun Battalion*, Amistad Research Center, Tulane University, New Orleans, LA.
8. U.S. Headstone Applications, ancestry.com.
9. U.S. Passport Applications, 1795–1925, ancestry.com.
10. *1921–1923, 1924, Durham, NC*, U.S. City Directories, 1821–1989 (Beta) ancestry.com.
11. Kappa Alpha Psi (ΚΑΨ) is a collegiate Greek-letter fraternity with a predominantly African-American membership. Since the fraternity's founding on January 5, 1911, at Indiana University Bloomington, the fraternity has never limited membership based on color, creed or national origin. en.wikipedia.org/wiki/Alpha_Kappa_Psi.
12. "Liberians Are Grandly Feted by Carolinians," *Chicago Defender*, October 21, 1922, 5.
13. "Philadelphia, PA," *Pittsburgh Courier*, August 18, 1923, 13.
14. "Raleigh, N.C.," *New Journal and Guide* (1916–2003), August 2, 1924, 8.
15. "North State Dental Assn in Session," *Pittsburgh Courier*, April 25, 1925, 5.
16. "Rocky Mount, N.C.," *New Journal and Guide* (1916–2003), May 30,1925, 8.
17. *Retirement of World War Officers, March 29, 1928*, Committed to the Committee of the Whole House on the State of the Union, www.genealogybank.com (accessed July 31, 2012).

Rufus S. VASS

23 May 1887–1 June 1957
Leonard Medical School, 1918

Roots and Education

Rufus Vass was born in Raleigh, North Carolina, to the Reverend Samuel N. and Mary Eliza (Haywood) Vass. His father was a "nationally known educator, minister and author" who was born, educated and spent his life in Raleigh. The Reverend Vass received honorary degrees from several universities and among his most notable books was "How to Study and Teach the Bible."[1] He was well regarded in his nine years of teaching the classics and history at Shaw University. "Some have spoken of him as possessing a mind of unusual brilliancy, but he himself has always looked upon himself rather as a mediocre, and he attributes his success as a teacher to hard work."[2]

In recognition of his Bible scholarship, Shaw University and Livingstone College at Salisbury, North Carolina, conferred upon Rev. Vass the honorary degree of doctor of divinity in 1901.[3]

Rufus Vass and his sister Maude grew up in an environment where education and religion were highly valued. Rufus followed in his father's footsteps and received his A.B. from Shaw University in Raleigh in 1908. He earned his medical degree from Shaw's Leonard Medical School in 1912.

Leonard was established in 1880 when medical schools were professionalizing. It was the first medical school for African Americans in the United States to offer a four-year curriculum.[4] During the 40 years of its existence, it graduated more than 400 physicians. Many of Raleigh's white medical professionals taught at the school on a part-time basis.[5]

After graduating, Dr. Vass married Sarah Clarke Green. She was a graduate of St. Augustine School in Raleigh and a teacher in the church mission schools in North and South Carolina. Dr. and Mrs. Vass settled into Smithfield, North Carolina, near Raleigh. They were there when Sarah suddenly became very ill. She went to stay with her parents who lived nearby and died in her sleep on March 22, 1916.[6]

Military Service

As America entered the First World War, Dr. Vass volunteered for the U.S. Army and was called into active service on August 3, 1917. He reported to Fort Des Moines for training on September 7, 1917. First Lieutenant Vass was then assigned to Camp Funston, Kansas, where he was assigned to the 367th Ambulance Company of the 92nd Division. Once in France, he was reassigned to the 368th Field Hospital.

His hospital reports cover infectious diseases, including tuberculosis (a medical condition that could send a soldier home) and sexually transmitted diseases such as gonorrhea and syphilis. The most significant disease that struck during World War I was influenza. Many of the soldiers and general public who died during the 1918–1919 pandemic actually died of pneumonia.[7] Antibiotics for the treatment of such infections were not available at this time in history.

The hospital was actually set up for casualties from the trenches in the Vosges region where the 92nd Division had its baptism by fire. There was only light fighting there and the hospital was then moved to serve the unit in the Meuse-Argonne battle.[8] After his participation in the battle of Metz, November 10 and 11 (the last two days of the war) Lieutenant Vass was promoted to the rank of captain in the Medical Corps. Captain Vass served overseas from June 19, 1918, to February 24, 1919.

Career

Dr. Vass returned to his practice in Smithfield, North Carolina, and on November 3, 1920, he married Luatle (Lucille) M. Jeffries. "Luatle's mother was a slave until the end of the Civil War; however, Luatle and her two sisters managed to graduate from Shaw University."[9] The couple would have no children. For the rest of their lives, Vass and his wife served the African American population in and around Smithfield. She served as his secretary and nurse at his home office.

The influenza pandemic raged in North Carolina at the end of 1919. By February 1920 it was abating and the order that closed schools and churches in the towns was lifted. Rural churches never closed and work at the tobacco companies never stopped. By March 1920 it was estimated that there were 90 to 100 deaths in nearby counties caused by the flu. The majority of the fatalities were among the African American community. It was thought this happened because they did not see a doctor in the very early stages of the disease. The doctors in this part of North Carolina reported attending more than 500 flu patients. During one two-week period in late February all of the doctors were working 20-hour days.[10]

In 1921 the state of North Carolina spent money on better roads. In fact a $50-million bond was issued and two paved state highways were built through Johnston County. East-west North Carolina 10 (later renumbered as U.S. 70) and a north-south North Carolina 22 (redesignated in the early 1930s as U.S. 301) passed through Smithfield. Smithfield became a bustling small town, and Dr. Vass was able to travel easily to more of his patients.[11]

In early 1923 Dr. Vass joined Drs. McCauley, Robert and Perry at McCauley Private Hospital at 513 South Wilmington Street in Raleigh. Even with the new highways into town, Smithfield to Raleigh was a 30-mile drive.

The African American community was mostly poor. Despite good fortune in commercial centers, farmers in the 1920s were suffering under a postwar agricultural depression that brought dramatic fluctuations in cotton and tobacco prices. Farms operated by tenants also jumped from an already high 51 percent in 1920 to 59 percent in 1930. Cotton farmers tried to make up for their losses by overproducing—a practice that only served to drive market prices even lower.

The stock market crash of 1929 and Great Depression that followed intensified the hard times farmers were experiencing. Most banks closed, and wealthy families in practically every town saw their fortunes disappear. The boll weevil joined forces with federal crop controls in dethroning "King Cotton" in Johnston County. While many farmers then turned to tobacco, market prices for the golden leaf remained low through the 1930s. Nevertheless, a combination of federal programs, conservatism, and firmly entrenched interdependence among families and neighborhoods saw people through this difficult era.[12]

Dr. Vass was interviewed in July of 1939 as part of the Federal Writers' Project. The Project was created in order to provide writers with jobs during the Great Depression. William S. Cramer, author of *The Federal Writers' Project Life Stories: An Iconoclast Among the True Believers*, included an interview with Dr. Vass. Although Dr. Vass lived in a time when African Americans were treated unequally, he and his wife owned a very large home with nine rooms and fine furniture. Most of his patients came to his office there. He made house calls if they were very ill. Many of his patients worked labor jobs in Raleigh.

Dr. Vass said, "I simply cannot see why a white man should be paid $18 a week for the very same work that a Negro is paid $10 per week. That is exactly what is being done in Raleigh." His outlook, however, was very positive. He believed that "in the future, whites and blacks would be able to live side by side, respecting one another's culture and receiving equal opportunity."[13]

In addition to his general practice, Dr. Vass was the medical director for Eagle Life Insurance Co. in Durham and on the staff of St. Agnes Hospital. He was active in the National Medical Association (NMA), the Raleigh chapter (L. A. Scruggs Medical Society) and North Carolina's Old North State Medical Society.[14] He was a lifelong Baptist. Later in his career he joined the NAACP and the North Carolina Tennis Club. When a summer camp for 350 of Raleigh's African American girls was organized in 1939, Dr. Vass was there with several other local doctors to provide medical examinations for each of them.[15]

At the 60th annual convention of the National Medical Association, he was among 199 members recognized for 40 years of service as general practitioners. He had actually served his patients for 43 years since his graduation from Leonard.

Dr. Vass died at the age of 70 in his home at 417 South Person Street in Raleigh of a coronary thrombosis. He was buried with a military headstone at Mount Hope Cemetery in Raleigh.

President Barack Obama once observed, "The best way to not feel hopeless is to get up and do something. Don't wait for good things to happen to you. If you go out and make some good things happen, you will fill the world with hope, you will fill yourself with hope."

This was certainly a philosophy that also guided Dr. Vass, and his community was richer for it.

Notes

1. "Veteran Religious Leader Passes at Home of Daughter in Raleigh," *Pittsburgh Courier*, October 8, 1938.
2. Ruth Anita Hawkins Hughes, "Dr. Samuel N. Vass," *Contributions of Vance County People of Color* (Sparks Press, 1988) 163.
3. *Ibid.*, 167.
4. *Leonard Hall (Shaw University)*, en.wikipedia.org/wiki/Leonard_Hall_(Shaw_University) (accessed July 13, 2012).
5. ncpedia.org (accessed April 3, 2015).
6. "Obituary," *The Warren Record*, April 14, 1916, 2.
7. minnpost.com (accessed April 3, 2015).
8. *Dr. Rufus Samuel Vass*, en.wikiversity.org/w/index.php-Federal_Writers_Project_-_Life Histories (accessed July 26, 2013).
9. *Ibid.*
10. Francis B. Hays, "Worked Night and Day," *Oxford, NC Health Doctors, Hospitals, Nurses*, Vol. 62, a collection of newspaper clippings.
11. *History of Johnston County*, www.johnstonnc.com/mainpage.cfm?category_level_id=649 (accessed Sept 4, 2013).
12. *Ibid.*
13. *Ibid.*
14. "Final Rites Held for Noted NC Physician," *New Journal and Guide*, June 22, 1957, 2.
15. "Camp for Raleigh Girls," *New Journal and Guide*, July 22, 1939, 5.

Henry Harvey WALKER

13 June 1882–14 July 1962
Meharry Medical College, 1913

Roots and Education

Records of Henry H. Walker's family or early life have evaded discovery. He was born in Davidson County, Tennessee, and his year of birth has been reported variously as 1882, 1883 and 1888. It is most likely between 1882 and 1884. He was educated in the state's most important city, Nashville. His college years were spent at Walden University in Nashville where he was awarded his A.B. He remained in Nashville and earned his M.D. from Walden's Meharry Medical College in 1913.

After graduation from Meharry, Dr. Walker married Elizabeth Fletcher, a local music teacher. The couple lived in Nashville for the rest of their lives. He was a first surgical assistant to Dr. John H. Hale at Hale Hospital. Dr. Hale had worked, studied, and travelled to the Mayo and Crile Clinics to advance his skills. He passed the knowledge he gathered on to Dr. Walker. Walker succeeded him in 1917 and joined the Meharry faculty, teaching anatomy as well as minor and orthopedic surgery.[1] He was also a clinical obstetrician at Meharry and an active member of the National Medical Association (NMA) and Rock City Academy of Medicine and Surgery in Nashville.[2]

The Walkers were active in the African American community. His medical office was in their home at 81 Claiborne Street. Their daughter Mary Ann was adopted while they were there. Dr. Walker was a member of the AME Church and became especially involved in the Masons, Kappa Alpha Psi, the Knights of Pythias, and the Republican Party.

Military Service

Before America's entry into the First World War, Dr. Walker served two years and six months in the State Militia of Tennessee (National Guard) as a first sergeant in the only black company in the south. In 1917 he responded to Meharry's World War I recruitment appeal for doctors. He was commissioned in the Medical Reserve Corps and received his training at the Medical Officers Training Camp (MOTC) at Fort Des Moines. His early training in the National Guard gave him an advantage over the other doctors. He was elected a section chief and by the end of camp was promoted to captain, Medical Corps. His wife Elizabeth was so proud of his promotion that she had their listing in the Nashville phone book changed to Captain and Elizabeth Walker.

At Camp Funston, Walker was named commander of the 368th Ambulance Company of the 317th Sanitary (Medical) Train. His company included five physicians and 153 medical enlisted men.[3] The company was sent to Camp Upton, New York, en route to its final departure to France.

Captain Walker was involved with providing lighter moments for his men. The Jesse Moorland Papers at Howard University include a March 9, 1918, YMCA newspaper column about some of the Camp Funston activities. One night he and Lieutenant Bates threw a party for the men. At other times, they organized basketball games or provided movies. There was often music (especially when the women visited from nearby Manhattan, Kansas), and the men played checkers until lights out.[4] Captain Walker also took an interest in the religious side of camp life by leading Bible study.

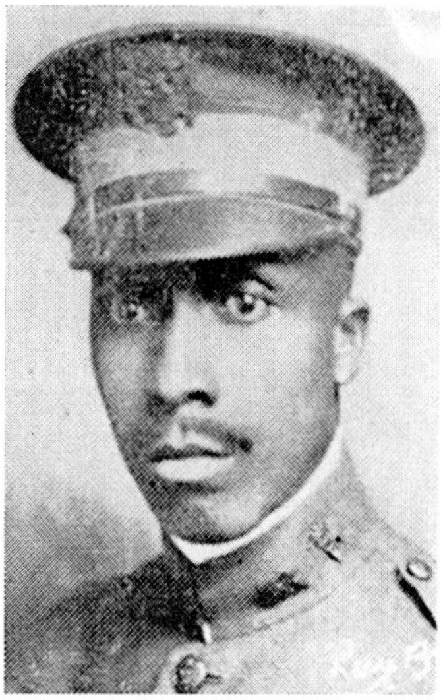

Major H. H. Walker (courtesy Meharry Medical College Archives).

Once in France, his responsibilities included much more than healing sick or wounded soldiers. As the unit commander, Captain Walker reported to Lieutenant Colonel Downing on his doctors' efficiencies, numbers of various kinds of illnesses, money spent for supplies, and a host of other matters judged important by the army. He also took time to defend one of his doctors (Lieutenant E. W. Bates) when he believed Bates was unfairly declared inefficient. Bates later proved his mettle under fire and received an award for his bravery.

Captain Walker commanded his ambulance company throughout the war. He was promoted to major before his return to the United States.

Career

After the war, Dr. Walker returned to Nashville and Hale Hospital. The 1920 Census reported the family now lived at 1024 First Avenue South. Elizabeth taught music there. Dr. Walker returned to Meharry's faculty. When Dr. Hale closed his hospital in 1923 to become chairman of the Department of Surgery at Meharry and Hubbard Hospital, Dr. Walker continued to work with him.[5] At this time, Dr. Walker moved his office out of his home and into a medical office in the Morris Memorial Building in downtown Nashville.

On March 14, 1933, a tornado swept through East Nashville. Among the buildings it destroyed was the Branden Memorial ME Church. The committee to rebuild consisted of pastors and bishops from Tennessee as well as those connected with Meharry. Dr. Walker worked with this group to raise the necessary funds to rebuild the church.

In 1934 Dr. Walker ventured into politics. "He was asked to withdraw from his run for city council in favor of a white candidate. He refused. Dr. Walker was leading the white candidates, but the ballot box was stolen. Judges declared the election void because expense accounts were not filed five days before the election."[6] In spite of this sad experience, he remained active with the Republican Party for the rest of his life.

In the late 1930s he became involved in the Nashville Negro Board of Trade, Community Chest Fund and the City Baby Clinic. The Walker family now owned their own home at 924 First Avenue in Nashville.

By 1940 Dr. Walker was chosen grand chancellor of the Knights of Pythias of Tennessee. He was also past commander of the Colored Legionnaires of Tennessee. He spoke at their meeting in Chattanooga urging support for Wendell Willkie for president because the Republican plank held "more assurance for Negroes than any other plank I've ever seen in my lifetime."[7]

While Dr. Walker was commander of the local American Legion Post in 1943, a special dinner honoring veterans of both races was held at Patterson Methodist Church in Nashville. Dr. Walker spoke and urged all men who were eligible to join the American Legion.[8]

Nashville had its share of racial disturbances in 1943. Dr. Walker witnessed an African American soldier ejected from a bar by the city's white military police. The incident escalated so much that the city's riot squad was called and a "large group of innocent Negroes were badly beaten." Dr. Walker was respected for his military service and when he approached

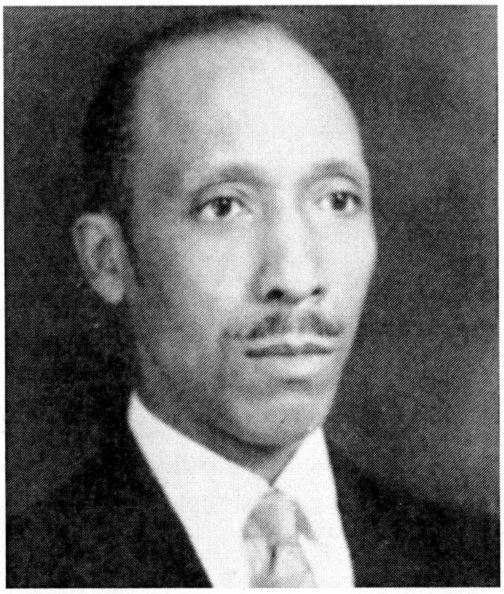

Dr. H. H. Walker, president, National Medical Association, 1950–51 (courtesy Meharry Medical College Archives).

Chief of Police Griffin about the incident, the chief agreed to a meeting. After some investigation of the police action, Griffin agreed to replace some of the white members of the military police with black men. A community council on human relations was formed. Dr. Walker was one of its appointed members.[9]

Dr. Walker was also active in the Meharry Alumni Association. In 1946, he donated $1,000 to its building fund.[10] In 1948 he did some fundraising with the NAACP that resulted in a $9,000 check for Meharry's Hubbard Hospital building fund.[11] At one time he served as president of its alumni association, and for a number of years, he was a trustee of the medical college.

In 1949 Dr. Walker was a member of a new hospital authority of the city of Nashville. It was responsible for a contract between Meharry's Hubbard and Vanderbilt hospitals to open both facilities to treat African Americans in the city of Nashville. Under the program, Meharry would receive $255,000 annually from the city. The city's general hospital would also keep a ward open for black patients. This was an extraordinary victory for health services for African Americans in the city of Nashville.[12]

His work in the National Medical Association (NMA) included his presidency in 1950–51. He led the 50th annual meeting in Philadelphia where more than 1,500 African American physicians from all parts of the United States were in attendance. Surgical clinics at that meeting included ones by the city's rescue squad in early treatment of burns, fractures and gas cases. Eye clinics were also offered. The members were urged to seek legislative action in their states to establish institutions to care for drug addicts. During this meeting he also made his official and personal endorsement of the March of Dimes campaign.[13]

In 1954 Tennessee Governor Frank Clement appointed Dr. Walker to the State Penal Institutions Improvement Committee. The Governor formed this group to study the state of the prison system and make recommendations to improve security.[14]

Dr. Walker died in 1962 in Nashville's Veterans Administration Hospital. He was 78 and suffered from arteriosclerotic heart disease, a rapid heart rhythm that is treated today with pace makers and beta-blockers. The funeral was held at Scay-Hubbard Methodist Church in Nashville. He was survived by Elizabeth, his wife of 49 years, daughter Mary Ann and his sister Mattie Shane, all of Nashville.[15]

Dr. Walker was buried at Nashville's Greenwood Cemetery. The following year *Jet Magazine* reported that Elizabeth gave a $2,000 grant to Meharry in honor of her husband.[16]

Martin Luther King, Jr., said, "The first question which the priest and the Levite asked was: 'If I stop to help this man, what will happen to me?' But ... the good Samaritan reversed the question: 'If I do not stop to help this man, what will happen to him?" Throughout his life H. H. Walker lived by this example. He stepped up and took leadership roles to help his fellow man.

NOTES

1. Thomas Yenser, *Who's Who in Colored America*, Sixth Edition (New York, 1944), 532.
2. John L. Thompson, *History and Views of Colored Officers Training Camp for 1917 at Fort Des Moines, Iowa* (Des Moines: *The Bystander*, 1917) 92.
3. Yenser, *Who's Who in Colored America*, Sixth Edition (New York, 1944), 532.
4. Russell S. Brown, *YMCA No. 11 (Colored Service)*, March 9, 1918, Jesse Moorland Papers, Box 126–72, Howard University Manuscript Archives,Washington, D.C.
5. AMA Deceased Physician Card, National Library of Medicine, Bethesda, MD.
6. "Wouldn't Sell Out, Ballot Box Stolen," *Afro-American*, April 14, 1934, 23.
7. "Memphis Leader Says Willkie to Bag Tenn." *Atlanta Daily World*, August 24, 1940, 4.
8. "Honor to Men in Service," *Pittsburgh Courier*, Sept 11, 1943, 15.
9. "Nashville Solves Race Problem with Negro MP's," *Kingsport Times*, July 22, 1943, 12.
10. "Lauded," *Chicago Defender*, July 13, 1946, 7.
11. "$9,000 More for Hubbard Hospital," *Afro-American*, October 30, 1948, 5.
12. "Meharry Deal with City of Nashville Completed," *Atlanta Daily World*, August 10, 1949, 4.
13. "Dr. Walker Endorses March of Dimes," *New Journal and Guide*, January 27, 1951, 8.
14. "Gov. Clement Names Three to Penal Unit," *Kingsport News*, February 26, 1954, 7.
15. "Dr. H. H. Walker of Meharry Dies," *Pittsburgh Courier*, July 28, 1962, 4.
16. "Meharry Grad's Widow Presents School $2,000 Grant," *Jet Magazine*, February 28, 1963, 17.

James Carroll WALLACE

25 September 1891–6 August 1957
Howard Medical College, 1917

Roots and Education

James Wallace was born in Gainesville, Texas, a small town 70 miles north of Dallas. In 1908 he graduated from Beaumont High School in Beaumont, Texas. Then in 1912 he graduated from Wiley College in Marshall, Texas. He was salutatorian in high school and college. Wiley was founded in 1873 by the Freedmen's Aid Society of the Methodist Episcopal Church for the purpose of providing education to the "newly freed men" and preparing them for a new life. It was named for Bishop Isaac T. Wiley, an outstanding minister, medical missionary and educator. Wiley is currently affiliated with the United Methodist Church. It lays claim to the title "first Black college west of the Mississippi River."[1]

After graduation from Wiley College, Wallace went on to medical school and graduated in 1916 from Howard University College of Medicine in Washington, D.C. He was awarded that year's Dean Bolloch prize as most outstanding student in surgery.[2] From Washington he went to Kansas City, Missouri, where he interned from July 1, 1916, to July 1, 1917, at Kansas City Hospital No. 2.

Military Service

While still in his surgical residency at the Kansas City Hospital, Dr. Wallace registered for the draft. He was single and living in Kansas City at 22nd and Cherry Street. He then volunteered and was accepted into the Army Medical Reserve Corps in July. Lieutenant Wallace reported for training at Fort Des Moines on August 24, 1917. His home address became 306 Park Street in Beaumont, Texas.[3] After basic training, Wallace was transferred to Camp Funston, Kansas, where he joined the 368th Field Hospital. He was one of five physicians from Fort Des Moines who were assigned there.

Once in France, in addition to battle wounds, they treated soldiers for exhaustion, appendicitis, influenza, pneumonia, and a host of other problems. The rapidity with which patients were evacuated to and from field hospitals varied widely and was dependent on the type of casualty, enemy fire, as well as weather and road conditions. Since the field hospitals rarely could accommodate more than 200 patients, it was impossible to hold patients in the division. Beds were needed for later casualties.

The average time men were held in the field hospitals was four days. They were either returned to duty or moved to a hospital further in the rear.

Physicians and medics became specialists. They kept the commanding officer informed of patients who were ready to be evacuated. In periods of stress (high military activity), non-transportable patients were only those with hemorrhage, aspirating chest wounds, severe abdominal wounds, amputations, and deep shock.[4]

In addition to his medical duties, First Lieutenant Wallace was named supply officer of the hospital, responsible for requisitioning its medical supplies. Following the armistice on November 11, 1918, a field report just before Christmas in 1918 noted doctors saw their patients and operated in a "dark, crowded, cold barn with a leaky roof, no facilities for heating and with only one window."[5]

Career

After the war, Dr. Wallace married Maude Thomas. The couple initially lived in Jefferson, Texas, with his aunt Boshie Swindon and stepbrother Charles Wilson. Later he and Maude moved to the house at 2890 Houston Street in Beaumont where they raised their four sons—James Jr., Spurgeon (Virgil), William and Charles. All four sons went to his alma mater, Wiley College. Two went on to medical school, James Jr. (dental school at Meharry) and Charles (Prairie View A & M University).[6]

Dr. Wallace was a practicing physician in Beaumont for more than 35 years. He was on the staffs of both the Beaumont Municipal and Hotel Dieu hospitals. His office was located upstairs at 465 Forsythe Street. He and Maud were members of the AME Church. He was always active and prominent in civic life.

In 1934 *Pittsburgh Courier* reporter Albert White wrote an article about the booming Texas city of Beaumont. In it he cites the boom was being shared with the black community in a large part due to the civic involvement of its leadership. One of the leaders mentioned was Dr. Wallace. Reporting on the success of National Negro Health Week, White called Wallace "one of the foremost members of his profession, a progressive and public-spirited citizen."[7] Wallace also served in several leadership positions of his professional organizations including the local Oil City Medical, Dental and Pharmaceutical Association. In fact, he was treasurer of that organization while helping develop an operational local chapter of the NAACP.[8] When the NAACP membership drive opened in Beaumont in April of 1935, Dr. Wallace was one of the first to join.[9] He was active in the local chapter for the rest of his life.

Maud died in 1951. Six years later, Dr. Wallace died suddenly at home at the age of 66 of a coronary occlusion (heart attack).[10]

Dr. and Mrs. Wallace were proud of all four sons. Dr. James C. Wallace, Jr., probably received the most press coverage. He set up his first dental practice in Cairo, Illinois, married Annetta Lucas and had two children. He became one of the leaders in the fight to end segregation in the schools.[11] In 1952 a cross was burned in his yard. A shot was fired into his home. It was a dangerous place for an activist. Cairo had named him Citizen of the Year in 1950.[12]

He also followed his father into the Army Medical Corps. During the Korean War, Major Wallace served in Korea and then in Bamberg, Germany as the dental officer-in-charge in the dependent's dental clinic.

After his military service, he relocated his family to Chicago. Dr. Wallace, Jr., was dental director of the Martin Luthur King, Jr. Neighborhood Health Center, providing dental care for the center from the Lincoln Dental Society. He was also president of the National Dental Association (NDA) and was involved in a host of Chicago civic activities. By 1965 he had received NDA's President's Award for outstanding service to his community for three years in a row.

NOTES

1. www.wileyc.edu/history (accessed April 30, 2012).
2. "Texas Medical Men," *Chicago Defender*, June 28, 1941, 7.
3. John L. Thompson, *History and Views of Colored Officers Training Camp for 1917 at Fort Des Moines, Iowa* (Des Moines: *The Bystander*, 1917) 93.
4. U.S. Army Medical Department, Office of Medical History, Vol. VIII Field Operations, Chapter IV, Medical Service of the Division in Combat (Washington, D.C.:

GPO, 1925) history.amedd.army.mil (accessed April 23, 2015).

5. Field Hospital 368, 317 Sanitary Train, 92d Division, Amer. E. F. Mobile, December 23, 1918, Declassified Holdings, National Archives, College Park, MD.

6. Crawford, Mary Greer, "Wiley by the Week," *Pittsburgh Courier*, April 11, 1941, 19.

7. "Beaumont Is Making Rapid Civic Progress," *Pittsburgh Courier*, September 8, 1934, A6.

8. *Ibid.*, 16.

9. *Ibid.*, "Beaumont Opens NAACP Drive," Apr, 13, 1935, 7.

10. "Obituary 2—Rites Held in Beaumont for Dr. J. C. Wallace," *Chicago Defender*, August 13, 1957, 6.

11. *Ibid.*, "Air Cairo Violence," March 15, 1952, 5.

12. "Violence Running Rampant in Cairo, Ill. Community," *Atlanta Daily World*, February 3, 1952, 1.

William WALLACE

1874–15 June 1933
Meharry Medical College, 1905

Roots and Education

William Wallace was born in Shreveport, Louisiana, to Mr. and Mrs. Joseph Wallace. After completing studies at the local elementary school, William enrolled for two years of college preparatory studies at Bishop College in Marshall, Texas. The school was founded in 1881 by the Baptist Home Mission Society to serve black students in east Texas.[1] He went on to Straight University in New Orleans, Louisiana. The school was founded by the American Missionary Association of the Congregational Church. Throughout its history, Straight offered courses of study ranging from elementary to college level courses in music and theology. In 1934 financial difficulties led to its merger with Dillard University.[2]

After graduating from Straight, Wallace went on to Meharry Medical School and received his medical degree at the age of 31 in 1905. He returned to Shreveport, established a medical practice, married, and had a son (William Jr.). His wife was a teacher.

Military Service

At the age of 43, Dr. Wallace volunteered for the U.S. Army Medical Reserve Corps. He reported to the Medical Officers Training Camp (MOTC) at Fort Des Moines on September 18, 1917. He was one of the older physicians there. He must have been physically fit because he made it through all the physical aspects of the training. On November 3 First Lieutenant Wallace was transferred to Camp Funston, Kansas, where he was assigned to the 92nd Division's 317th Sanitary (Medical) Train. Just prior to his departure for France, he was assigned to the 366th Field Hospital. Some of the MOTC graduates spent their entire time in France assigned to the same medical unit. Others were moved as medical needs changed. On July 18, 1918, Lieutenant Wallace was transferred to the medical detachment of the 317th Engineers.

In October 1918 he wrote (apparently to his mother), "Officially I am identified with numerous problems for physicians are scarce in this country [France], so besides my regimental duties, I have quite a number of civilians to look after. The French people are very kind and grateful to the American soldiers, and nothing is too good for the 'Sammies.' Every second woman is wearing mourning. The ravages of war stand out vividly everywhere. The 'survival of the fittest' theory is being worked out admirably in this war ... the tide seems to be turning in our favor.... The colored soldier is keeping up his standard of bygone days, and we have already won the love and respect of the French people. We know how you are working at home, and we are determined to keep pace with you over here, for we mean to make you feel proud of us."[3]

Career

In early 1919, Dr. Wallace returned to his wife and his medical practice in Shreveport. He was active in the Louisiana Medical, Dental and Pharmaceutical Society and was the local Examining Physician for the Knights of Pythias and Odd Fellows.[4]

In 1919 he bought Mercy Sanitarium from Dr. Fred K. T. Jones. It was the first black hospital in Shreveport. In 1921 he moved the hospital to a larger building at 1218 Pierre Avenue. He was perhaps the most popular doctor at the hospital. He and other members of the Shreveport Colored Medical, Dental and Pharmaceutical Association volunteered for two hours every Wednesday to see indigent citizens. They saw 100 people on the first day of operation.[5]

In an appeal for funding in 1930, Dr. Wallace wrote about the work of Mercy Sanitarium. It was a "two-story frame building provided with beds for sixteen patients (two for charity cases) and space for the accommodation of nine more." In addition to the medical staff, there were "four competent employees, a registered nurse, a practical nurse, a trained cook and a utility maid." There was also a Veterans Club offering medical services. In closing he made an appeal: "This sanitarium is owned entirely and exclusively by two individuals, only one of whom, Dr. Wm. Wallace, is actively engaged in its management, which is absolutely too cumbersome for one person with limited resources. But, with some financial assistance from some persons imbued with the spirit of altruism, giant strides can be instantly made towards establishing this institution upon a firm and progressive basis, which will reflect honor upon the benefactor."[6]

In 1931 he and about 100 who served in the First World War attended the first annual convention of the National Association of Race War Veterans. He addressed the meeting about the needs of veterans, especially those wounded in the war.[7] At the time of his death in 1933, he was serving on the executive board of the National Medical Association (NMA).[8]

Dr. Wallace died at the age of 57. After his death, the clinic and the hospital could not financially continue to operate. They both closed in 1936.[9] It is interesting to speculate on whether the burden and effort he expended in keeping it going contributed to his death. His dedication and love for the African American community in Shreveport was heartfelt, and his passing was a very sad day. His funeral was at C. M. E. Temple in Shreveport. He was buried in the city's Zion Rest cemetery with a military headstone.

In 1945 his widow Mrs. M. M. Wallace participated (in honor of Dr. Wallace's World War I service) in a ceremony in Nashville honoring Meharryites who served in World War II.[10] She was then supervisor of the elementary schools in Shreveport. Their son William graduated from the University of Michigan and was on the faculty of Grambling College.[11]

NOTES

1. www.tshaonline.org/handbook/online/articles/kbb11.
2. wikipedia.org/wiki/Straight_University (accessed August 12, 2014).
3. Unsourced clipping from unknown newspaper dated October 24, 1918.
4. AMA Deceased Physicians Card, National Library of Medicine, Bethesda, MD.
5. Willie Burton, *Mercy Hospital and Other Doctors, on the Black Side of Shreveport*, 1983, 24.
6. "Mercy Sanitarium," *Journal of the National Medical Association (JNMA)*, Fall 1930, Vol. XXII, No. 3, 134.
7. "War Vets in First Annual Convention," *Chicago Defender*, November 28, 1931, 2.
8. "Dr. Bousfield Takes Office as NMA Head," *Chicago Defender*, August 19, 1933, 2.
9. www.caddohistory.com/mercy_sanatorium.html (accessed September 14, 2014).
10. "Meharryites Honored in Shreveport," *Chicago Defender*, May 26, 1945, 15.
11. "Baton Rouge," *Chicago Defender*, January 15, 1957, 18.

Joseph Henry WARD

26 August 1872–12 December 1956
Indiana University, 1900

Roots and Education

Ward was born in Wilson, North Carolina, to Mittie Roena Ward and Napoleon Hagans. His father had been born a free man of color on August 22, 1840, in Nahunta, Wayne, North Carolina. Napoleon's mother was Louisa Hagans and his father is unknown. Ward's mother Mittie and her sister Apsoline were born in the 1850s. They were slaves to Sarah Darden and David G.W. Ward. Mittie and Napoleon did not marry, but he did marry her sister Apsoline.

Ward was illiterate at age 13 when he left home and traveled to Indianapolis, Indiana, where he found work cleaning stables. He made a most fortunate connection there with Dr. George Hasty. Hasty hired him and then took a special interest in young Ward. He helped him get an education that set him on his medical path for the rest of his life.

Dr. Hasty was the founder of the Physiomedical College of Indiana.[1] Physiomedicalism is a system of natural herbal medicine that developed during the early 19th century.[2]

Dr. Hasty must have seen the possibility for greatness in young Ward. He moved Ward into his home and provided him with employment as a servant and driver while Ward attended and graduated from his Physiomedical College of Indiana. Soon after Ward completed his training, he set up his own medical practice on Indiana Avenue in Indianapolis.

By the mid 1890s the Indianapolis Freeman newspaper described Dr. Ward was a "very promising young physician of this city ... a man of ability and aggressiveness" when it reported his appointment as deputy supreme chancellor of the Colored Order of Knights of Pythias for the state of Indiana.[3]

The Knights of Pythias was a fraternal organization and secret society founded at Washington, D.C., on February 19, 1864. It was the first fraternal organization to receive its charter under an act of the U.S. Congress. Members of the Knights of Pythias subscribe to the ideals of loyalty, honor and friendship and are dedicated to benevolence and charity.

Thomas W. Stringer later founded the Colored Knights of Pythias with similar goals, but this society also offered a service that was not found in any other social organization of the times: life insurance.[4] Ward was an active member all of his life.

Ward continued his education and in 1900 at the age of 30, he received his medical degree from Indiana University Medical College. Soon after, he traveled to New York to complete post-graduate work in surgery.

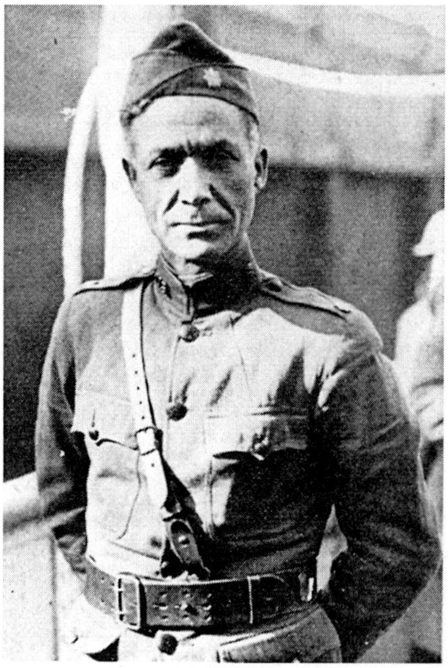

Major Joseph H. Ward standing aboard ship (Emmett J. Scott, *Scott's Official History of the American Negro in the World War I*, 1919).

Early in the 1900s Dr. Ward helped found the Senate Avenue YMCA in Indianapolis. He served as chairman of its management committee. The institution became one of the country's outstanding African American branches and a cultural hub. Leading scholars such as Charles S. Johnson, William Pickens, Walter White and W.E.B. Du Bois lectured there.

Zella Louise Locklear was a free black woman who arrived in Indianapolis in the late 19th century. She and Ward met and married on November 23, 1904. Zella also became involved in community health care. In 1905 she worked with Lillian Thomas Fox to found the Women's Improvement Club, an organization that ran a tent city for African American tubercular patients.

By 1909 Dr. Ward was well known in Indianapolis when he opened the Ward's Sanitarium and Nurses' Training School. It was a large brick structure adjoining a large house on Indiana Avenue. It was renovated to include a white-tiled operating room, attached sterilization and preparation rooms, and modern surgical equipment. "The entire place was lighted by electricity and heated by steam." There were many women who applied for training as nurses at the hospital. Amazingly, Ward was able to make a deal with the white City Hospital to have his nurses attend lectures there. He required those completing training at his hospital to pass the same state examinations as nurses at the white hospital.[5]

Dr. Edmund Clark, president of the City Board of Health, proclaimed he "would not hesitate to take surgical or medical cases to this [Ward's] institution for treatment." Dr. W. N. Wishard, a leading white Indianapolis physician, said of Ward, "His progressive spirit is farther shown in his purpose to maintain a training school for colored nurses ... and his methods in the general practice of medicine, which I would say, equal the best."[6]

Dr. Ward had an interesting connection to Madam C.J. Walker (born Sarah Breedlove) who is widely thought of as the Mother of African American hair care products. When Madam Walker moved to Indianapolis in 1910, she knew the Wards through the women's auxiliary of the Knights of Pythias. She and her husband stayed with the Wards, and initially she used the Wards' home as her salon to demonstrate her products. Soon she bought a house around the corner from the Wards on North West Street.

Walker's business was booming by 1911 so she purchased an income rental property, then a salon, and ultimately built a manufacturing facility for her growing company. She soon became a millionaire and built a mansion in New York. She moved there, but her manufacturing company remained in Indianapolis. Dr. Ward continued to serve as her personal physician for the rest of her life. He kept telling her to slow down, but she wasn't having any of it. She built her multi-million dollar business, her mansion, and her manufacturing plant all within the course of nine years.

Military Service

When the United States entered the First World War in 1917, Ward had a wife and two children, and a profitable medical practice. He was 44 years old. He had practiced surgery for 18 years, had been the city school inspector in Indianapolis for eight years, and was very active in the Indianapolis branch of the YMCA. Yet, he put his practice on hold and volunteered for service as a medical doctor in the U.S. Army. "This is a history-making period, and I want to be connected with it," was the simple explanation offered by Dr. Ward and reported in the *Washington Bee* on August 4, 1917.[7] He was commissioned a first lieutenant in the Medical Reserve Corps.

When Lieutenant Ward reported to Fort Des Moines for the Medical Officers Training Camp (MOTC) on August 8, 1917, he was second oldest of the 118 physicians who reported to camp. Fourteen of the original physicians didn't complete the program, but he did.[8]

By the end of camp he had been recommended for promotion to captain by the MOTC commander Lieutenant Colonel Bingham. Ward would become the army's highest-ranking African American medical officer. He was assigned to Camp Sherman, Ohio, with the 92nd Division's 325th Field Signal Battalion. He was sent to France in mid–1918 where he ultimately commanded a base hospital. There he had the distinction of being one of the only two African American officers in the Medical Corps to attain the rank of major.[9] The other was his fellow Hoosier, Dr. Arthur Henry Wilson. Ward continued his service in the Medical Reserve Corps after the war, and in September 1924, he was promoted to lieutenant colonel.

Career

With Ward's return from France, he and Madam Walker found time to meddle in her daughter's life. They did not like her suitor, Wiley Wilson. Their preference was "Gentleman Jack" Kennedy, a pharmacist and physician who had served in France with Ward and who was considered his "prodigy."[10] They won out, and A'Lelia married Kennedy, but not until 1926, and the marriage only lasted two years.

In 1919 when Harlem's Hellfighters (the 369th Infantry Regiment) returned from World War I and marched through Manhattan, nearly a million New Yorkers cheered. Among them were Colonel Ward and his wife Zella, who were visiting Madam Walker. Walker's daughter A'Lelia was in the parade, driving her Luxury Pathfinder. Ward noted Madam Walker's kidney disease had advanced significantly.[11] He insisted that she curtail her speaking engagements, but resting was not her style. It was not Ward's style either.

Dr. Ward returned to Indianapolis in 1919 and resumed his practice. In June 1922 the press reported, "The Ward Sanitarium of Dr. Joseph H. Ward, 231 Indiana Avenue, has moved to its new home on Boulevard Place. Dr. Ward announces a grand opening this week. The Sanitarium is now modern from every angle. Visitors are asked to come and see the new home."[12]

Following World War I, African American leaders demanded medical care for disabled African American veterans as a reward for the wartime service of an estimated 385,000 men. Public hospitals in the South often refused to treat black soldiers or provided only limited care. In 1921 the National Veterans Hospital System had its beginnings. "Organized and financed by the federal government, these hospitals were to serve veterans with service-related diseases and injuries." The Consultants on Hospitals who were responsible for plans for this hospital system recognized the imperative demand for some separate provision for the African American veterans living in the South. They decided on a separate national hospital for African Americans.

To be sure, there was opposition from various groups on the location, the segregation and the whole premise, but the chairman of the consultants, William Charles White, stood his ground.[13]

Tuskegee Institute donated 300 acres and construction was underway. The Veterans Hospital housing was constructed by skilled African American labor from the Tuskegee training school. The property was described as a picturesque campus.

The dedication took place at that site on February 12, 1923, Abraham Lincoln's birthday. President Calvin Coolidge was the keynote speaker.[14]

Tuskegee's U.S. Veterans Hospital No. 91 for African American veterans opened with an all-white staff. General Frank T. Hines was Administrator of the Veterans Bureau. After a year of lobbying lead by Robert R. Moton, president of Tuskegee Institute, the National Medical Association (NMA) and leaders from the African American and white communities, a controversial decision was made to transition the facility to an entirely African American staff.[15] There were protest marches by the Ku Klux Klan and various white state politicians rose to object.[16]

General Hines was responsible for the ultimate selection of competent African Americans to replace the white personnel. He chose a white man, Colonel Robert H. Stanley, as the first medical officer. Dr. Stanley was not sympathetic to the idea of African American staffing. It took major lobbying and assistance in the search for the right doctors, led by Dr. Michael O. Dumas of the National Medical Association. General Hines gradually found African American doctors from all over the United States to come to Tuskegee.

Colonel Ward was appointed medical officer in charge on July 7, 1924.[17] It wasn't an easy transition. In March before his official appointment, white personnel were ordered to vacate their quarters and move into the town of Tuskegee. Dr. Ward didn't issue the order. It came from the Veterans Administration, but he did express satisfaction over it.[18]

In April 1924, just as he was planning his move from Indianapolis to Tuskegee, Ward and his wife rushed to Washington, D.C., to be at the bedside of his mother, who had suffered a paralyzing stroke while visiting Ward's sister.[19] His mother, Mrs. Mittie Ward, had lived with the Wards for many years and was known as "Mother Ward" to many of their friends. She died on April 24, 1924, at 70, and was buried at the Crown Hill Cemetery in Indianapolis.[20] While home for the funeral, he took the time to recruit Dr. Frederick A. Stokes (who served with him in France) to serve as his executive officer at Tuskegee.

Under Dr. Ward, more than 6,000 were admitted to Tuskegee Veterans Hospital for treatment of diseases in every branch of medicine. The initial African American staff consisted of 21 physicians and dentists and numerous assistants. Services would grow to include medical, tuberculosis, surgical and neuropsychiatric divisions, as well as completely equipped departments for clinical laboratory work, radiology, physiotherapy, occupational therapy, dietetics and library.[21]

"Firm in purpose, alert in demeanor and fair in his dealings with subordinate personnel, Colonel Ward amassed an enviable reputation in the Tuskegee community. His legendary inspection tours on horseback and his manly fearlessness in dealing with community groups at a time when there was a fixed subordinate attitude in Negro-White relations are two of the more popular recollections of associates."[22] This was Dr. Eugene Dibble's description of Ward in the 1920s.

In 1925 President Coolidge wrote that he and General Frank T. Hines, director of the Veterans Bureau, had confidence in Ward's administration of the hospital, and they recommended the construction of a recreation and assembly building. Expansion was underway.

Dr. Ward continued his active involvement with the National Medical Association

(NMA). At its 1925 Chicago meeting, he presented "Medullary Sarcoma of the Tibia."[23] He also published a report on the progress of the V.A. hospital in Tuskegee in the January 1926 Veterans Bureau's medical bulletin. He was elected chairman of the new National Hospital Association. At its third annual meeting in 1926, Dr. Ward is listed as vice president of Veterans Bureau Hospital, Tuskegee, Alabama.[24]

Dr. Ward likely used his attendance at these meetings to recruit staff. After passing his civil service examination in 1926, Dr. James Arthur Kennedy moved to Tuskegee to become Ward's assistant medical officer in charge.[25]

In his 1930 National Medical Association article about the Tuskegee hospital, Dr. Ward was proud to report the hospital was rated as Class "A" without reservation by the American College of Surgeons and the American Hospital Association.[26] By this time, the hospital was treating about 1,000 patients annually. To help with the patient load, and help African Americans graduating from medical school, Colonel Ward recommended that his Veterans Hospital No. 91 be used for internships and residencies for young African American physicians. The idea was favorably received in Washington and elsewhere.[27] In a testament to Ward's successful operation of the hospital, the Veterans Bureau at various times published at least six contributions to medical science by physicians who worked under Colonel Ward during his 12-year tenure at the Tuskegee V.A. hospital.[28]

During the 1930s Ward was recognized for his outstanding service to medicine and his race. In June 1931 he was awarded an honorary degree of doctor of laws from Howard University.[29] In August 1934 he participated in a program of the National Hospital Association at the NMA annual meeting in Nashville.[30] Then in December he spoke to the Kappa Alpha Psi fraternity annual conclave in New York City. Kappa Alpha Psi is a prestigious, predominately African-American collegiate fraternity formed in 1911 in Indiana. Dr. Ward was a lifelong member.

Dr. and Mrs. Ward are mentioned in numerous society columns of the time. In 1935, for example, they hosted his sister and several educators from Indianapolis at their home in Tuskegee. His guests took time to visit veterans at the hospital.[31]

One of the biggest social events of the time was the wedding of the Wards' only child, daughter Mary. She and Erskine Goode Roberts of Boston, an architectural engineer, were married at the Wards' home in Tuskegee on January 1, 1936.[32]

In February 1937, after 12 years as head of the Tuskegee Veterans Hospital, Dr. Ward was dismissed from the hospital amidst charges of mishandled funds. Once before charges had been made in 1925 by chief engineer W. L. Jones that Ward and members of his staff used government gasoline in his private car and entertained influential citizens at government expense. These were dismissed as trivial, and Dr. Ward was given a clean bill of health. Jones was dismissed. But in 1937 Ward, his secretary, Mrs. L. M. Patterson, and 14 other employees were charged with conspiring to convert government property for their own sake.[33]

The *Chicago Defender* reported the specific charges were using hospital food for his personal use and misappropriating funds of war veterans. He and his staff had also disregarded regulations that prohibited neuropsychiatric patients from paying for their own special barbering services. He was also accused of paying too much attention to the advice of Tuskegee Institute officials, a private institution, in the running of the Federal hospital.[34]

It is interesting that these charges came on the heels of the Republican Administration's statement that the Tuskegee Veterans Hospital was one of the best managed in the country. Race and politics certainly were involved in Ward's dismissal. He had been appointed by a Republican administration, and jobs were needed for deserving Democrats in the new administration.[35] "The trouble at Tuskegee had its inception in internal difficulties. Here was one of the most important governmental institutions in the entire country manned and controlled by Negroes. White Alabama grinned and bore it, ... but never got accustomed to it. When Dr. Ward left Tuskegee there were 500 employees at the hospital, 24 physicians, 60 nurses, 2 dentists and other specialists." It was judged by white Alabamans as "too much money ($450,000 per year in payroll alone) to be going to African Americans."[36]

In April 1937 he and his staff pled guilty to charges related to misuse of funds and were fined $250 for each charge.[37]

It was not until 1954 that segregation ended in all veterans hospitals. White patients who applied directly to the hospital at Tuskegee were being admitted for some time before the integration order was made.[38]

Dr. Ward returned to Indianapolis in 1936 and re-established his medical practice. From the *Chicago Defender* we learn, "Wards in Indianapolis—Dr. and Mrs. Joseph H. Ward, now residing in Indianapolis, look natural amid the surroundings of the city rich with tradition in the progress and professional career of the Ward family."[39]

He picked up where he left off in his community activities. He was elected vice-president and grand chancellor of the board of trustees for the YMCA Metropolitan Board. He was a 33rd degree Mason, and he was also a member of the American Legion. In 1936 he was elected its local commander. The Wards were again congregants of the Bethel AME Church. During the January 8, 1937, meeting of the Kappa Alpha Psi fraternity, Dr. Ward was awarded the Trophy Cup by the Indianapolis, Indiana Alpha chapter of Indiana University.[40] Ward was also elected to office in the Supreme Lodge of the Knights of Pythias and served as Supreme Medical Registrar.

On November 4, 1937, Dr. Ward (at age 67) was seriously injured when he was struck by a car when crossing a road. The white driver's car came around the corner and knocked him down with his left fender. Dr. Ward suffered various injuries, including severe scalp lacerations, a wound on the neck and leg, concussion of the brain, and spinal injuries.[41] After a short time in the local hospital, he was transferred to the VA Medical Center in Indianapolis. After a time, he recovered enough to continue his activities.

Dr. Ward was in touch with his half-brothers and their children throughout their lives. Wanda Mercer, whose great-grandfather William Scarlett Hagans (1869–1946) was Dr. Ward's half-brother, shared this story from her uncle, Leroy T. Barnes regarding Dr. Ward in his early 80s. "I'll never forget Uncle Joe. He and his wife Zella visited and stayed with Mama on Baring Street [in New York]. They were in their early 80s, but lively and used to being catered to. Uncle Joe ordered everybody around as if we were army privates. Later, when I was living in Jamaica [New York] on South Road, Uncle Joe came to visit us. He was in town for a Dodger baseball game, among other things. He did not know our address so he told the bus driver to 'take me to Dr. Barnes' office' (no doubt in his typical colonel's tone). Without hesitation, the driver delivered Uncle Joe to the corner of South Road and New York Blvd. where my sign was visible on the second floor over the funeral home."[42]

Zella Ward passed away in 1954. Dr. Ward joined her and his mother at Crown Hill Cemetery in Indianapolis in 1956.

Colonel Ward was a lifelong community activist. He and Zella had a lasting impact on the Indianapolis African American community and all veterans. Granddaughter Alice Palmer (née Roberts) embraced the Wards' legacy and went on to make a difference in her community, the city of Chicago.

Alice Roberts graduated from high school in Indianapolis at age 16 and enrolled at Indiana University. She dropped out for a number of years, but ultimately received her B.S. in English and sociology from Indiana University in 1965.[43]

She began her teaching career in Indianapolis then moved to Chicago to teach at Malcolm X College, one of the City Colleges of Chicago. She earned an M.A. in urban studies from Roosevelt University, and a Ph.D. in educational administration from Northwestern University. While working on her Ph. D. degree at Northwestern, Palmer co-authored two books and tutored. She then took a position at Northwestern as associate dean and director of African American Student Affairs for five years.

She married Edward L. "Buzz" Palmer, a Chicago police officer and activist, and became involved in a national voter education movement. She was one of the founders of the Chicago YMCA Youth and Government Program in 1986. She was also executive director of Chicago Cities in Schools.

A veteran of Mayor Harold Washington campaigns, Palmer had support from the civil-rights activists in Chicago. She was well known for her efforts to improve Chicago schools. Her husband Buzz was another source of her popularity. He had been leader of the Afro-American Patrolmen's League.[44]

Mrs. Palmer was appointed to the Illinois State Senate in June 1991 to fill the remainder of the term of retiring state senator, Richard J. Newhouse, Jr.[45] She successfully ran for election in 1992 and served a full four-year term that ended on January 8, 1997. She was succeeded by Barack Obama.

After leaving public office, Palmer became an associate professor in the College of Urban Planning and Public Affairs at the University of Illinois, Chicago, and she was a special assistant to the president of the university before retiring.[46] She was an active force in Chicago politics.

In 2010, Senator Richard J. Durbin paid tribute to the Palmers from the floor of the Senate. "Mr. President, today I recognize Alice and Edward 'Buzz' Palmer for their service and dedication to Chicago's African American community. The Palmers have worked for many years in a variety of capacities to build a strong, involved, and educated African-American community in the city of Chicago."[47]

Notes

1. David Bodenhamer and Robert G. Borrows, *Encyclopedia of Indianapolis* (Bloomington: Indiana University Press, 1994).
2. "History of Physio Medicalism," www.toddcaldecott.com (accessed June 3, 2010).
3. "Dr. Joseph H. Ward; Deputy Supreme Chancellor Knights of Pythias," *Indianapolis Freeman*, October 23, 1897.
4. Michael Tow, *Secrecy and Segregation, Murphysboro's Black Social Organizations 1865–1925*, NIU.edu (accessed October 15, 2012).
5. "New Sanitarium, Operated by Dr. H. H. Ward with Training School for Nurses at the Hoosier Capital," *Indianapolis Freeman*, June 19, 1909.
6. *Ibid.*
7. "The Training Camp," *Washington Bee*, August 4, 1917, Howard University Manuscript Archives, TM Gregory Collection, newspaper articles, Box 37–1.
8. *Ibid.*
9. Emmett J. Scott, *Scott's Official History of the American Negro in the World War* (Chicago: Homewood Press, 1919) 304.
10. *Ibid.*, 268.
11. *Ibid.*, 267.
12. "The Hoosier Capital by Alvin D. Smith," *Chicago Defender*, June 24, 1922, 18.
13. *Journal of the National Medical Association (JNMA)*, Vol. 54, No. 2, 1962.
14. *Tuskegee Veterans Administration Hospital*, www.alabama.travel/things-to-do/attractioncs/tuskegee_veterans_administration_hospital (accessed October 12, 2012).
15. *Ibid.*
16. "Tuskegee Hospital in Negro Control," *The Baltimore Sun*, July 14, 1924, 1.
17. "U.S. Veterans' Hospital," *Journal of the National Medical Association (JNMA)*, July–September 1930, Vol. 22, No. 3, 133.
18. "Whites Vacate Tuskegee," *Pittsburgh Courier*, March 8, 1924, 1.
19. "Mother of Major J.H. Ward, Tuskegee Hospital Head, Dies," *Pittsburgh Courier*, April 19, 1924, 3.
20. "Col. and Mrs. Ward Celebrate Anniversary at Tuskegee, Ala," Philadelphia Tribune, December 12, 1929, 5.
21. "U.S. Veterans' Hospital, Tuskegee, Alabama," Col. J. H. Ward, MD, *Journal of the National Medical Association (JNMA)*, July–September 1930, 133–134.
22. "Historical Notes on Tuskegee Veterans Hospital," *Journal of the National Medical Association (JNMA)*, March 1962, Vol. 54, No. 2, p. 133–138.
23. "Colored Doctors Have Convention in Chicago Soon," *The Washington Post*, July 26, 1925, R10.
24. "National Hospital Association," *Journal of the National Medical Association (JNMA)*, Vol. 18, No. 3, 152.
25. "Order Reigns at Veterans' Hospital; Threat Rumors Unfounded: Ward Placed in Charge. Race War Over. Director Hines Acts," *Pittsburgh Courier*, July 19, 1924, 1.
26. *Ibid.*
27. "Ward Wants Vet's Hospital to Unite with Tuskegee," *Pittsburgh Courier*, July 4, 1925, 3.
28. *Journal of the National Medical Association (JNMA)*, Vol. 21, No. 2, 1929.
29. "Howard University Gave Them Honorary Degrees Friday," *Afro-American*, June 13, 1931, 6C.
30. "National Medical Association Holds Greatest Meeting" *Atlanta Daily World*, August 23, 1934, 1.
31. "Visit Embraces Social and Educational Phases," *Chicago Defender*, April 13, 1935, 7.
32. "Tuskegee Institute Scene of Two Pretty Weddings," *Atlanta Daily World*, January 14, 1936, 1.
33. "Indict Col. Ward, 13 Other at Tuskegee," *Chicago Defender*, July 18, 1936, 1.
34. "Tuskegee Hospital," *Baltimore Afro-American*, July 11, 1925, A9.
35. Who'll Be Glad When?" *Baltimore Afro-American*, February 15, 1936, 4.
36. "Sixteen Indicted at Veterans' Hospital," *Baltimore Afro-American*, July 18, 1936, 2.
37. "Col. Ward, Secretary Guilty in Tuskegee Hospital Theft Case," *Chicago Defender*, April 10, 1937, 1.
38. "Veterans Hospital at Tuskegee," *Journal of the National Medical Association (JNMA)*, March 1954, 140.
39. Nahum Brascher, "Random Thoughts—This and That Along the Way," *Chicago Defender*, December 11, 1948, 9.
40. "National Problems Analyzed at CONFAB," *Chicago Defender*, January 9, 1937, 6.
41. "Colonel Ward Seriously Hurt in Auto Mishap," *New Journal and Guide*, November 13, 1937, 1.
42. Telephone Interview with niece, Wanda Mercer, July 12, 2013.
43. *Alice Palmer Biography*, The HistoryMakers, Au-

gust 9, 2000, www.historymakers.com (accessed November 29, 2011).
44. *Ibid.*
45. David Remnick, *The Bridge, the Life and Rise of Barack Obama* (New York: Vintage, 2010), 278.
46. *Alice Palmer Biography,* The HistoryMakers (accessed November 29, 2011).
47. *Congressional Record*, Sept. 20, 2010, vol 156, number 126, p. s7197–s7198.

Sylvanus Holsey WARFIELD

17 November 1885–28 February 1970
Meharry Medical College, 1904

Roots and Education

Sylvanus was born in Guthrie, Kentucky. His father was the Reverend W. I. Warfield, a minister in Colored Methodist Episcopal (CME) churches in several different towns including Princeton and Hopkinsville, Kentucky, Topeka, Kansas, and Louisiana, Missouri. Sylvanus' middle name honored Bishop L. H. Holsey, an AME pastor in Augusta, Georgia, who advocated for institutions of higher learning for the training of African American ministers in Kentucky and Tennessee.

Sylvanus initially attended local elementary school in Hopkinsville, Kentucky. In 1889 at about six years of age he was enrolled in the scientific course at Central Tennessee College's Preparatory Course at Nashville, Tennessee.[1] It is likely that his father's connections helped with his acceptance at the school. While he attended prep school, he was a tenor in the choral society.

During his early years in prep school, Meharry Medical College was a part of Central Tennessee. By the time he entered medical school in 1900, the school was under the auspices of Walden University and the Methodist Episcopal Church, North (the church had split over slavery before the Civil War and would not reunite until 1939).[2] Dr. Warfield received his medical degree in 1904. He married in 1905 but the marriage did not last, and once divorced he never remarried. By 1910 he was living and practicing medicine in Dayton, Ohio, at 43 West 6th Street.

During the first half of the 20th century, black-owned businesses thrived in Dayton. One block from Dr. Warfield's office, along West Fifth Street, was the major shopping thoroughfare. Locals could stop at Ben's Hamburgers, Hiram Poore's Service Station, Lloyd Lewis' Furniture, Cal's Barbershop, the Palace Theatre, Harris' Cocktail Bar, Pop Mason's Flamingo Club, William's Cleaners, Preston Drugs, the McFall Hotel, the Owl Club, or Mac's Chicken Shack.[3] It should have been a good neighborhood for a new doctor, but there were others already there. Dr. Charles Johnson's office, for example, was on West 5th Street.

Whatever the reason for his departure, by 1912 Dr. Warfield had moved across the Ohio River and set up a practice in Bowling Green, Kentucky. There was no hospital in Bowling Green that accepted African American doctors so when two of his patients, Mrs. L. B. Bradley and Mrs. J. T. Porter, needed special operations, he took them 70 miles south to Meharry Hospital in Nashville.[4]

By 1915, Dr. Warfield left Kentucky and moved to another promising town, Louisiana, Missouri. Louisiana is located on the Mississippi River, 90 miles northwest of St. Louis. In addition to river traffic, Louisiana had two railroads whose tracks ran parallel to the Mississippi and crossed the Mississippi on one of the oldest bridges on the river, the Louisiana KCS Rail Bridge, first put in service in 1873.[5]

Dr. Warfield passed the Missouri State Medical Licensing Examination and opened a practice, but he wasn't there long. Two years later, when he entered the army in 1917, he gave his address as that of his brother, the Reverend M. J. Warfield who lived at 1409 South Jackson Street in Topeka, Kansas. His father was also in Topeka and pastor of a local CME Church.[6]

Military Service

Dr. Warfield was 32 when he was called to active service on August 3, 1917. He reported for duty at Fort Des Moines on September 17. First Lieutenant Warfield was in training camp for 49 days until his transfer on November 3, 1917, to Camp Funston. He was then assigned to the 372nd Infantry Regiment (93rd Division) and sent to Camp Stuart, Newport News, Virginia, for transport to France.

On February 21, 1918, his future in the military was finished when he joined a group of soldiers at a public dance hall in Hampton, Virginia. According to his general court martial, Lieutenant Warfield was drunk and boisterous, and when ordered to do so, refused to leave the hall. The military police were called, and Warfield was insulting and without a pass to be out after 11:00 p.m. Warfield was placed under arrest. His unit sailed for France without him at the end of March 1918. He faced a general court martial on June 7, 1918. He was found guilty of being "so drunk and disorderly while in uniform, in the presence and hearing of a large number of enlisted men and civilians, as to disgrace the military service." He was dismissed from service and the final order was signed by President Woodrow Wilson.[7]

Career

After his military experience, Dr. Warfield settled in Detroit, Michigan. His choice of Detroit is easily explained in light of the Great Migration. During the war, Detroit manufacturers sent agents to the South to recruit African Americans and others to work in Ford's and other factories. These migrants established social and fraternal orders, churches and social welfare organizations to accommodate their needs. Health care professionals were recruited.[8]

Warfield remained there for the next 50 years, the rest of his long life, practicing medicine from a series of rental houses. In 1920 Dr. Warfield was 36, divorced and renting a house at 60 Riopelle Street; his office was up the street at 1041 Riopelle.

According to the 1930 U.S. Census, he was still in Detroit, still single and renting, but had moved to 1703 Chene Street. There his rent was $50 a month. By 1940 he had moved again, this time to a rental house at 560 East Adams. His private practice was located at 3263 Joy Road.[9]

His addresses were in an area of the city known as Paradise Valley. Much has been written about the prosperity of its business people, the creativity of its musicians and the dynamic black community that emerged there, despite the Jim Crow practices that pervaded Detroit. The area was, however, densely populated and probably had one of the higher death rates in the city. Criminal activities were also common there.[10]

Other than his addresses, nothing more has been unearthed about his medical or personal activities in Detroit. No evidence was found of his association with any of Detroit's major African American hospitals.

Dr. Sylvanus H. Warfield died in the Detroit General Hospital on February 28, at age 84 of metastatic carcinoma (cancer).[11]

Notes

1. *Catalogue Central Tennessee College, Nashville, 1889–1890* (Nashville: Marshall & Bruce Stationers & Printers, 1890).
2. en.wikipedia.org/wiki/Meharry Medical_College (accessed October 18, 2013).
3. www.daytondailynews.com/news/news/a-timeline-black-history-in-the-miami-valley (accessed April 26, 2015).
4. "Bowling Green, KY," *Indianapolis Freeman*, February 3, 1912, 4.
5. Louisiana-mo.com (accessed April 25, 2015).
6. "C.M.E. Annual Conference," *Plaindealer*, November 13, 1914, 8.
7. National Personnel Records Center, National Archives, St. Louis, MO.
8. daahp.wayne.edu (accessed March 3, 2015).
9. 1920, 1930 and 1940 U.S. Federal Census.
10. detroit1701.org, *Paradise Valley Marker* (accessed April 14, 2015).
11. Christyne M. Douglas, MLIS, Meharry Medical College Library, Chief Archivist.

Leo Edward WELKER

1881–2 March 1937
Harvard University, 1908

Roots and Education

Welker was born in 1881 in Cambridge, Illinois, to Freeman O. and Alice Battle Welker. Cambridge is a village in western Illinois, about 30 miles from Moline, Illinois. The town was founded in 1843 when the Reverend Ithamar Pillsbury, a Yankee settler from New England, donated the land to the town council for the community. From its beginnings, the center of community activities was the school. Even today, this town of about 2,000 (less than one percent African American) boasts a blue ribbon elementary school.[1]

After public school in Cambridge, Welker attended Fisk University where he was a star of its football team. After graduation, he studied biology and chemistry at Iowa College (now Grinnell). The co-ed, multi-racial college was established in 1846 to educate its students "for the different professions and for the honorable discharge of the duties of life."[2] In 1903, he was awarded his PhD.

Welker next enrolled in Harvard Medical School. He was awarded the Hayden Scholarship for two years. Hayden, an escaped slave who eventually made his way to Boston, was a prominent abolitionist and a state representative. His widow, Harriet, donated their estate on her death in 1893 to establish a scholarship at Harvard Medical School for African American students.[3] This enabled Welker to complete his medical degree in 1908.

By 1910 Dr. Welker had moved to Hamilton, Tennessee, where he set up his medical practice with a friend, Dr. Herbert E. Simms. In 1912 he moved to Nashville where he worked as Director of Physical Culture at Fisk University. He continued his involvement with Fisk's athletic program long after his graduation, coaching at the alumni games and even writing a column for the *Chicago Defender* on the outcome of Fisk football games with Morehouse and Meharry.[4]

By 1917, Dr. Welker was married to Frances (Frankie) Effie Caldwell, a teacher. The couple and their two daughters (Constance and Winifred) lived near Fisk University at 1710 Jefferson Street, in Nashville.

Military Career

At the age of 37, Welker left his wife, two daughters, his medical practice and his involvement with Fisk's athletics. He volunteered for service in the U.S. Army Medical Reserve Corps. In August 1917 he reported to the Medical Officers Training Camp (MOTC) in Fort Des Moines for basic training. Lieutenant Welker was one of two Harvard Medical School graduates at the MOTC. The other was Louis T. Wright, who later became known as "Mr. Harlem Hospital."[5]

Welker completed training camp on November 3, 1917, and reported to Camp Dodge, Iowa. When large numbers of men are gathered from all over the country (such as in the training camps), contagious diseases can be a problem. The first epidemic was measles. The outbreak began right after Christmas in 1917. It spread through the camps until late spring 1918. It had just passed when the scarlet fever outbreak reached its height.

Both had passed by the time troops sailed to France in June 1918.[6] In France, in September of 1918 the influenza pandemic struck. By the time it had worked its way through the army, more men had died from influenza and the accompanying pneumonia than from war wounds. Influenza would run its course through the troops until March 1919, well after the war ended.

Lieutenant Welker was assigned to the medical detachment of the 366th Infantry Regiment of the 92nd Division. By August 23 his front-line unit was sent to the Vosges Mountains in the Saint-Dié "quiet" sector for further training. His medical detachment saw its first combat there when the Germans counterattacked trying to recover (unsuccessfully) the town of Frapelle from the Americans. It had been taken by troops of the 5th Division just before the 92nd moved in to replace them. Welker remained there until September 20, when the division moved to the Meuse-Argonne for the fall offensive. In the final fighting of the First World War, November 9–11, the 92nd division suffered 498 casualties; 186 were soldiers of the 366th Infantry who had been wounded in action. Of these, 16 were killed in action and 10 more died of their wounds.[7]

Welker had certainly experienced the horror of war by the time he returned from France on March 5, 1919. He was assigned for several months at Camp Upton to care for returning soldiers until his discharge on August 3, 1919.

Career

After the war, Dr. Welker and his family moved from Nashville to Detroit, Michigan. Henry Ford's plant had opened in 1910. Ford's first hospital opened in 1915. By 1918 Dunbar Hospital opened as the first hospital owned and operated by and for the African American community. By 1919 there were 2600 manufacturing plants in the area, all needing workers. In 1920 alone 5,000 immigrants (of every race and nationality) arrived in the city.[8] There was great need for medical care for these workers.

In 1920 Dr. Welker, his wife Frankie, their two girls and his mother Alice were part of this bustling community. In 1921 son Leo Edward Welker, Jr., was born. The family lived at 602 Pennsylvania Avenue, and his office was at 3501 St. Antoine Street.

During the 1920s Detroit's educated African American community was doing well financially, but there were problems. On September 8, 1925, a white mob attacked the 2905 Garland Street home of Dr. and Mrs. Ossian Sweet, an African American doctor and family that had moved out of the African American community called Paradise Valley to an otherwise all-white East Side neighborhood. As the growing crowd moved towards the house, someone inside shot, wounding one man and killing another. After one acquittal, the court ruled in a subsequent trial that the Sweets were defending their lives and property.[9]

In 1926 Mayor John Smith formed the Mayor's Interracial Commission after a number of violent racial clashes occurred because of rampant police brutality of African American citizens.[10] In spite of the city's racial problems, Dr. Welker's practice and his involvement in Detroit's African American community grew during the late 1920s and early 1930s.

By the 1930 census, Frances was working for the city's recreation and welfare departments. She was also president of the Detroit Study Club and had held leadership positions in Alpha Kappa Alpha sorority. She entertained her sorority sisters with bridge parties in her home.[11]

In 1937 Dr. Welker was admitted to the U.S. Marine Hospital for symptoms related to arteriosclerosis or hardening of the arteries. The hospital was a federal hospital built in Detroit to care for sick and wounded seaman. Its role was expanded to provide for any military veterans sometime after the First World War. Dr. Welker died there at the age of 57.

After his death, Mrs. Welker and the family moved to a house at 503 Chandler Street. She taught in the Detroit public schools for many years. In 1963, more than 25 years later, Frankie joined her husband in Detroit's Woodlawn Cemetery.

Notes

1. en.wikipedia.org/wiki/Cambridge,_Illinois#Geography (accessed March 16, 2015).
2. www.Grinnell.edu (accessed March 18, 2015).
3. news.harvard.edu/gazette/story/2015/02/legacy-of-resolve/ (accessed March 16, 2015).
4. "Fisk Univ. Wins Over Morehouse," *Chicago Defender*, December 5, 1914, 6.
5. Robert C. Hayden, *Mr. Harlem Hospital* (Littleton, MA: Tapestry Press, 2003).
6. history.amedd.army.mil/booksdocs/wwi/communicablediseases/chapter12.html (accessed March 12, 2015).
7. www.kaiseracross.com (accessed March 11, 2015).
8. wikipedia.org/wiki/History_of_Detroit#Rise_of_industry_and_commerce (accessed March 14, 2015).
9. www.daahp.wayne.edu/1900_1949.html (accessed March 3, 2015).
10. *Ibid.*
11. Russell Cowans, "Detroit, Mich," *The Afro-American*, August 5, 1935, 21.

Herndon WHITE

20 May 1876–8 September 1943
Massachusetts College of Physicians and Surgeons (Boston), 1907

Roots and Education

Herndon was born in Fredericksburg, Virginia, to Elizabeth (Beasley) and Richard White. His father was a farmer, and his mother stayed home to care for Mildred, Joseph, Edwin, Barton and Herndon. The Whites adopted another son, Henderson Addison. All the boys were expected to help in the fields.

After public school in Fredericksburg, White graduated from Hampton Normal School in 1890. The school's most illustrious graduate was Booker T. Washington. Its website tells the story of Washington's acceptance. "By 1872 Hampton Normal and Agricultural Institute was flourishing and drawing students from all over the country. One day that year, a young man met with the assistant principal to request admission. His clothing and person were so unkempt from his long journey he was nearly turned away. The assistant principal asked him to sweep the recitation room. The young man, excited at the prospect of work, not only swept the floor three times but thoroughly dusted the room four times, thereby passing a rigorous 'white glove' inspection. Upon seeing the results of his work, the assistant principal said quietly, 'I guess you will do to enter this institution.'"[1]

White chose Livingstone College in Salisbury, North Carolina, for his undergraduate work. It had been founded by the African American Methodist Episcopal Church in 1879. From there, he went to Shaw University in Raleigh.

At the age of 34, he was lodging with many other students as he attended the College of Physicians and Surgeons of Boston. He received his medical degree in 1907. During his internship in Portland, Maine, he met Katrine P. Nelson. In 1917 as the United States entered the First World War, Dr. White volunteered for service with the U.S. Army Medical Reserve Corps.

Military Service

First Lieutenant White was 41 when he reported to Fort Des Moines for active duty on September 18, 1917. The camp was in operation for 110 days, but actual intensive instruction and training was only conducted between August 27 and November 13, 1917. There were many defects of the camp that needed to be corrected before the real training began. Changes affected its physical aspects (installing wood flooring in the stables which were used as barracks), its instructors (only three were provided, so additional ones were pulled from the new medical officers) and the ill-fitting shoes.[2] The last may seem so basic, but the officers and enlisted (1,000 medics) were expected to drill, so shoes that fit well were absolutely necessary.

After basic training, Lieutenant White was assigned to Camp Funston, Kansas. While on leave on April 11, 1918, he married Katrine Nelson. The wedding was in Providence, Rhode Island, at the home of the bride's mother, Mrs. S. E. Roby. Only a few friends were on hand, but there was all the usual music, flowers and presentations of wedding gifts. After the wedding they were going "home" to Manhattan, Kansas, near Camp Funston. About 30 friends were at the station to bid them goodbye.[3]

Lieutenant White left for France on June 15 and served with the 92nd Division's 367th Field Hospital. The Portland newspaper got word of his safe arrival in France and included it in the newspaper.[4]

In August 1918 Lieutenant Colonel David B. Downing determined First Lieutenant White did not "have the necessary adaptability for service in a Sanitary Train."[5] He was listed to appear before an efficiency board.[6] White was then transferred out of the 317th Sanitary Train, and he likely served in a camp hospital in France until the end of the war. The camp hospitals were set up in existing old French structures and were complemented with tents to increase capacity to 100 or 200 beds in the smaller ones, thousands in the larger. The sick or wounded would be evaluated and cared for until they could be shipped home or sent back to the battlefronts. After the Armistice, he sailed from Brest, France on January 4, 1919, for Hoboken, New Jersey.

After receiving his honorable discharge, Dr. White returned to Portland, Maine, to resume his practice. He stopped in his wife's hometown of Providence, Rhode Island, on the way to Maine and spoke at an AME Zion Church about his war experience.[7]

Career

A few years after the war, the Whites decided to move to Baltimore. By May 1925, Dr. White had opened his own maternity hospital with accommodations for 24 patients at 1029 Madison Avenue. He allowed all doctors to bring patients, and he had two nurses in attendance at all times. "According to Dr. White, this is the first hospital in the city specializing in maternity cases."[8]

The hospital took care of other ailments. When Ralph Matthews, city editor of the *Afro-American*, had an eye problem, he went to White's Hospital for treatment.[9]

Unfortunately, Dr. White did not choose the quietest location for his hospital. In a humorous article in the *Afro-American*, Ralph Matthews described his stay. The children of the neighborhood ignored the "Hospital Zone Quiet" sign and set off firecrackers. "Dr. White's institution was as peaceful and quiet as a base hospital at the front line in the middle of a bombardment."[10]

When the National Medical Association's annual convention met in Baltimore in 1928, many of its members took the opportunity to tour Dr. White's Hospital and his recently opened nurses' training school. The nurses were trained to work in hospitals, medical offices and nurseries. The hospital was good for the community, but it was not a financial success. It closed about 1929.

Katrine White worked beside her husband in his practice and in the community. In 1926 she was in charge of the annual Better Baby Contest held in conjunction with Baltimore Health Week. During the week a variety of classes in improving the health of children were offered to local residents.[11] Mrs. White was also an accomplished pianist. She was called upon by various African American organizations to entertain with piano selections. On June 11, 1927, she played Mendelssohn's "Scherzo" from Opus 16 and "The Sextet from Lucia" for the Afro-American Club as its "guest artist."[12]

Throughout his lifetime, Dr. White was active in Baltimore social circles as well as his professional organizations. He was a member of the National Medical Association as well as the local Wayland Medical, Dental and Pharmaceutical Association. He was active in the Masons, Odd Fellows, Knights of Pythias, and the Ancient Order of Moses. He was also examining physician for two Elks chapters.

For 10 years he was sponsor of the Young People's Forum. This local group was organized under the auspices of the NAACP. During the Great Depression of the 1930s, it helped to find jobs for young African Americans.[13]

By 1930 he and his wife Katrine had two children, Herndon Jr., and Katrina. For many years, the family rented a house at 1344 Druid Hill Avenue in Baltimore. In the 1940 census, he estimated he worked 60 hours a week for all 52 weeks a year.[14]

He and Katrine were lifelong members of Grace Presbyterian Church where he served as a trustee.

In 1943 after a three-week illness at the U.S. Marine Hospital in Baltimore, Dr. White died at 67. He was buried in Baltimore National Cemetery.

Throughout his life he was an entrepreneur who wasn't afraid to try a new venture, and he encouraged others to make the most of their lives. His maternity hospital and nursing training introduced true medical care for women. His Young People's Forum educated and found employment for many of the city's young African Americans. Dr. White's entrepreneurial lifestyle contributed to the well-being of his community and was a stellar example to the young people of Baltimore.

Notes

1. www.hamptonu.edu/about/history.cfm (accessed August 7, 2014).
2. Bispham, William N., Col. M.C., *The Medical Department of the United States Army in the World War*, Vol. VII, Training, 266–268.
3. "Wedding in Providence, RI," *The New York Age*, April 20, 1918, 2.
4. Providence, RI, *The New York Age*, July 13, 1918, 2.
5. 317th Sanitary Train, 92nd Division holdings of the National Archives, Box 210, 27 August 1918.
6. *Ibid.*, "Supplemental List of Officers for Reassignment."
7. "Providence, RI," *The New York Age*, March 1, 1919, 7.
8. "Maternity Hospital Opened Here," *Baltimore Afro-American*, May 16, 1925, 18.
9. "On the Sick List," *Baltimore Afro-American*, July 14, 1928, 11.
10. *Ibid.*, "In Darker Baltimore," 15.
11. "Champion Babies to Be Chosen Health Week," *Baltimore Afro-American*, March 27, 1926, 10.
12. "Music Notes," *Baltimore Afro-American*, June 11, 1927, 18.
13. "Dr. White Dies in Baltimore at Age of 67," *Afro-American*, September 18, 1943, 16.
14. 1930 and 1940 U.S. Federal Census.

James Thomas WHITTAKER

15 October 1876–3 March 1931
Louisville National Medical College, 1898

Roots and Education

J. T. Whittaker was born in Carrollton, Kentucky, a small city located on the Ohio River midway between Cincinnati and Louisville. He was one of six children of Scott and Cecelia Whittaker. He was educated in the local Louisville African American school before entering medical school. His younger brother Richard followed in his footsteps.

Whittaker received his medical degree in 1898 from Louisville National Medical College (LNMC). The independent medical school opened in 1888 to all races. It was one of a few medical schools in the nation to offer medical degrees to African Americans.[1] The school grew to have 40 students, a teaching staff of 17 part-time professors, an eight-bed hospital and minimal laboratory facilities. By 1902 the school's newspaper ad in *The Freeman* claimed 100 graduates.[2] It was too small to meet the new standards established after the 1910 Flexner Report and closed in 1912, having trained 150 physicians.[3]

Dr. Whittaker opened his first medical practice in Pittsburg, Kansas, a coal-mining town. At the turn of the century, Pittsburg had 55 coal companies employing nearly 12,000 workers. It was there he met Odella Turner. Odella graduated from high school in Pittsburg. She went on to Hobson Norman Institute in Parsons, Kansas, and graduated with her teaching degree in 1895. She taught for several years, and by the time she and Dr. Whittaker were married, she was principal of the grammar school in Yale, Kansas, about eight miles from downtown Pittsburg.[4] They married on April 2, 1902, and she was "an inspiring helpmate to him" for the rest of his life.[5] There would be no children.

He apparently struggled with his practice in Pittsburg and saw greater promise in Coffeyville (another coal mining town about 75 miles southwest of Pittsburg). The couple relocated there.

The Whittakers were well received by the Coffeyville community. His entrepreneurial spirit took flight. In 1904, he ran for county coroner. It was a contentious election. The *Coffeyville Weekly Journal* reported on the Republican ticket, "Dr. J. T. Whittaker, the next coroner, is a colored practitioner who stands well with the medical fraternity. He is a well-educated young man."[6] Just before the election the *Journal* endorsed him: "He is a colored man, one of the brainy shrewd ones of the county, and is representative of the better class of his race. He is a capable physician, possesses judgment and tact, and is well fitted to fill the office. He has gained the respect of the citizens of the community for his industry and his quiet, unassuming manners. His wife is a teacher in the Coffeyville schools, and on the whole, doctors stand high among their race. He will make a good coroner, and should and will be elected."[7] He won the position.

It may have been his experience with the power of the press that led him to get involved in the newspaper business. Right after his election, he agreed to be manager (and financer) of a new newspaper to cover the African American community. The first issue came out in mid–December 1904.[8]

In 1905 he joined with a group of 28 citizens to charter Oriental Lodge No. 29 of the Knights of Pythias. Dr. Whittaker was appointed their examining physician, and pronounced them "the healthiest bunch of K.P's in the Jurisdiction."[9] The same year, he and M. E. Woods opened the city's first African American pharmacy, W. & W. Drug Company, on Walnut Street. In addition to filling prescriptions, customers could buy sundries and stop at the "thoroughly modern" soda fountain.[10]

His personal financial reverses likely began when he became involved with the newspaper, *The Vindicator*. In 1905 the newspaper was purchased by the American National Development Co, a new local organization funded by 25 of the city's leading African American citizens.[11] At its November 1905 meeting Dr. Whittaker was elected business manager because the previous manager had left.[12]

During 1906 several unflattering articles about Dr. Whittaker appeared in the *Coffeyville Daily Journal*, now a competing newspaper. In June an article appeared about the doctor being "drunk and disorderly" and firing a gun while inside his drug store. He was fined $10 and court costs.[13] In August Dr. Whittaker felt compelled to announce that a stranger who came and offered to cure leprosy for $30 (to a person who had smallpox) was NOT one of the local black doctors.[14] In November in his role as coroner, he took a case to the coroner's jury to ensure there would be no doubt about his call that the death was in fact a suicide.[15]

By 1906 "the [newspaper's] financial liabilities several times rested solely upon the shoulders of Dr. J. T. Whittaker."[16] The newspaper closed. Before the end of the year W. & W. Drug Store moved to cheaper quarters, taking over two rooms over Foster Williams' grocery store. With the strain on his finances greatly reduced, he could focus on his practice.

In addition to all of his entrepreneurial undertakings, he continued to improve his medical skills and kept up with new surgical techniques. In 1907 he spent six weeks in Washington, D.C., taking a post-graduate course in surgery at Freedmen's Hospital.[17]

By March 1908 the *Coffeyville Weekly Herald* reported Dr. Whittaker sold his interest in the drugstore to his partner M. E. Wood so he could devote more time to his practice.[18] He was then out of the newspaper and pharmacy businesses.

In the early 20th century, many people (black and white) saw migration to California as a golden opportunity. The real estate market offered inexpensive housing and jobs were open to African Americans in civil service and at many factories. There were very few African American doctors in the Los Angeles area so Dr. and Mrs. Whittaker left Kansas. Los Angeles was "widely regarded among the nation's African Americans of that era as an oasis where they could co-exist with whites in a less intolerant and violent atmosphere and where the racial laws were less humiliating and oppressive. Consequently thousands of African Americans migrated to Los Angeles, beginning in the early 20th century."[19] Pasadena is an outlying suburb of Los Angeles. Its history reports Dr. James Whittaker was the town's first African American doctor.[20] He arrived there in 1917 and was later joined by his brother Richard and his family.

Military Service

In 1917 as the United States entered the First World War, Dr. Whittaker volunteered for service in the U.S. Army's Medical Reserve Corps. On September 4, 1917, at the age of 41, First Lieutenant Whittaker reported for basic training at the Medical Officers Training Camp (MOTC) in Fort Des Moines. On November 3 he was assigned to the 366th Field Hospital of the 317th Sanitary (Medical) Train at Camp Funston, Kansas. He was detailed to report on surgery at medical meetings and put in charge of the officers' mess between November 1917 and April 1918. That latter duty involved financial activities including collecting money and paying bills owed, which proved useful to him in later years.

On May 20, 1918, Lieutenant Whittaker was deemed "not physically capable of performing field service at the present time" by his supervisor Lieutenant Colonel David Downing.[21] He submitted his resignation and was honorably discharged from the army in June, shortly before his unit was sent to France.

Career

Dr. Whittaker returned to his wife Odella and his Pasadena practice. By 1923 he, his brother Richard and Dr. Charles S. Diggs established the Dunbar Hospital on East 15th Street in Pasadena. It was the first hospital for African Americans in the history of Los Angeles. He was named surgeon-in-chief.

The *California Eagle* reported on the hospital's progress in 1927, "Other dark moments faced the trio who, had they not been of the caliber that sticks to and fights for what they feel is right and an absolute social need, would have quickly given up in the attempt." The hospital was declared as good as any white hospital and meant black patients would no longer have to go the back-door route and pay extra to a hospital where they weren't welcome.[22]

Although it was small, the hospital had all the facilities of the larger white hospitals. The laboratory was capable of all kinds of tests. Its sterilizing plant took care of instruments and laundry. The delivery room could handle three patients. There were even quarters for night nurses on site. Most important for black physicians in Los Angeles, "any physician who is a member of the Medical Association is privileged to operate" as well as local white physicians.[23]

In addition to surgery, Dr. Whittaker continued his medical training at the University of Southern California and specialized in pulmonary diseases. "At one time he had a record of attending hundreds of pneumonia cases without losing one of them."[24]

In 1929 he founded the Citizens Cooperative Council. The organization was lead by the "fearless and formidable" Dr. Whittaker, Attorney C. Jones and Attorney J. T. Philips. Their goal was to "protect the rights and best interests of the Negroes of Pasadena." They started by lobbying city officials to end city restrictions involving race.[25]

In addition to his medical practice and duties at the hospital, Dr. Whittaker also took time to sponsor a health program. He spoke to the community from the pulpits of the local churches on good health practices.

The community was shocked at the sudden death of Dr. Whittaker. He began to hemorrhage at his home at 577 North Fair Oaks Avenue and was taken to Dunbar Hospital. He died of acute nephritis less than 24 hours later. Friend and fellow MOTC graduate Dr. Frank A. Pearl signed his death certificate. He was survived by his wife Odella, three brothers and two sisters.[26] His funeral service was at the Pasadena AME Church and he was buried with full military honors.

Dr. Whittaker's entrepreneurial instincts were always strong. We learn from his obituary that he operated a 30-acre fox ranch. It was in San Bernardino County near Big Bear Lake and housed more than 200 foxes, some valued at $1500 per pair."[27] His "Silver Black Foxes" business actually engaged a staff of 15 salesmen.[28]

Not long after his death, Dr. Charles Diggs, a partner in the hospital, died. After the deaths of both men, Richard Whittaker closed the hospital.[29] The Pasadena community suffered a significant loss.

NOTES

1. Henry Fitzbutler, *The Encyclopedia of Louisville* (Lexington: University Press of Kentucky, 2001) 293.
2. "Study Medicine at Louisville National Medical College Ad," *The Freeman*, August 2, 1902, 4.
3. Todd L. Savitt, *Race and Medicine in Nineteenth- and Early-Twentieth- Century America* (Kent, OH: Kent State University Press, 2007) 190–198.
4. "Mrs. O'della Turner Whittaker," *Vindicator*, Coffeyville, Kansas, February 10, 1905, 1.
5. "Dr. J. T. Whittaker, Veteran Pasadena Physician and Surgeon, Dies Suddenly!" *California Eagle*, March 6, 1931, 1.
6. "Republican Ticket," *Coffeyville Weekly Journal*, July 15, 1904, 4.
7. "Marking the Ballot," *Coffeyville Weekly Journal*, November 4, 1904, 5.
8. *Ibid.*, "New Negro Paper," December 19, 1904, 2.
9. "K.P. Lodge Organized," *Vindicator*, January 13, 1905, 1.
10. "Negro Business in Coffeyville," *Vindicator*, April 28, 1905, 1.
11. "To Establish Laundries," *Coffeyville Weekly Journal*, November 7, 1905, 5.
12. "An Important Meeting," *Coffeyville Weekly Journal*, November 10, 1905, 6.
13. *Ibid.*, "Shot at the Stars," June 8, 1906, 1.
14. *Ibid.*, "*Case of Smallpox,*" August 31, 1906 1.
15. *Ibid.*, "*Suicide the Verdict,*" November 24, 1906, 1.
16. *Ibid.*, "*New Year's Greeting*," January 5, 1906, 4.
17. *Ibid.*, "*News/Opinion,*" June 28, 1907, 4.
18. *Ibid.*, March 21, 1908, 1.
19. www.whitewashedadobe.com/2012/08/las-oasis-for-african-americans-val-verde (accessed October 18, 2014).
20. Ann Scheid, *Historic Pasadena: An Illustrated History* (HPN Books, 1999), 89.
21. Declassified Holdings of the National Archives, 92nd Division, Box 193, College Park, MD.
22. "Dunbar Hospital," *California Eagle*, December 23, 1927, D.
23. *Ibid.*
24. "Dr. J. T. Whittaker Passes," *California Eagle*, March 6, 1931, 3.
25. *Ibid.*, "A New Organization," February 27, 1925, 3.
26. "Dr. J. T. Whittaker Dies in Pasadena," *Chicago Defender*, March 14, 1931, 1.
27. "Dr. J. T. Whittaker Passes," *California Eagle*, March 6, 1931, 3.
28. "Pasadena Section," *California Eagle*, February 21, 1930, 2.
29. nkaa.uky.edu/all.php?sort_by=W (accessed August 23, 2014).

James Malachi WHITTICO, Sr.

22 September 1886–10 August 1975
Meharry Medical College, 1912

Roots and Education

Whittico was the last of 10 children born to Hezekiah J. and Letitia Pace Whittico. His father had inherited 500 acres of land near Ridgeway, Virginia, from his grandparents,

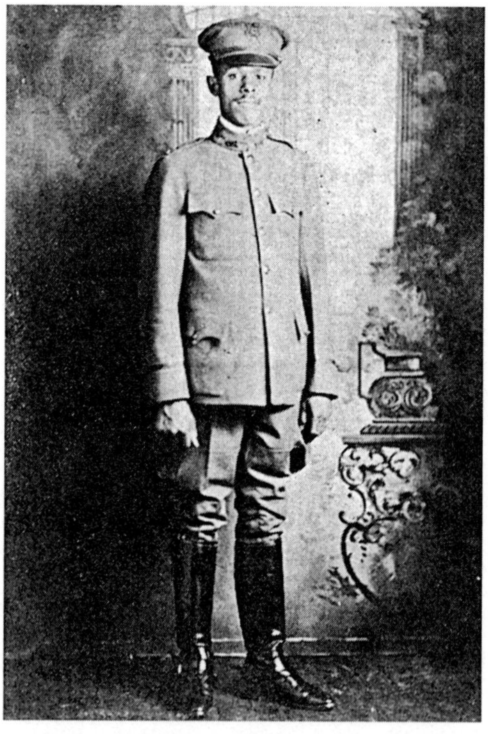

Lieutenant James M. Whittico (courtesy Meharry Medical College Archives).

Thomas and Catherine Whittico. All of the children worked the farm and went to public school.

When it came to securing his early education, young Whittico had the usual experiences of a farm boy. He divided his time between the farm and the local African American public school. His initial schooling was done in Martinsville, Virginia. He was able to leave and go on to three years of secondary education at Mary Potter School at Oxford, North Carolina, not far from Ridgeway.[1] After his mother died, he went to work in the mines of West Virginia to finance his education. He then did hotel and railroad work to pay his way through Walden University in Nashville, Tennessee.[2]

After earning his undergraduate degree, he enrolled at Meharry Medical College in Nashville, where he worked in the hospital. Whittico also found time to play college baseball and football.

At the time of his graduation in 1912, West Virginia faced a crisis. There were not enough physicians to serve all of the miners and railway workers coming to the state for jobs. Dr. Whittico saw the possibilities of a secure medical practice there and moved to the mining town of Williamson in southern West Virginia on the banks of the Tug Fork River. The railroad was new to the town, and the population was increasing rapidly, from 688 in the 1910 Census to 6,819 in 1920. The African American population was only about 10 percent of the total, but it would be enough for a new doctor. He established his practice there and met Nannie Lena Cobbs from Keystone. She was a graduate of the West Virginia Collegiate Institute and an accomplished teacher.

On December 24, 1914, Dr. Whittico married Nannie. They had one child, James Malachi Whittico, Jr., who also graduated from Meharry and become a remarkable surgeon in St. Louis. Early in Dr. Whittico's medical career he recognized the importance of continuing education offered through the medical societies. In 1915 he made his first presentation to the West Virginia Medical Society annual meeting in Huntington.[3]

Military Service

When the United States entered the First World War, Meharry was involved in a major recruiting effort among its alumni. As a result, more African American physicians volunteered from that school than any other (34), including Howard University (16) in Washington, D.C. Dr. Whittico joined the Army Medical Reserve Corps and was called to active service on August 9, 1917.

First Lieutenant Whittico reported to the Medical Officers Training Camp (MOTC) at Fort Des Moines on August 25 and received 71 days of training. He did well during training. In fact, he received special recognition from his superior officers for his initiative, efficiency and tact.

Lieutenant Whittico was transferred to Camp Meade, Maryland, in November 1917 as a member of the medical detachment of the 368th Infantry, 92nd Division. He served there for six more months before his unit was transported to France. He continued to serve with the 368th infantry as a surgeon for the remainder of the war. Fellow MOTC graduates Lts. Ponder, Harris and Jones served with him.

In August 1918 the 92nd Division was sent to St. Dié for additional training and its first experience in the trenches. It relieved the 5th Regular U.S. Army and was later brigaded with the French army in September 1918 at the outset of the Meuse-Argonne campaign. His inexperienced regiment was the only one in the division that was chosen to attack and engage the Germans. During their first days in heavy combat, the men of the 368th were not supplied with heavy-duty wire cutters, flares or grenade launchers. There was immediate communications breakdown between units. Despite repeated calls, there was no artillery barrage. Enemy artillery fire was unexpectedly heavy. It was chaos for those first five days until they were withdrawn and labeled failures. Casualties were 42 killed in battle, 16 more died of their wounds. More than 200 were wounded.[4] It was a poorly planned, poorly supplied and disorganized start to U.S. involvement in the war. Lieutenants Whittico, Ponder, Harris and Jones experienced enough gore to last them a lifetime. The 92nd Division was also chosen to attack toward Metz in October and November 1918 as part of the AEF Second Army. His unit, the 368th, was held in reserve in that battle while the 365th, 366th and 367th infantry regiments were committed to it. Following the war, Lieutenant Whittico was returned to the United States in early 1919 and discharged. He had served honorably and experienced some of the worst that war presents.

Career

Dr. Whittico returned to Williamson, his family and his practice. He continued his involvement in the state and national medical societies as well as the local organization, Flat Top Medical Society.

Politically, he was a Republican and took an active interest in the local African American organization. He served as superintendent of the Sunday school at the local Presbyterian Church. Among the secret and benevolent orders, he belonged to the Masons, Pythians, Odd Fellows and St. Luke's. He was the local medical examiner for the Pythians.[5]

His marriage to Nannie ended in divorce in 1936.[6] On January 10, 1939, he married Lafadie Belle Dickerson. They had a son, Matthew Thomas. She helped the doctor in his practice and in the Whittico Drug Store he opened in Williamson soon after the war.[7]

Dr. Whittico's son and grandson followed him into the medical profession. His son grew up in Williamson. He enjoyed telling stories about his father. One involved an unexpected event that caused his father's reputation to rise. Dr. Whittico became a friend of the Hatfield family, known for its legendary feud with the McCoys.

"One day, the matriarch of the Hatfield family was ready to deliver a baby, and the white doctor could not be found. Some of Hatfield's sons summoned Dr. Whittico, the only other doctor in town.

"It was nearly dark when they took him up into the mountain. And when they got to the clearing old man Hatfield was sitting on the porch. He was upset when he saw that the doctor was black and insisted that he wasn't about to let no black doctor touch his wife. Well, the story is that the boys tied the old man to a tree to allow my father to tend to the wife. They then untied the father to see the baby (a boy). From that day on, my father and the Hatfields were good friends."[8]

When the National Association of Life Insurance Medical Examiners met in Philadelphia at the 1926 annual meeting of the National Medical Association (NMA), Dr. Whittico was listed as treasurer of the organization. He was a lifelong member of the NMA and held various offices in the organization for 35 years. In 1955, at NMA's 60th convention, he was "one of 199 physicians who received an award for 40 years or more of service to the medical profession."[9]

At the West Virginia Medical Society meeting in 1966, the main topic was once again the crisis in the state's medical care. The majority of practicing doctors were at retirement age. In 1965 the society "made a determined effort to get some of the younger doctors and dentists to practice in West Virginia. Not one answered the appeal."[10] Dr. Whittico summed up this medical crisis: "There simply is not enough dynamics in West Virginia for professional trained Negro young people. They pass us up like a passenger train passes the freight.... Our problems continue to outrace the solutions. Maybe the tide will turn."[11]

Dr. Whittico died where he had lived most of his life, in Williamson, West Virginia. He served all citizens of his town, black and white, for more than 60 years. This modest, unassuming man made his mark on the politics, health, and wellness of the entire community. A lengthy and colorful three-page tribute to Dr. Whittico appeared in the *Journal of the National Medical Association* in 1976. He is shown astride his horse "Fancy" along with the observation that his career spanned a remarkable time in human history from horseback to the jet age. "His influence will long survive him over a much broader area. The NMA will cherish his memory."[12]

Dr. DeHaven Hinkson, another World War I medical corps veteran, wrote of being privileged to meet Whittico's son James during his service in the Second World War at a large army station hospital at Fort Huachuca, Arizona. James Whittico, Jr., served in the Southwest Pacific Theater with the 93rd Division and rose to the rank of lieutenant colonel. He was awarded a Bronze Star for his combat service. Dr. Whittico Jr. later became president of the National Medical Association.[13] He is described as a living legend and was still practicing medicine in St. Louis, Missouri, as recently as 2012 at the age of 97.[14]

NOTES

1. *James M. Whittico*, www.wvculture.org/history/histamne/whitticj.html (accessed June 1, 2014).
2. "James Malachi Whittico, Sr, MD, 1893–1975," *Journal of the National Medical Association (JNMA)*, 1976 September; 68(5): 441–443.
3. "The Diagnostic Significance of Localized Pain," *Journal of the National Medical Association (JNMA)*, July–September 1915, Vol. 7, No. 3, 239.
4. Arthur Barbeau and Florette Henri, *The Unknown Soldiers* (Philadelphia: Temple Press, 1974), 151.
5. "James Malachi Whittico, Sr, MD, 1893–1975," *Journal of the National Medical Association (JNMA)*, 1976 September; 68(5): 441–443.
6. *Ibid.*
7. www.clantonadvertiser.com/2011/07/15 (accessed March 13, 2015).
8. *By Just Doing His Job, Dr. Whittico Helps Make Sure Other Blacks Could Enter Medicine,* www.stlbeacon.org, 3 (accessed June 22, 2012).
9. "The Forty Year Practitioners," *Journal of the National Medical Association (JNMA)*, November 1955, Vol. 47, 412.
10. "Negro Medical Society Faces Uncertain Future," *Charleston Daily Mail*, June 18, 1966, 6.
11. *Ibid.*
12. "James Malachi Whittico, Sr, MD, 1893–1975," *Journal of the National Medical Association (JNMA)*, 1976 Sep; 68(5): 441–443.
13. DeHaven Hinkson, MD, "The Role of the Negro Physician in the Military Services from World War I Through World War II," *Journal of the National Medical Association*, January 1972, Vol. 64, 75.
14. "97th Birthday Blessing for a Lifetime of Service," *The St. Louis American*, stlamerican.com (accessed March 27, 2015).

John Henry WILLIAMS

23 July 1879–5 December 1959
Meharry Medical College, 1902

Roots and Education

John H. Williams was born in Bagdad, a small community in Shelby County, Kentucky. Located east of Louisville near Frankfort, it was founded at what is currently the intersection of Kentucky routes 12 and 395. The name of the tiny community came from the name of an old railroad station named "Daddy's Bag" after a colorful railroad worker who lived there. The name was eventually shortened to "Bagdad."[1]

Williams first answered his country's call in 1898. At the age of 19 he was a medical student at Meharry Medical College, but he left his studies on July 19 and enlisted in the U.S. Army at the beginning of the Spanish-American War. The African American community strongly supported the rebels in Cuba and American entry into the war. Thirty-three African American sailors died in the battleship USS *Maine* explosion in Havana harbor.

Booker T. Washington promoted enlistment. In fact, he promised the secretary of war "at least ten thousand loyal, brave, strong black men in the south who crave an opportunity to show their loyalty to our land."

White officers and news reports offered praise of the Negro regiments. A Lieutenant Roberts, who had been shot in the abdomen, later said: "The heroic charge of the Tenth Cavalry saved the Rough Riders from destruction; and, had it not been for the Tenth Cavalry, the Rough Riders would never have passed through the seething cauldron of Spanish missiles."

When Colonel Theodore Roosevelt returned from the command of the famous Rough Riders, he delivered a farewell address to his men, in which he made the following reference to the gallant black soldiers: "Now, I want to say just a word more to some of the men I see standing around not of your number. I refer to the colored regiments, who occupied the right and left flanks of us at Guásimas, the Ninth and Tenth cavalry regiments. The Spaniards called them 'Smoked Yankees,' but we found them to be an excellent breed of Yankees. I am sure that I speak the sentiments of officers and men in the assemblage when I say that between you and the other cavalry regiments there exists a tie which we trust will never be broken."

Unfortunately, these heroes of Cuba returned home to discrimination, segregation, and even a revision of the importance of their contribution from Roosevelt himself. In 1899 writing for *Scribner's* magazine, Roosevelt revised his earlier comments to criticize the performance of African Americans in the taking of San Juan Hill. He wrote that they were "peculiarly dependent on their white officers," and that they ran when encountering heavy enemy fire. Only when he threatened to shoot them, Roosevelt said, did they return to the line.[2]

Private John Henry Williams received an "excellent" rating and was honorably discharged on May 24, 1899. He returned to Nashville to resume his medical studies.

After graduation from Meharry Medical College in 1902 Dr. Williams moved to Buxton, Iowa, and set up his medical practice. Buxton was a coal-mining colony with a large African American population that grew quickly in southern Iowa at the beginning of the 20th century. There was no overt segregation in Buxton. The Consolidated Coal Company created the town and treated blacks and whites equally in employment and housing. Schools were racially integrated and taught by black and white teachers.[3] Dr. Williams married Marietta (Mary) and their daughter Gladys was born there in 1905. They remained in Buxton for several years.

In 1910 the family moved to Des Moines, Iowa. Dr. and Mrs. Williams lived at 819 Thirteenth Street with five-year-old Gladys. Again, they only stayed a few years. The family's next stop was Jeffersonville, Indiana, located just across the Ohio River from Louisville, Kentucky. Then in 1917 they moved into Louisville proper. From their home at 1007 West Chestnut Street, Dr. Williams answered his country's call once again. As America entered the First World War, he volunteered to serve in the U.S. Army Medical Reserve Corps. He received a commission as an officer on August 15, 1917.

Military Service

First Lieutenant Williams reported to Fort Des Moines to the Medical Officers Training Camp (MOTC) on August 20, 1917. After completing his training on November 3, 1917, he was transferred to Camp Meade, Maryland, with the medical detachment of the 368th Infantry Regiment of the 92nd Division. He was later sent to France where he was reassigned as a medical officer with the 365th Infantry Regiment. His unit suffered significant casualties during October and November 1918 during the AEF Second Army major offensive attack on German positions near Metz.

Many years later, Lieutenant Williams' payroll records survived the fire at the St. Louis Archives. From them we learn that a military doctor initially earned $166.67 a month. By early 1918, his monthly pay increased to $183.33, and later in the year to $240.48. With his return from France following war's end, he had completed his second round of military service. Lieutenant Williams was honorably discharged from the 365th Infantry Regiment at Camp Grant, Illinois, on March 13, 1919.

Career

He returned to his family in Louisville, where he lived and worked for the next 40 years. Over the next several years, five news items about Dr. Williams appeared in the *Chicago Defender* newspaper. In August 1924 it reported he had taken a flying trip to Nashville, Tennessee, to attend the funeral of Dean Hubbard of Meharry Medical College. He carried with him resolutions of sympathy from the Meharry alumni of Louisville. In September 1924 he drove his daughter from Louisville to Bloomington, Indiana, where she was re-entering Indiana University.

In September 1925 he and Harry Dugan purchased a sandwich shop on West Walnut Street in Louisville. By June 1927 his daughter Gladys graduated from the Collegiate Department of Indiana University. In July 1928 Dr. Williams, described as a "prominent physician" of Louisville, was initiated into the Alpha Lambda chapter of the Alpha Phi Alpha fraternity.[4]

In 1930 Dr. and Mrs. Williams and Gladys lived at 1932 Chestnut Street in Louisville. He was active in the Blue Grass State Medical Society, taking time to run a surgical clinic at its annual meeting in Lexington.[5] A brief news item from June 1933 said that Dr. Williams had been slightly injured but was once again able to resume his medical practice. A year later, in June 1934, the paper reported that Dr. Williams, a well-known surgeon, had returned home after being confined at the U.S. Veterans Hospital at

Tuskegee. He was in much better health except for his eyesight.[6]

In 1940 Dr. Williams and his wife and daughter, Gladys, still lived on Chestnut Street. Gladys was working as a teacher.

On November 29, 1959, Dr. Williams passed away at his home in Louisville at the age of 80, having served his country in two wars, the Spanish American and World War I. He was buried at the Zachary Taylor National Cemetery in Louisville. A brief obituary appeared in *Jet*, the national African American news magazine, reporting his passing.[7]

NOTES

1. en.wikipedia.org/wiki/Bagdad,_Kentucky (accessed September 26, 2013).
2. www.authentichistory.com/1898–1913 (accessed September 26, 2013).
3. Online Encyclopedia—www.BlackPast.org Buxton, Iowa (accessed September 8, 2012).
4. "Kentucky State News: Louisville News," *Chicago Defender*, August 30, 1924; September 20, 1924; September 26, 1925; June 11, 1927, and July 7, 1928.
5. "Kentucky Medical Society Holds Annual Convention," *Chicago Defender*, June 6, 1931, 11.
6. *Ibid.* July 1, 1933, and June 23, 1934.
7. "The Week's Census-Died," *JET Magazine*, December 24, 1959.

Arthur Henry WILSON

4 September 1876–3 August 1943
Indiana University, 1907

Roots and Education

Wilson was born in Indianapolis, Indiana, to Charles Henry and Mary E. (Moore) Wilson. He graduated in 1896 from Franklin High School in Franklin, Indiana, 25 miles south of Indianapolis. He remained there and attended Franklin College in 1896–1897. He taught school from 1898 to 1901 and continued his studies. He married Mary Hugel on February 12, 1900. Their daughter Martha was born on May 12, 1901.

Wilson was always involved in athletics. He was a star football player (left half-back on the 1898 team) and a member of Franklin's baseball team. He was also a member of the debating and glee clubs. In 1902 he became Franklin's first African American graduate. Throughout his life, Wilson was proud of his college and seldom missed an alumni day or homecoming event.[1]

Following his graduation, he worked as the head of the Colored High School in Franklin where he was known as Professor Wilson. He also entered the Indianapolis Medical College of Purdue University and graduated in 1907.[2]

The Wilsons owned a home at 1264 North Sheffield Avenue in Indianapolis. Daughter Martha was born there. He established his of-

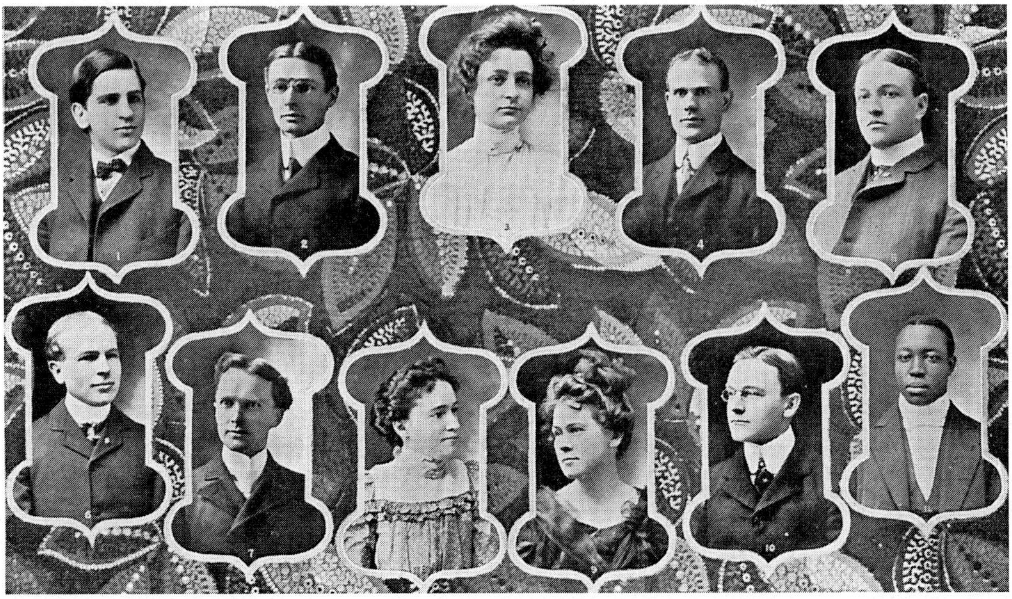

Arthur H. Wilson (bottom right) graduation picture 1902 (courtesy B.F. Hamilton Library, Franklin College).

fice at 543½ Indiana Avenue and became active in local professional organizations. When the Indiana Medical, Dental and Pharmacy Association had its first annual meeting in 1908, Wilson worked with its chief organizer, Dr. Joseph Ward, to ensure its success.

Wilson was also a member of the American Legion, Masons, Shriners, and NAACP. He was a Baptist and both he and his wife were active in the Ebenezer Baptist Church where he was choir master.[3]

He was more than a member of the YMCA. After his college days when he was a member of the football and baseball teams, Dr. Wilson continued to enjoy sports. When the local chapter held its first athletic meet for African American youths in 1912, he was one of he officials at the event which drew 500 citizens to Indianapolis' Northwestern baseball park. The event included music from the YMCA band and lots of students in their high school colors.[4]

There were African American doctors in the city, but the black population often failed to receive proper health care. Indianapolis City Hospital until the late 1940s was the only municipal institution that admitted African American doctors. Unable to gain admission to existing hospitals, African Americans established their own. In August 1909 Wilson joined nearly all the African American doctors in the city in the incorporation of the Lincoln Hospital Association. The medical consulting staff consisted of a number of the city's leading physicians who worked together to cover special patient needs. Dr. Wilson was the group's surgical specialist in genito-urinary and venereal diseases.[5] Other small hospitals followed, including Charity Hospital (1911), Dr. Ward's Sanatorium, and Provident Hospital (1921). All these institutions were short-lived because they lacked adequate money and proper facilities to practice modern medicine.

Topics at the September 1912 meeting of the Indiana Association of Negro Physicians and Dentists and Pharmacists included " The Quack Doctor and How to Suppress Him." Dr. Wilson was elected president that year. The meetings in the association's early years were all held at the YMCA in Indianapolis. The location of the "annual banquet" gives a clue to the size of the organization. It was set in the YMCA's café.[6]

By the fall of 1912, Dr. Wilson had separated from his wife and left her and his daughter at the home on North Sheffield Avenue. He moved 172 miles away to Evansville where he rented a house at 410 Lincoln Avenue and took in two boarders.

He joined the Second Baptist Church in Evansville where he directed its musical programs. As early as June 1913, he directed the Sangerfest, a competition of musical groups. It was the church's chief fundraising activity.[7]

When the Indiana Association of Negro Physicians, Dentists and Pharmacists met in Indianapolis in 1913, Wilson was serving as its president. The main topic of the meeting was about continuing education, "Observations of the Mayo Clinic."[8] Dr. Daniel Williams, famed surgeon at Chicago's Provident Hospital, conducted a clinic during the meeting.[9]

By 1914 he was president of the tri-state (Indiana, Ohio, and Kentucky) medical association. This meeting drew about 100 delegates to Indianapolis for its annual meeting. Among the session topics were "The Duty of the Physician to the Public" and "The Business Side of the Physician."[10]

Wilson was obviously politically active in his community. He was a Republican, as were most of the Evansville African Americans. In the November 1916 election, he and William Williams, a fellow Republican, were arrested as a result of a fight at the polls with attorney Thomas Higgins, a Democrat. Republicans charged that Democratic workers were intimidating Republican African Americans and buying votes. It was reported "revolvers and knives were freely flashed at the polls in the city without interference by the police."[11]

Military Service

In 1917 Dr. Wilson volunteered to serve his country during World War I. After completing training at the Fort Des Moines Medical Officer Training Camp (MOTC) in November 1917, he was stationed at Camp Funston, Kansas, with the 92nd Division. He was assigned to the 368th Field Hospital, where he was a urological specialist.

First Lieutenant Wilson went with his division to France in June 1918. Toward the end of August 1918, the division left the 11th Training Area at Bourbonne-les-Bains and moved east to trenches in the St. Dié sector of the Vosges mountains, a so-called "quiet sector." This was the first real taste of combat for the division. The 368th Field Hospital was held in reserve in La Salle, a small village northwest of St. Dié, where Wilson was billeted in the rectory. Several of the doctors from his time at the Fort Des Moines MOTC were also assigned to the field hospital: James C. Wallace, Romeo A. Johnston, Frank P. Raiford, and Jackson Smitherman.

At the end of August 1918, Lieutenant Wilson was transferred to the 317th Sanitary (Medical) Train just a few weeks before the great Meuse-Argonne offensive began in late September. He was appointed assistant division urologist. Urology was not a separate medical certification in those years, but was important. Bladder infections could be severe and incapacitating. Soldiers who suffered spinal injuries could die from bladder infections related to paralyzed bladders.

His division was engaged in active combat in the Argonne for a week at the end of September and suffered numerous casualties. In early November 1918, as the end of the war drew near, Wilson was attached to the 366th Field Hospital and promoted to the rank of captain. In 1919 his division returned to the United States.

Wilson continued to serve in the Medical Officers Reserve Corp well into the 1930s, and was assigned to the Ohio National Guard's 372nd Infantry at Camp Perry, Ohio. He was a charter member of the Otis Stone Post of the American Legion of Evansville.[12] He became the second African American from Indianapolis to rise to the rank of lieutenant colonel (Dr. Joseph H. Ward of Indianapolis was the first).[13]

Career

Following his return from France and discharge from active service, Dr. Wilson returned to his medical practice in Evansville.

In 1921 he was once again president of the Indiana Medical Association. He led a group of Indiana doctors to the National Medical Association convention in Louisville where they

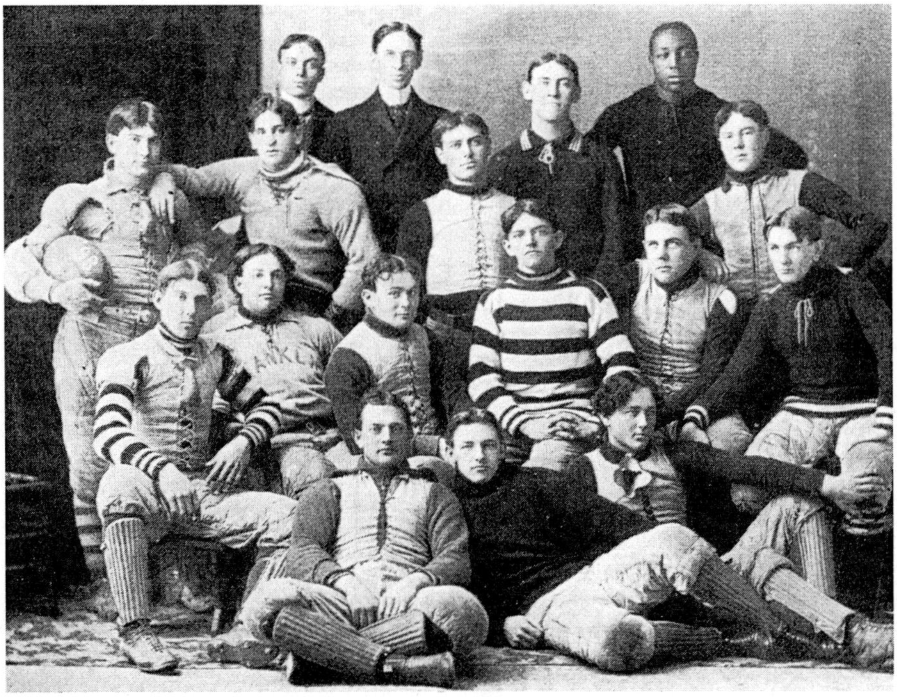

Arthur H. Wilson (upper right) on Franklin College football team (courtesy B.F. Hamilton Library, Franklin College).

participated in four days of programs.[14] In 1929, when the African American Boy Scout troops of Indianapolis needed physicians to give physical exams to those attending summer camp, Dr. Wilson volunteered.[15]

When the "Colored" Pythians held their 25th annual national convention in Indianapolis in 1929, Dr. Wilson was elected to one of its positions. In addition to the fraternal order, and the parades in uniforms (more than 3,000 participated in that year's parade), the Pythians brought baseball to African American youths. The Pythians' founders viewed baseball as more than just a pasttime; they believed the game could be a vehicle for black self-improvement. It was a place where young African Americans could assert their skills and gain leadership experience. The games were held at the state fairgrounds.[16]

In January 1931 the *Indianapolis Recorder* reported Dr. Wilson's divorce from his wife was finalized in the Vanderburgh Probate Court. The charge was abandonment.[17] Also in January, Dr. Wilson was appointed medical examiner for the U.S. Veterans' Bureau in Evansville and county physician for Vanderburgh County.[18]

Wilson continued to be active in the military reserves. On April 11, 1931, the *San Diego Evening Tribune* reported that Lieutenant Colonel Arthur H. Wilson was in California at the Ninth Corps of the Citizens' Military Training Camp (CMTC). It was the first year California had invited Easterners to come for training.[19] Attending that year's training camp appears to have been one of the benefits of his continued involvement in the military.

By 1935 Wilson had purchased a nearby house at 419 Lincoln Avenue in Evansville. He was always extremely active in his professional societies. In 1936 the Indiana State Medical, Dental and Pharmaceutical Association met in Muncie on June 10 and 11, and Dr. Wilson was chairman of the resolutions committee "and presented well-timed resolutions respecting the excellent manner in which the citizens of Muncie took care of the visitors."[20]

The 1940 U.S. Census lists him still at the house on Lincoln Avenue. At 63, he was still practicing medicine.

At the age of 67, Dr. Wilson passed away at his daughter Martha's home in Indianapolis from hypertension. Martha and her husband John Q. Martin lived in the same house on Sheffield Avenue the doctor had shared so many years ago with his family. Dr. Wilson's body was returned to Franklin where he was buried in Greenlawn Cemetery.[21]

NOTES

1. "Franklin College," *The Indianapolis Star*, February 2, 2007.
2. *Who's Who in Colored America*, 1928–1929 (Second Edition), 403.
3. *Ibid.*
4. "Flanner Guild Holds First Athletic Meet Before 500," *The Indianapolis Star*, August 9, 1912, 16.
5. George H. Rawls, MD, *Lincoln Hospital, History of the Black Physicians in Indianapolis*, 1870 to 2000, October 1984, 29.
6. "Quack Doctors Discussed," *The Indianapolis News*, September 5, 1912, 7.
7. "Indiana News in Brief," *The Indianapolis News*, May 6, 1913, 8.
8. "Colored Association Meets," *The Indianapolis Star*, October 15, 1913, 14.
9. "Sessions at the Y.M.C.A.," *The Indianapolis News*, October 4, 1913, 3.
10. *The Indianapolis Star*, September 6, 1914, 10.
11. "Vote in Indiana Passes Quietly," *The Indianapolis Star*, November 8, 1916, 4.
12. "Dr. A. H. Wilson War Veteran Succumbs Here," *Indianapolis Recorder*, August 7, 1943, 7.
13. Thomas Yenser, *Who's Who in Colored America*, 1941–1944 (Sixth Edition) (New York, 1944) 573.
14. "Will Attend Convention," *The Indianapolis News*, August 20, 1921, 27.
15. *The Indianapolis News*, August 17, 1929, 33.
16. www.PhilaPlace.com (accessed April 6, 2015).
17. "Physician Granted Divorce from Wife," *Indianapolis Recorder*, January 1, 1931.
18. "Dr. Wilson Appointed Medical Examiner," *Chicago Defender*, January 24, 1931.
19. "Training Camps Attracting Easterners," *San Diego Evening Tribune*, April 11, 1931, 8.
20. "Indiana Medical Men Hold Meet in Muncie," *Chicago Defender*, June 20, 1936.
21. "Dr. Arthur Henry Wilson (D. 8-3-1943)," *Journal of the Indiana State Medical Association*, Vol. 36, No. 9, 1943, 528.

James Lancelot WILSON

27 July 1890–18 October 1969
Columbia University, 1916

Roots and Education

Dr. Wilson was born on Estate Enfield Green in 1890 near Frederiksted, St. Croix, in what was then the Danish Virgin Islands. (In 1917 the Danish Virgin Islands were purchased by the United States and became the U.S. Virgin Islands.) His father William Wilson was born in Ireland, and came to St. Croix in 1855. He managed sugar plantations on the island. His mother was Charlotte Petersen, a native born in St. Croix in 1852. She was a field laborer who met William at a very young age.

Dr. Wilson was the last of eight children born to this couple. His mother passed away in 1895 while he was still a very young child. He lived then with his older sister, a dressmaker, at their family home #01 King Street in Frederiksted. He attended a Danish school, the city's Government Boys High School.[1]

As a young man, he immigrated to the United States via Jacksonville, Florida, in 1905. He lived with older siblings in the New York area and went to public schools in New Jersey. He graduated from Jersey City High School in January 1910. At that time, there was only one high school in Jersey City and four black graduates in that class.[2] Wilson was one of two boys who made front-page headlines in the Jersey City newspaper when they led their class of 80 pupils. Wilson had the highest grade point average, 93.84.[3]

In 1910 he was accepted into a special program that enabled students to complete their A.B. at Columbia College and their medical degrees at Columbia's College of Physicians and Surgeons in six years. The 1910 U.S. Census lists 20-year-old James L. Wilson, living at 162 York Street, Jersey City, Hudson County, New Jersey.

Wilson worked at least one summer at the Hotel Maryland in Asbury Park, New Jersey, to help pay for his medical education. He also received a modest, but critical, scholarship of $175 during his medical school years. He lived in Jersey City and commuted to Manhattan. Wilson received his A.B. from Columbia College in 1914, and his M.D. from the College of Physicians and Surgeons in 1916. After his graduation from Columbia's medical school he obtained a one-year internship (July 1916–July 1917) at Freedmen's Hospital in Washington, D.C.[4]

Military Service

Following the U.S. entry into the First World War in April 1917, Wilson volunteered and was commissioned a first lieutenant in the Army Medical Reserve Corps. He arrived at Fort Des Moines, Iowa, on October 3, 1917. When he completed his training there on November 11, 1917, he was assigned to the 92nd Division at Camp Funston, at Fort Riley, Kansas.[5] He worked in the division infirmary.

On December 26, 1917, he was examined for pulmonary tuberculosis at the Fort Riley Base Hospital. A small but healed lesion was found in the upper right apex, but it did not immediately incapacitate him for military duty. A March 1918 army report lists him working as the medical officer assigned to the division's 317th Supply Train. On May 20, 1918, shortly before his division left Kansas for New York and France, Wilson was declared one of several officers "not physically capable of performing field service at present time."

He was recommended for base hospital work. At that time he was assigned to the 367th Field Hospital at Camp Upton, Long Island, New York. A July 10, 1918, report, "Daily Report of Casualties and Changes," lists First Lieutenant James L. Wilson, F.H. 367 as "absent, sick at base hospital." His division had already sailed for France. He completed his wartime military service in the United States and was honorably discharged with the rank of captain in 1919 in New York.[6]

Career

In August 1919 Dr. Wilson assisted his good friend Dr. Louis T. Wright in performing an abdominal operation, which according to Wilson, was the first major operation controlled by an African American in New York State.[7]

In 1920 Dr. Wilson partnered again with Dr. Wright, a fellow MOTC graduate and veteran, in establishing the original Booker T. Washington Sanitarium in Harlem. It provided inpatient treatment for those with tuberculosis. Drs. "Jimmie" Wilson and "Louie" Wright were close friends and professional associates throughout their lives. An excellent 2003 biography of Dr. Wright says, according to Mrs. Wright, that Wilson was "one of Louie's most loyal, devoted and trusted friends and colleagues."

Wilson had settled in New York in Harlem at 216 West 137th Street in 1920. He owned his home and had his medical office there. His sister, Alice Westcott, lived with him and was his housekeeper. He also had two boarders whose rent helped him pay his mortgage.[8] Wilson was an active member of the New York African American medical community and a member of the North Harlem Medical, Dental and Pharmaceutical Association.[9]

In 1925 he and a group of black doctors formed a corporation to create the Edgecombe Sanitarium.[10] That December they purchased the Brunor Sanitarium at 137th Street and Edgecombe Avenue, and merged it with the Booker T. Washington Sanitarium, which had been operated on Seventh Avenue by Dr. Wilson. He became superintendent of the combined Edgecombe Sanitarium. The hospital had 15 beds.

During its first year of operation the hospital handled 278 cases, 188 of which were surgical cases; some were described as of "rare major proportions." There were 47 medical and maternity cases, with 21 transient cases. "The sanitarium was open to all, regardless of race, creed, or color." The sanitarium's board of directors was composed of many distinguished Harlem physicians including its officers, as well as Drs. James T. Granady, C.A. Edwards and Louis T. Wright. Dr. H. J. Oliver, a fellow army veteran, was Treasurer.[11] Wright was also a staff physician at Harlem Hospital.

Because Harlem Hospital was municipal and not private, it "existed primarily to care for the indigent or those unable to meet the expenses of private medical care." Wright was not allowed to use it for the care of his private patients, so he would use Edgecombe Sanitarium to treat them, as did the other doctors who had helped form and support it.

In 1925 Dr. Wilson was living at his home in Harlem with his older brother, Alexander Wilson, a waiter (age 45) and his older sister, Alice Wescott, a housekeeper (age 47).[12] He was single and remained so until 1928.

We are fortunate that the African American press carried a number of stories mentioning Dr. Wilson during the 1920s–1950s. Their articles paint a wonderful picture of Wilson as a physician, businessman, hospital director and community activist. On February 17, 1927, a formal banquet was given by the Edgecombe Sanitarium Corporation with the Nursing Staff and Ladies Auxiliary, to celebrate the successful first year of operation of the hospital. Dr. Louis T. Wright, a director, praised the work of its Superintendent, Dr. James L. Wilson.[13]

On March 21, 1928, in Jersey City, Dr. Wilson married a fellow Columbia University graduate, Miss Shamray Bryant. She was from Asheville, North Carolina, where her father was successful and prominent African American physician Dr. Reuben H. Bryant. Her father passed away in 1929, shortly after she married Wilson. In 1943 her former family home, a two-story, ten-room residence, became the Asheville Colored Hospital.

Shamray had graduated from Talladega College in Alabama and taught at Stephens-Lee High School in Asheville. She was awarded a master's degree in English from Columbia in October 1924.[14] Her master's essay was published in 1925 and entitled "Lord Byron in Venice."[15] A newspaper article in June 1928 carried her photograph and described her as the "charming wife of Dr. James Lancelot Wilson ... a recognized leader in Harlem's smart set."[16] Shamray later attended the Columbia School of Library Service from 1932 to 1934, graduating with a B.S. in library service in June 1934.

Their home in Harlem was in a fashionable area noted for housing artists, academics, businessmen and professionals. The house is still standing. It is a large four-story stone house near the middle of the block, surrounded by similarly fine homes. His medical office was there too. Wilson lived and practiced there for more than 40 years.

In August 1928 Wilson was one of the community leaders who brought about the formation of a new New York-based insurance association in Harlem that would provide life insurance to its members.[17]

In 1929 the newspaper referred to Dr. Wilson as one of Harlem's leading physicians[18] and he was busy performing surgery at his Edgecombe Sanitarium.[19] In November he was one of the hosts for a large social event that drew 1,100 people to a blue ribbon ball given by members of the Kappa Alpha Psi fraternity.[20]

The Wilson's son, James L. Wilson, Jr., was born on August 4, 1929, in New York City.

In 1930 one Harlem newspaper reported that during 1929 Edgecombe sanitarium treated 249 patients; 165 were surgical, 58 medical and 30 were obstetrical. It had 17 beds and employed 4 day nurses and 1 night nurse. Although it paid no rent to the doctors who owned it, it reported a successful year with net income of $2,330.[21]

There was a political split in New York's black medical community and by 1930, 55 physicians, including Drs. Wilson and Wright, had left the North Harlem Medical Association and established a new organization called the Manhattan Medical Society. Wilson, president of the society, said in an interview the reason for the new organization was the desire of many physicians in and outside the old body to halt internal dissension. They wanted to devote themselves to promoting medical science and combating disease. "There is too much to be done in Harlem to be wrangling."[22]

When a well-known private philanthropist from Chicago named Julius Rosenwald proposed to fund a survey to determine the need for an African American hospital in New York City, Wilson, Wright and their supporters opposed it. They rejected the notion that such a survey be done or that a separate hospital be established. They took the position that equality of care and opportunity in hospitals was the goal, not the creation of a Jim Crow type of separate institution. Wilson and Wright fought consistently for that equality principle throughout their lives.

In January 1933 a newspaper reported that Columbia Medical School records indicated there were still only 11 "colored" graduates, and just 3 of them, including Wilson, were practicing in New York City.[23]

Not everything in Wilson and Wright's life was deadly serious. On Saturday, April 8, 1933, the *New York Age* newspaper covered a humorous program in which the doctors of Harlem stepped out for two nights at the YWCA Auditorium on West 137th Street. They showed off their theatrical talent on behalf of the Edgecombe Ladies Auxiliary. Drs. James L. Wilson, Godfrey Nurse, Louis T. Wright, Aaron MacGhee, Vernon Ayer and James Granady were among the physicians who performed. It also reported "on both nights the auditorium was jammed to capacity by those who came to see the doctors perform, and those who came went away satisfied that the theatrical profession lost many excellent artists when these men threw in their lot with science."[24] The *New York Amsterdam News* also carried an amusing story about the same event headlined "Pu-Leeze, Doctor! You're Surprising."[25]

In another example of his civic mindedness during the 1930s, Dr. Wilson served on the Advisory Council of the Birth Control Clinical Research Bureau (BCCRB) Harlem Branch. The group was started by Mrs. Margaret Sanger, the eminent birth control authority. The Harlem branch served a mostly African American clientele with birth control services and operated in conjunction with the New York Urban League. It provided contraceptive instruction for married women and couples, a range of gynecological services, and trained African American physicians and students.[26]

Wilson and his Edgecombe Sanitarium remained busy. During 1933, 46 physicians treated 178 patients there. One hundred and five were surgical admissions.[27] A society column in November 1934 reported Wilson was the attending physician at Edgecombe for the birth of a six-pound baby girl.[28]

By 1935 the Great Depression had begun to take its toll and Edgecombe was on the verge of financial collapse. Its financial structure was changed from a closed corporation to a broader membership corporation and a committee of citizens rallied to the side of the sanitarium to save it for Harlem.[29] A major fundraising benefit, supported by stars and celebrities, was held December 12, 1935, at the Renaissance Casino in Harlem.[30] Other fundraisers followed in 1936 and 1937, and the hospital remained open.

In 1936 Wilson returned to St. Croix for the first time since leaving. There on September 17, 1936, he made a presentation to the Citizens Progressive League. He was introduced by its president, a well-known businessman and civic leader, Axel Schade.[31] He returned to St. Croix a number of times in later years. He even brought his good friend, Dr. Louis T. Wright, with him in the early 1950s.

In 1937 Wilson joined with 27 other physicians in support of Dr. Wright's formation of the Harlem Surgical Society. It raised surgical specialty standards, and Wilson participated actively in its activities.[32]

Early in 1939, Dr. Wilson was called to Havana, Cuba, to perform a special operation. His interpreter for the occasion was his friend W. W. Smith, president of the Le Cercle Victor Hugo, the French club at City College.[33] In May 1940, Wilson, identified as honorary president of El Circulo Antonio Maceo Spanish Club, was one of three guest speakers at the formal opening of the Henri Christophe School of Languages, whose director was W. W. Smith.[34]

In September 1939 Wilson's close friend, Louis Wright, was hospitalized for tuberculosis treatments. He remained hospitalized for nearly three years, until May 1942. During that time Wilson corresponded regularly with Wright and kept him apprised of activities at Edgecombe Sanitarium. Wilson led the effort, with Wright's counsel from bed, to turn Edgecombe into a full-fledged, voluntary, state-approved hospital. When the application was made to state and city authorities, at Wilson's request, Wright drafted the rationale and purpose that was required. The application was approved and the medical welfare of the people of Harlem was enhanced.[35]

His Edgecombe Sanitarium continued to be the beneficiary of charitable fundraising, and in 1942 it was able to add an x-ray machine and a modern "sterilizery." The entire top floor of one of its buildings had become a complete maternity ward, including a baby formula room.[36]

A tragic but amusing letter by Wilson to the editor of the *New York Amsterdam News* appeared on April 3, 1943. He reported he was in Harlem Hospital with a broken leg, a victim of a Seventh Avenue taxi driver who hit him and a woman on the next corner and escaped. He offered to help the journalists in a campaign against "miscreant" hit and run "cowboy" drivers.[37]

He recovered from his injury and a later 1943 *New York Age* newspaper reported, "Dr. James L. Wilson Saves Woman's Life After Hope Was Lost." "In addition to his long list of accomplishments Dr. James L. Wilson ... proves once more his great ability and skill in the medical profession when he performed a major operation on a patient for whom all hope was completely lost." He performed the lifesaving surgery at his Edgecombe Sanitarium where he was still serving as the medical director.[38]

In 1948 Dr. Wilson was made a fellow of the American College of Surgeons (ACS), the highest honor attainable in his profession. Twelve African American surgeons were given that honor at an impressive ceremony. It was the largest number of African American doctors ever admitted at one time into the college, and it brought the total number of African American Fellows to 27. The first was admitted in 1913.[39]

The ceremony ended a three-year fight against discrimination that began in 1945 when one of the doctors, George D. Thorne, applied and was rebuffed with a letter that stated in part "that fellowship in the college is not being conferred on members of the Negro race at the present time." The significance of the change of the discriminatory policy went beyond simply recognizing the professional achievements of the individuals, because admission to ACS was often a prerequisite for staff advancement at leading hospitals.[40]

In 1951 Dr. Wilson received a similar honor when he was one of five eminent surgeons admitted into the International College of Surgeons (ICOS) as certified fellows at its annual meeting in Chicago. More than 2,200 surgeons from Canada, the United States and many foreign countries were in attendance.[41] Four black doctors in New York City were members and less than a dozen in the entire country.

On March 19, 1954, the *New York Times* carried a photograph of Dr. Wilson in a lengthy article entitled "Surgeon Pays Off Forty-Year Debt, Harlem Doctor Is Putting Up $10,000 for Scholarships at Columbia College." It describes the $175 scholarship he received in 1913 that enabled him to complete medical school. The article described him as a successful specialist in traumatic surgery who, except for his military service in World War I, practiced medicine in Harlem. He was then an associate visiting surgeon at Harlem Hospital, Fellow of the American College of Surgeons, and fellow and diplomat of the International College of Surgeons. At that time he and his wife still lived on 137th Street. His only child, the Reverend James L. Wilson, Jr., was 25 years old and a traveling missionary for Jehovah's Witnesses in Oklahoma and Arkansas.

Dr. Wilson also enjoyed owning a home in his birthplace, St. Croix, U.S. Virgin Islands. In 1941 he wrote inviting his good friend Dr. Louis Wright, who was recovering from a serious case of pulmonary tuberculosis, to come and rest at his "modernistic mansion with garden by the sea." It was not until the spring of 1951 that Wright came to St. Croix for a long-delayed and nearly month-long vacation with his friend and confidante. Dr. Wilson arranged for Wright, who was not well, to be chauffeured around St. Croix. Wright was comfortable and enjoyed his stay in Wilson's "paradise."[42]

In 1955 the *Virgin Islands Daily News* newspaper carried a report that he had spoken in July about the health situation in the islands at a mass meeting of the American Virgin Islands Civic Association in New York.[43] Wilson was an officer of the association and a close friend and associate of its leader, Ashley Totten. When Totten died in 1963, Wilson was grief stricken. He and Totten had worked together for many years to improve conditions for people in Harlem and the Virgin Islands. In 1955 Wilson was 65 years old, and approaching retirement. He slowed his activities, but his name continued to appear in the published list of Fellows of the American College of Surgeons. In 1968, at age 78, his name appeared at a different address at 2460 Seventh Avenue, located around the corner and a few blocks from his long time home on West 137th Street. He was still shown as an associate visiting surgeon at Harlem and Montifiore hospitals.[44]

Wilson died of a strangulated hernia at age 79 at the St. Barnabas Hospital in New York.[45] With his passing New York City and America lost a brilliant, able and devoted citizen.

NOTES

1. "A Biographical Sketch of Dr. James Lancelot Wilson," *St. Thomas Daily News*, September 28, 1936, St Croix Landmarks Society Research Library & Archives.
2. Cynthia Harris, Librarian, Jersey Room, Jersey City Free Public Library, Main Library, 472 Jersey Ave, Jersey City.
3. "Two Colored Boys Lead January '10 High School Class," *The Jersey Journal*, February 12, 1910, 1.
4. Stephen E. Novak, Head, Archives and Special Collections, A.C. Long Health Sciences Library, Columbia University Medical Center, New York, NY.
5. Table of Medical Reserve Corps—Colored—Receiving Instruction, Medical Training Camp, Fort Des Moines, Iowa, RG-112, Records of the Army Surgeon General, National Archives, College Park, MD.
6. RG-120, Records of the American Expeditionary Forces (World War 1), 1918–1919, 92nd Division, National Archives, College Park, MD.
7. Robert C. Hayden, *Mr. Harlem Hospital, Dr. Louis T. Wright: A Biography* (Littleton, MA: Tapestry Press, Ltd., 2003) 75.
8. 1920 U.S. Federal Census.
9. "Tuskegee Hospital Head Honored by Physicians," *Chicago Defender*, August 23, 1924, 20.
10. "Edgecombe Sanitarium Open for Inspection Sunday," *New York Amsterdam News*, December 9, 1925, 3.
11. "Edgecombe Sanitarium Corporation Is Host to Ladies' Auxiliary and Nurse Staff at Formal Banquet, February 17," *The New York Age*, February 26, 1927, 2.
12. New York, State Census, 1925, James L. Wilson, ancestry.com.
13. "Edgecombe Sanitarium Corporation Is Host to Ladies' Auxiliary and Nurse Staff at Formal Banquet, February 17," *The New York Age*, February 26, 1927, 2.
14. "Miss Shamray Bryant and Dr. Jas. L. Wilson Wed," *New York Amsterdam News*, March 28, 1928, 6.
15. Bryant, Shamray, *Lord Byron in Venice*, www.worldcat.org/title/lord-byron-in-venice (accessed March 20, 2014).
16. "Gotham Matron, Mrs. James L. Wilson," *Pittsburgh Courier*, June 23, 1928, 7.
17. "Forms Fraternal Insurance Society," *Chicago Defender*, August 25, 1928, 11.
18. "Stage Set for Tennis Champs," *New York Amsterdam News*, August 7, 1929, 8.
19. "In Hospital," *New York Amsterdam News*, August 14, 1929, 4.
20. "Kappas Sponsor Kostume Karnival," *New York Amsterdam News*, November 13, 1929, 5.
21. "Harlem Sanitarium Treats 249 in 1929," *New York Amsterdam News*, January 8, 1930, 4.
22. "Thirteen More Doctors Quit Harlem Hospital," *New York Amsterdam News*, June 11, 1930, 1.
23. "11 Medicos Are Columbia Grads," *Pittsburgh Courier*, January 21, 1933, 3.
24. "Doctors Show Their Theatrical Talent," *The New York Age*, April 8, 1933, 2.
25. "Pu-Leeze, Doctor!" *New York Amsterdam News*, April 5, 1933, 3.
26. *About Margaret Sanger, Birth Control Clinical Research Bureau (BCCRB)*, www.nyu.edu/projects/sanger/secure/aboutms/organization_bccrb.html (accessed March 3, 2014).
27. "Edgecombe Hospital Treated 178 in 1933," *New York Amsterdam News*, January 24, 1934, 3.
28. "Society," *New York Amsterdam News*, November 3, 1934, 6.

29. "Harlem Medics Fight to Save Its Hospital," *Chicago Defender*, November 9, 1935, 2.
30. "Thousands Expected Out for Worthy Charity," *New York Amsterdam News*, December 7, 1935, 12.
31. "A Biographical Sketch of Dr. James Lancelot Wilson," *St. Thomas Daily News*, September 28, 1936.
32. "27 Doctors in Surgical Association," *New York Amsterdam News*, April 24, 1937, 2.
33. "Surprised," *New York Amsterdam News*, March 4, 1939, 9.
34. "School Opens; Purpose Told," *New York Amsterdam News*, May 25, 1940, 10.
35. Robert C Hayden, *Mr. Harlem Hospital, Dr. Louis T. Wright: A Biography* (Littleton, MA: Tapestry Press Ltd., 2003) 130–138.
36. "Edgecombe Auxiliary Aids Dr. Brook's Room," *New York Amsterdam News*, February 7, 1942, 20.
37. "Dislikes Cab Drivers, Wild and Reckless," *New York Amsterdam News*, April 3, 1943, 10.
38. "Dr. James L. Wilson Saves Woman's Life After Hope Was Lost," *The New York Age*, August 28, 1943, 2.
39. "College of Surgeons Initiates 12 Negroes," *Los Angeles Sentinel*, October 28, 1948, 9.
40. "3-Year Discrimination Fight Ends in College of Surgeons," *New York Amsterdam News*, October 30, 1948.
41. "International Surgeons Cite Five," *Chicago Defender*, September 22, 1951, 5.
42. Robert C. Hayden, *Mr. Harlem Hospital, Dr. Louis T. Wright: A Biography* (Littleton, MA: Tapestry Press Ltd., 2003) 174–175.
43. "Speakers Denounce Virgin Islands Administration," *The Daily News*, Charlotte Amalie, Virgin Islands, USA, July 15, 1955, 1.
44. American College of Surgeons Directory (Chicago: The Lakeside Press, R. R. Donnelley and Sons Company, 1968), 858.
45. AMA Deceased Physician Card, National Library of Medicine, Bethesda, MD.

Roscoe (Rosko) Jerome WILSON

12 April 1888–14 December 1965
Howard Medical College, 1912

Roots and Education

Roscoe Wilson was born in Charleston, South Carolina, to the Reverend Joshua Eden and Evelyn Gordon Wilson. He grew up in a large family in Florence, where his father was a clergyman and district superintendent with the AME conference as well as a community leader. His father served on the Florence City Council in 1873, during Reconstruction.[1]

Great grandson Michael Lythcott wrote that the Reverend Wilson was also "one the first Trustees of Claflin College. During Reconstruction, he won election to the U.S. House of Representatives for Darlington County, South Carolina. He actually made the trip to Washington. Meanwhile the state white politicos invalidated many of his votes and protested his election. There was a trial in the U.S. Senate and Great Grandfather lost the seat." Racism was apparent. "He was re-nominated by the president, but a white Jim Crow senator from South Carolina protested and the Senate refused to confirm him."[2]

The most prestigious federal post in Florence was that of postmaster. During most of the 1890s, the Reverend Wilson held that position. There were a number of white citizens who wanted the post, but Congressman George Dargan endorsed the Reverend Wilson for the position as the "least displeasing of the black Republicans."[3] Rev. Wilson was religious, a conservative leader, and an industrious businessman. As a result, he received the political appointment and held it for 10 years. In 1899 John Norton, the new Democratic congressman, convinced President McKinley not to confirm the Florence postmaster, so Wilson's term in office ended. Black political activism all over the South had been dealt a sharp blow by *Plessy v. Ferguson*, the 1896 Supreme Court decision that sanctioned the "separate but equal" policies of the South. It would destroy

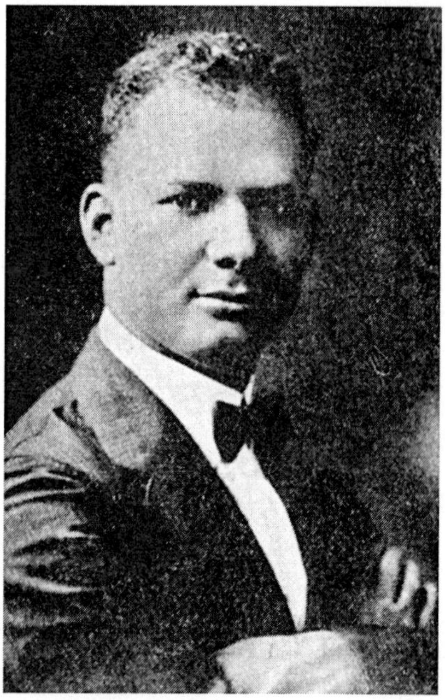

Dr. Roscoe J. Wilson (national pictorial, members of the National Medical Association, 1925, courtesy Kansas City Public Library).

whatever progress had been made in civil rights since the Civil War.[4]

In his youth, Rev. Wilson's son Roscoe served as a general delivery and money order clerk at the Florence Post Office.[5] The family lived in downtown Florence on Coit Street. The 1900 U.S. Census reported eight children in the family, five sons and three daughters. Roscoe was the third youngest, with one younger brother and sister. The two oldest sisters worked as teachers.

Roscoe went to Wilson High School in Florence. The school was named for his father Joshua. He then attended Claflin College in Orangeburg before leaving the state for his medical education. In 1912 Dr. Wilson received his medical degree from Howard Medical College in Washington, D.C. He returned to Florence where his permanent residence was again listed at the family home. His youngest sister, Evelyn, was only 13 years old.[6] Evelyn grew up and married one of his friends from Claflin College and Fort Des Moines, Dr. George I. Lythcott.

Military Service

In 1917 as America entered the First World War, Howard University was actively involved in recruiting officers from its alumni to serve in the war. Physicians were particularly needed. Dr. Wilson registered for the draft in Florence and gave his address as the Coit Street family home. He was still single at the time.[7]

He volunteered and joined the U.S. Army Medical Reserve Corps where he was commissioned as a first lieutenant. He was ordered to active duty at Fort Des Moines. While there, he reconnected with other doctors from Howard Medical School. T. E. Jones and Frank Pearl had graduated with him in 1912. His friend George Lythcott from Claflin was also there.

The army wrote a comprehensive plan for training these physicians and medics. Unfortunately, as the final reports states, "at no time, except during the last few weeks of is existence, did this camp have adequate or satisfactory quarters for the instruction or accommodation of the officers and enlisted men."[8] Nevertheless, by the time the camp closed, 104 physicians and 948 medics had completed MOTC training and departed for further training with their units before sailing to France.

Lieutenant Wilson was sent to Camp Funston, Kansas, where he was assigned to the 366th Field Hospital as a Battalion Adjutant of the 317th Sanitary (Medical) Train, 92nd Division.[9] In this position, he was the administrative head of the field hospital. He was charged with developing and directing personnel systems including strength and personnel accounting, replacement operations, casualty reporting, awards, promotions and reductions. In June he took leave and married Miss Lillian McLain of Camden, South Carolina.

At the beginning of November 1918, he was working as a member of the Medical Detachment of 367th Infantry Regiment. There were seven physicians with this unit, and six were African Americans. The 367th saw combat, but much of Lieutenant Wilson's time during training and preparation for combat was spent caring for the general health of the regiment's almost 3,600 troops. Pneumonia, tuberculosis, influenza, venereal disease, measles and injuries were major concerns. The effects of air attacks, gas attacks, artillery bombardment and machine gun wounds were also serious. Lieutenant Wilson specialized in eye, ear and nose problems.

Medical services during World War I were primitive and antibiotics had not yet been discovered. Relatively minor injuries could prove fatal through onset of infection and gangrene. The Americans recorded that 44 percent of casualties who developed gangrene died. Fifty percent of those with head wounds died. Seventy-five percent of wounds came from shell fire. A wound resulting from a shell fragment was usually more traumatic than a gunshot wound.

A shell fragment would often introduce debris, making it more likely that the wound would become infected. These factors meant a soldier was three times more likely to die from a shell wound to the chest than from a gunshot wound. The blast from shell explosions could also kill by concussion. In addition to the physical effects of shellfire, there was the psychological damage. Men who had to endure prolonged bombardment would often suffer debilitating shell shock, a condition not well understood at the time.

As in many other wars, World War I's greatest killer was disease. Sanitary conditions in the trenches were quite poor, and common infections included dysentery, typhus, and cholera. Many soldiers suffered from parasites and related infections. Poor hygiene also led to fungal conditions, such as trench mouth and trench foot. Burial of the dead was usually a luxury that neither side could easily afford. The bodies would lie in no man's land until the front line moved, by which time the bodies were often unidentifiable.[10]

The war ended with the Armistice on November 11, 1918. On December 1, Lieutenant Wilson was reassigned to the 366th Ambulance Company. It took the division several cold and harsh winter months before it was returned to the United States in early February 1919, and the doctors were honorably discharged to return home.[11]

Career

After his military service, Dr. Wilson completed post-graduate work at Manhattan EENT (Eye, Ear, Nose and Throat) Hospital and the School of Refraction in New York City.[12]

By 1920 Dr. Wilson and his wife were back in Florence living with his mother at 310 Coit Street. During the 1920s, he worked about 20 miles east of Florence, in Marion, South Carolina.[13] He was a member of the National Medical Association (NMA), the Masons and the Palmetto Medical Association. He continued to serve in the army reserves, and by 1925 he held the reserve rank of captain.[14]

By 1930 Dr. Wilson had left his practice in Marion and settled back in Florence. He was, in fact, driven out of town for treating white patients.[15] In the most segregated regions of the Jim Crow South, African American physicians were not to compete with white ones for white patients.

In the 1930s and 40s he and wife, Lillian, owned a home in Florence at 619 North Coit Street. They later moved down the street to the home they would occupy for the rest of their lives at 614 North Coit.

In addition to his activities in fraternal and medical associations, he became a trustee of the Cumberland Methodist Church of Florence. His medical career included service as medical examiner for Florence and its branches of the Selective Service and a term as president of the state's Palmetto Medical-Dental-Pharmaceutical Association.

The list of his local community organizations is nearly endless. In the 1930s he served as chairman of the civic welfare committee that established a community center for black residents of Florence. He then worked with the WPA to bring a federal project to the city. It set up a training school for domestic workers and was located in that community center.[16] He chaired the city's first community center, was chairman of the city's tuberculosis auxiliary, and was the organizer of the first African American Boy Scout Troop.[17] During World War II, he chaired the African American Advisory Committee of the local USO clubs and got the local club involved in planning activities for returning soldiers, as well as gathering and disseminating food to needy servicemen's families.[18]

Dr. Wilson also appeared before the Florence City Council advocating recreational facilities in black playground areas. In 1950 he spoke at a health program encouraging citizens to clean up the neighborhood.[19] He was also chairman of the local African American division of the American Cancer Society and the local fundraiser.[20]

He and Mrs. Wilson were advocates of ending segregation. In 1950 the *Index-Journal* (newspaper in nearby Greenwood) reported that he had been warned three times and threatened with tar and feathering and had a cross burned in his yard by members of the Ku Klux Klan for his beliefs and involvement with white activists such as Federal Judge Julius Waties Waring. One of the judge's visits to the Wilson's home led to a phone call with one of the warnings.[21]

At the 1962 Howard University Medical Alumni Association Banquet, Dr. Wilson was one of the men honored for 50 years of medical service. The toastmaster of the event was Dr. Jack Kennedy of Tuskegee who had served with Dr. Wilson during the First World War.[22]

By early 1965 he and his wife had moved from downtown Florence westward to Fairfield

Circle. They had been married nearly 50 years when he died after an extended illness in 1965.[23] He was 77 years old and had suffered from arteriosclerosis for a long time.[24] Despite the large, extended family he enjoyed in Florence, he and Lillian did not have any children of their own. His funeral service was conducted in the Cumberland Methodist Church of Florence.

Dr. Wilson is buried in the Florence National Cemetery, Section C, Site 588-A, with a veterans headstone provided by the U.S. Army.[25] For seven years after his death, his wife Lillian ran an annual "In Memoriam" notice in the *Florence Morning News*. It said, "May your sleep be as sweet as my memories of you."[26]

NOTES

1. Udogu, E. Ike, "Economic, Social and Political Despair," African American Politics in Rural America (Lanham, MD: University Press of America, 2006), 57.
2. Family history provided to authors in written form by Michael Lythcott.
3. Udogu, E. Ike, *African American Politics in Rural America*, 62.
4. Ike, *African American Politics in Rural America*, 64.
5. "Funeral Services Held for Prominent Doctor," *Baltimore Afro-American*, January 2, 1966, 19.
6. 1900 and 1910 U.S. Federal Census.
7. World War I Draft Registration Card 1917–1918.
8. Bispham, William N., Col. M.C., *The Medical Department of the United States Army in the World War*, Vol. VII, Training, 267.
9. Table of Medical Reserve Corps—Colored—Receiving Instruction, Medical Training Camp, Fort Des Moines, Iowa, RG-112, Records of the Army Surgeon General, National Archives, College Park, MD.
10. en.wikipedia.org/wiki/Trench_warfare (accessed January 14, 2013).
11. Record Group 120, Records of the 92d Division, 317th Sanitary Train, Memoranda 1918, National Archives, College Park, MD.
12. "Florence Doctor Honored for Works," *Florence Morning News*, June 30, 1962, 2.
13. Joseph Boris, *Who's Who in Colored America* (New York: Who's Who in Colored America Corp., 1929), 224.
14. *National Medical Association Yearbook, 1925*, Kansas City Missouri Public Library.
15. Thomas J. Ward, Jr., "The Struggle for Patients," *Black Physicians in the Jim Crow South* (Fayetteville: University of Arkansas Press, 2003) 152.
16. "Domestic Training School of WPA," *Florence Morning News*, May 17, 1936, 2.
17. *Ibid.*, "Florence Doctor Honored for Works," June 30, 1962, 2.
18. *Ibid.*, "USO Notes," September 30, 1945, 2.
19. *Ibid.*, "Negro Cleanup Campaign to Wind Up Today," May 6, 1950, 8.
20. *Ibid.*, "Cancer Drive Negro Officers Elected," April 3, 1952, 3.
21. "Negro Doctor 'Warned' After Visit by Warings," *Index-Journal, Greenwood, SC*, December 16, 1950, 3.
22. "Howard Medical Alumni Banquet," *Pittsburgh Courier*, June 16, 1962, 10.
23. "Funeral Services Held for Prominent Doctor," *Baltimore Afro-American*, January 2, 1966, 19.
24. "AMA Deceased Physicians Card, National Library of Medicine, Bethesda, MD.
25. U.S. Veterans Gravesites Ca. 1775–2006 Ancestry.com (accessed December 8, 2012).
26. "Ad," *Florence Morning News*, December 14, 1972, 2.

Louis Tompkins WRIGHT

22 July 1891–8 October 1952
Harvard University, 1915

Roots and Education

Wright is the most nationally celebrated of the 104 African American physicians included in this history. The following story was compiled largely from several excellent sources of information about Wright that have been published in print and on the Internet. The best-known and most detailed biography is a 223-page work entitled *Mr. Harlem Hospital* written by Robert C. Hayden and published in 2003.

Wright was born in La Grange, Georgia, to Ceah Ketchum and Lula Tompkins Wright. His father was a prominent physician and among the first group in the United States to be known as the Black Elite. He left medicine to become a clergyman and then died when Louis was only four.[1] Wright's mother remarried in 1898 to Dr. William Fletcher Penn, a physician, who played an influential role in Wright's life. Dr. Penn provided Wright with an excellent example of what it meant to be a strong, successful African American in a time of extreme racial tension. He also showed young Wright what it was like to be a physician.[2]

Louis Wright received his elementary education through a Clark University-run school in Atlanta, where he later also received his secondary and college education. He eventually was valedictorian of his class at Clark. Dr. Penn and Wright both felt that Harvard Medical School was the best fit for Wright, so Dr. Penn paid for Wright's train ride to Boston. Wright made an appointment with the Dean of Harvard Medical and learned no one believed that a man educated by Clark University could pass the entrance exam for Harvard Medical School.

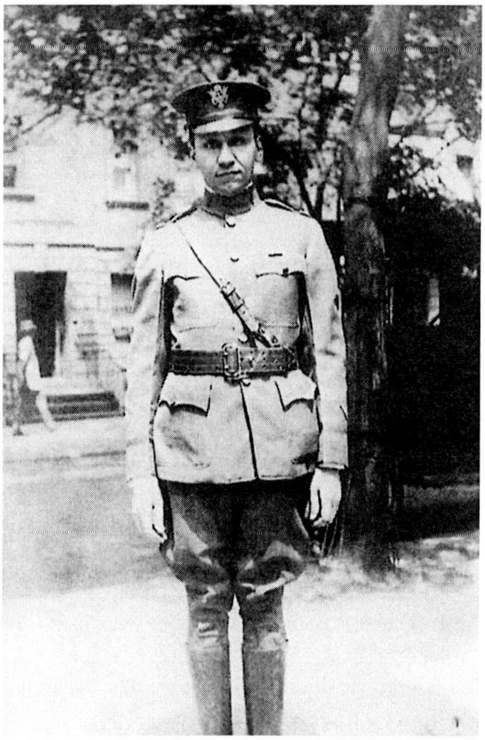

Lieutenant Louis T. Wright, before leaving for France, 1918, New York (in Robert C. Hayden, *Mr. Harlem Hospital*, courtesy Barbara Wright Pierce).

Wright was given an oral exam to test his knowledge of biology and chemistry. After the examination Wright was informed that he had sufficient knowledge and would be entering in the fall as one of two African Americans in the class.[3]

In May 1915 Wright received his Doctor of Medicine degree from Harvard, finishing fourth in his class. The next year, he interned in Washington, D.C., at Freedmen's Hospital. While there he conducted a study of the use of the Schick test for diphtheria and proved the color of one's skin did not affect the outcome of the test.[4] Following Freedmen's, he joined his stepfather in his practice in Atlanta. When the United States entered World War I, Dr. Wright decided to volunteer to serve in the U.S. Army.

Military Service

In April 1917 Dr. Wright went to Fort McPherson, Georgia, applied to become, and eventually received the rank of first lieutenant in the Army Medical Reserve Corps. In August Lieutenant Wright reported to Fort Des Moines for medical officer training. Although he scored 100 percent on all promotional examinations there, he was not promoted to the rank of captain because of what was considered insubordinate behavior. He did not respond well to condescending white officers. After 75 days of training, Wright was assigned to the 367th Infantry Regiment's medical detachment, part of the 92nd Division, at Camp Upton, New York. While stationed there he met his wife, Corinne M. Cooke. They were married on May 16, 1918, shortly before he went overseas.

In June 1918 Lieutenant Wright's unit was sent to France. On September 4, 1918, at Mt. Henri, Wright and his battalion were hit by a phosgene gas shell only 50 feet away from where Dr. Wright was operating. After three weeks of hospitalization, and attempts to recover from what would end up being permanent damage to his lungs, Lieutenant Wright received orders to report for duty to the 366th Field Hospital where he served until the end of the war.[5]

During the 92nd Division's last great offensive battle of the war near Metz, he commanded the surgical wards of the division's triage hospital at Millery near Pont-à-Mousson.[6] Numerous battle casualties flooded into his hospital and required immediate attention. After the war, Lieutenant Wright returned home. In April 1919 he was honorably discharged after receiving a Purple Heart for his service and injury.[7]

Career

Dr. Wright was a man of "firsts." He introduced the intradermal method of smallpox vaccination to the army while at Camp Upton. He was the first African American staff surgeon at Harlem Hospital and the first police surgeon for the New York City Police Department (NYPD).[8]

His other firsts and contributions to the medical world included devising "a splint for cervical fractures and he introduced a special plate for the repair of certain types of fractures to the femur. He also developed a plate out of an inactive material, tantalum, for repairs of recurrent hernias. He and his team of black and white physicians were the first to use the antibiotic aureomycin in clinical tests on a human."

His chapter on "Head Injuries" in *The Treatment of Fractures* by Charles Scudder (1938) was the first contribution by an African American to an authoritative medical symposium. In 1948 he established the Harlem Hospital Cancer Research Foundation, and he secured funds for its support from the U.S. Public Health Service and private sources. He encouraged younger associates to engage in research and publication: 89 of Wright's publications list 51 different persons as junior authors.[9]

His crowning achievement was as director of Harlem Hospital. He was intolerant of mediocrity. His motto was "Equal opportunity—no more, no less,"[10] but he was able to bring harmony to the various white and African American groups that comprised the staff of Harlem Hospital. He recognized the problems faced by other minorities, particularly Jewish and Italian physicians, and dealt with these with characteristic honesty and directness. "Shortly before his death he referred to the institution as the 'finest example of racial democracy in the world.'" While this was certainly an exaggeration, it expressed his basic philosophy.[11]

Wright was noted for his civil rights activism. Throughout his life Wright involved himself in civil rights efforts, beginning in college when he missed three weeks of school to join picket lines protesting D. W. Griffith's *The Birth of a Nation,* a film controversial for its sympathetic portrayal of the Ku Klux Klan. At Harvard he insisted on equal treatment when a professor prevented him from delivering white patients' babies.

He joined the NAACP after medical school and remained involved with the organization for the rest of his life, eventually serving as chairman of its national board of directors from 1934 until his death in 1952.

In 1920, early in his tenure at Harlem Hospital, he played a key role in fighting the precedent in New York whereby African American doctors and nurses were barred from serving in municipal hospitals. He was a frequent leader in the struggle for integration, pushing for equal standards in medical education and opposing segregated hospitals, including a successful effort in 1930 to stop the construction of the new segregated facility proposed by the Rosenwald Fund.[12]

While Wright was president of the Manhattan Medical Association in 1934, most of the physicians in Harlem were in favor of reuniting with the North Harlem Medical Society. Wright had led the split some years earlier because he did not believe all the doctors met the required standards of training. His critics said, "For too long a time Dr. Wright has acted like a little czar." The merger was approved and both presidents were replaced.[13]

In 1940, he was the recipient of the Spingarn Medal for his dedication to racial equality and "his contribution to the healing of mankind and for his courageous position in the face of bitter attack."[14]

Hayden's biography tells us Dr. Wright's health began to fail in 1939 when he contracted pulmonary tuberculosis and was bedridden for nearly three years. He was able to recover his health and resume work in the early 1940s. Though he returned to medicine and was appointed chief of surgery in 1943, he never fully recovered. The lung damage he suffered during

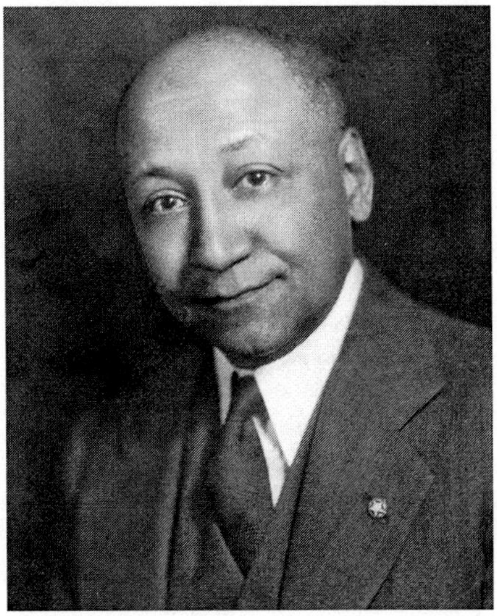

Dr. Louis T. Wright (in Robert C. Hayden, *Mr. Harlem Hospital*, courtesy Barbara Wright Pierce).

the First World War was always felt to have played a role.

One of his friends and colleagues in Harlem was Dr. James L. Wilson, a fellow army veteran with whom he had trained at Fort Des Moines in 1917. Wilson owned a home in St. Croix, Virgin Islands. In 1951, at 60 years of age, Wilson and Wright spent nearly a month there while Wright was recuperating from yet another problem with his lungs. Other than his army service, it was Wright's first and only trip outside the United States.

Many tributes were paid to Dr. Wright during his lifetime. In April 1952 Wright was feted at a big testimonial dinner at the Hotel Statler in New York City. First Lady Eleanor Roosevelt introduced him. Ten distinguished speakers spoke of his contributions as a scientist and humanitarian. Wright died of a heart attack five months later. More than 500 people attended his funeral in Harlem. He is buried in Woodlawn Cemetery in the Bronx.[15]

NOTES

1. *Louis Tompkins Wright, 1891–1952*, encyclopedia.com (accessed April 25, 2015).
2. Rayford W. Logan and Michael R. Winston, *Dictionary of American Negro Biography* (New York: W.W. Norton, 1982) 670–671.
3. Graduates of the 17th Provisional Training Regiment at Fort Des Moines, Iowa 15 October 1917, Dr. Louis T. Wright, www.fortdesmoines.org/officers/wright.shtml (accessed October 12, 2012).
4. Logan and Winston, *Dictionary of American Negro Biography*, 670–671.
5. Graduates of the 17th Provisional Training Regiment at Fort Des Moines, Iowa 15 October 1917, Dr. Louis T. Wright, www.fortdesmoines.org/officers/wright.shtml (accessed October 12, 2012).
6. Louis T. Wright, "I Remember," (unpublished autobiographical typescript) Moorland Spingarn Research Center, Howard University, Washington, D.C., Undated, 87.
7. Fredrick S. Mead, A.B., Editor, *Harvard's Military Record in the World War*, Boston:Harvard Alumni Association, 1921, 1048.
8. Vivian Ovelton Sammons, "Wright Louis Tompkins," *Blacks in Science and Medicine* (New York: Hemisphere Publishing Corp., 1990) 259.
9. Logan and Winston, *Dictionary of American Negro Biography*, 670–671.
10. George H. Rawls, Reviewer, *A Century of Black Surgeons: The USA Experience,* National Medical Association, December 1987 issue 79(12), 1305–1309.
11. Logan and Winston, *Dictionary of American Negro Biography*, 671.
12. en.wikipedia.org/wiki/Louis_T._Wright (accessed March 14, 2015).
13. "Dr. Wright Called 'Little Czar' as Harlem Medics Seek to Oust Him," *New Journal and Guide*, April 7, 1934, 14.
14. en.wikipedia.org/wiki/Louis_T._Wright (accessed March 14, 2015).
15. Robert C. Hayden, *Mr. Harlem Hospital, Dr. Louis T. Wright: A Biography* (Littleton, MA: Tapestry Press Ltd., 2003) 177.

Thomas L. ZUBER

16 July 1887–26 July 1956
Meharry Medical College, 1912

Roots and Education

Thomas Zuber was the eldest of three sons born to John D. and Alice (Miner) Zuber in Starksville, Mississippi. After graduation from Roger Williams College, his father became a teacher and a minister. Alice Zuber was a teacher in a normal (teachers' training) school. Alice died early and John married Annie Dunlap. They had one son, Walter. Both Thomas and his half-brother Walter would go on to become physicians. Walter set up his practice in Corinth, in northeast Mississippi.

Thomas Zuber completed his secondary education at Central Mississippi College and went on to earn his A.B. from Morehouse College in Atlanta. During those years he was quite a baseball player, playing with the Birmingham Black Barons before making his decision to go to medical school. He chose Meharry Medical College in Nashville and graduated in 1912. After Meharry, Dr. Zuber went home to West Point, Mississippi, and lived with his parents during his first year as a practicing physician.

He left West Point for two years for Carrollton, Alabama. While there, from 1913 to 1915, he was president of Lebanon Union Academy. In 1915, he returned to medicine, passing the Mississippi state medical boards and opening his practice back in West Point in Clay County.

Military Service

Meharry Medical College encouraged its graduates to volunteer for service in the Army Medical Corps. In fact, the largest contingent of medical school graduates at the training camp in Fort Des Moines was from Meharry (34 of the 104). Zuber volunteered and reported

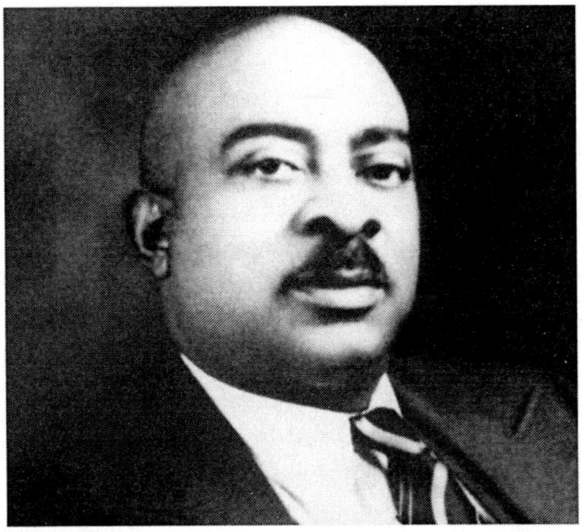

Dr. Thomas L. Zuber (courtesy Narva Perry, granddaughter).

to the Medical Officers Training Camp for basic training on August 7, 1917. By November 3, First Lieutenant Zuber was transferred to Camp Grant, Illinois, with the 365th Infantry of the 92nd Division.

Six months before he was sent to France in June 1918, he married Etta Augusta Deace on Christmas Eve 1917.

While in France, Zuber served as Battalion Surgeon with the medical detachment of the 365th Infantry. At Metz, one of the German's strongest points at the end of the war, he was gassed during the eight-hour battle that resulted in the capture of ground held by Germans. He ultimately would lose one lung as a result of the damage inflicted there. This was the final battle of the war. The "bugle sounded for the cease fire that ended the war at 11:00 am on November 11."[1]

Dr. Zuber was "declared totally and permanently disabled" and sent home in December 1918, earlier than most of the other troops. Despite the prognosis, he went on to practice medicine for another 40 years.[2]

Career

After the war, Dr. Zuber returned home to West Point and his new wife, Etta. Mrs. Zuber was born in Scooba, Mississippi. She attended Lincoln Academy in Meridian, and studied at Fisk University in Nashville for two years. She completed her undergraduate degree at Miles Memorial College in Birmingham and her master's at Columbia University in New York. The couple would go on to have six children—five girls and a boy. Mrs. Zuber would continue to work in education in Clay County.[3]

Dr. Zuber's practice and involvement in his West Point community expanded, just as his family did. He served as medical examiner for the North Carolina Mutual Life Insurance Company of Durham and National Benefit Insurance. He was active in the Mississippi Medical Association, serving a term as its president.[4]

He was a lifelong member of the National Medical Association (NMA). In 1923, he wrote an article for NMA's journal entitled "Possibilities of Medical Practice in the South." In 1925, he returned to school entering Columbia University, New York, where he specialized in internal medicine.[5]

He returned to his office upstairs at 39 West Main Street in West Point and became a leader in the Scottish Rite Masons (32nd degree). He was also Exalted Ruler of the Order of Elks and a deacon in his local Missionary Baptist Church.

Dr. Zuber took time from his busy schedule to work with the State Health Department. In 1934, for example, he spoke to the State Teachers Summer School.[6] In 1937, he addressed more than 200 students and teachers at a health program at West Point's Milton School.[7]

He believed in the importance of continuing medical training. In 1944, he was among five physicians given a state fellowship for special study in obstetrics and gynecology at Slossfield Health Center in Birmingham.[8] It had opened in 1939 to provide for African Americans living in a specified area, maternity and child health services, a tuberculosis control program, and diagnostic and therapeutic care to persons with venereal diseases. It was estimated that 50,000 Negroes, approximately half of the black population of Birmingham, lived within the area served by it.

In 1946, he was elected 4th district chair of Mississippi's Committee of 100, an organization of the Republican Party charged with seeking out potential candidates and raising funds for their campaigns. These state leaders discussed the poll tax, the need for additional black policemen, doctors, dentists, nurses and lawyers, and the need for improved teachers' salaries.[9]

By 1949, Dr. Zuber was historian of the local North Mississippi Medical, Dental, Pharmaceutical and Nurses Association. Topics at their March meeting included diagnosis of syphilis and the prevalence of gall bladder disease. The *Chicago Defender* noted in its coverage that Dr. Zuber had served as president of the organization "throughout its 16 years of existence." He gave up the office because he was elected president of the state medical association.[10]

On April 24, 1952, he became the Mississippi Medical and Surgical Association's "Man of the Year." At the same meeting, Dr. Zuber was appointed a new member of the organization's board of trustees.[11] The following year, the *Chicago Defender* included a photo of that board in its coverage of the National Medical Association's annual meeting, which drew 1,500 African American physicians to Nashville.[12]

In the summer of 1952, Dr. Zuber was among the delegates at the National Republican Convention in Chicago. The *Afro-American* newspaper said the black delegates could be the deciding factor between Taft and Eisenhower.[13] Dr. Zuber was also the only African American on a 106-person platform committee and was among delegates seeking to include a civil rights plank. That failed.[14] The convention also saw "bitter factional fights" over the seating of delegates in five states that included African Americans. Initially it looked as if the pro–Taft delegation from Mississippi (including Zuber) would prevail, but the other four state delegations lost out. The convention endorsement ultimately went to Eisenhower.

At the age of 69, Dr. Zuber died suddenly in his office of a heart attack while he was attending a patient.[15] He was survived by his wife, six children and his half-brother Walter.

It is difficult to image how different the lives of African American people of West Point would have been without the whirlwind that was Dr. Zuber. Throughout his life he worked to ensure that every aspect of the health of the African American citizens of his town got the best medical care. He fought for their human rights—veterans, civil, and moral.

In 1949, the Zuber's daughter Elmetra was valedictorian of her junior college class in West Point. She went on to Howard University for her degree.[16] In 1988, she contributed the biographies of her mother, uncle, father and grandfather to the *History of Clay County, Mississippi*.[17]

On February 10, 2015, Mayor Robbie Robinson and the West Point Board of Selectmen announced a plaque commemorating the doctor's achievements would be placed in Zuber Park, a six-acre municipal facility. The plaque, funded by the city and his family, was dedicated at a ceremony on July 18, 2015. Family friend Charles Ivy led the effort "to ensure younger residents and park visitors know the man behind the park's name." The bricks used on the monument came from Dr. Zuber's home.[18]

Notes

1. "Colored Unites Held Ground Where Others Had Failed Three Times," *New York Age*, January 11, 1919, 1, newspapers.com.
2. History of Clay County, Mississippi, The Clay County History Book Committee, 1988, 811–812.
3. "Mississippi," *Chicago Defender*, December 22, 1923, 23, ProQuest.
4. Boris, Joseph J., "Zuber, Thomas L.—Physician," *Who's Who in Colored America*, 1929, 417.
5. *Ibid.*
6. "Mississippi State News," *Chicago Defender*, August 11, 1934, 19, ProQuest.
7. *Ibid.*, "West Point, Miss," March 13, 1937, 26.
8. "5 Miss. Doctors Get State Fellowships," *Philadelphia Tribune*, July 29, 1944, 18, ProQuest.
9. "Committee of 100 Convenes in Mound Bayou," *Norfolk Journal and Guide*, May 16, 1946, 4, ProQuest.
10. "North Mississippi Medics Confer on Ailments Common Among Race," *Chicago Defender*, March 5, 1949, 26, ProQuest.
11. *Ibid.*, "Cite Mississippi Medic," May 10, 1952, 13.
12. "1500 Attend 58th National Medical Meet in Nashville," *Chicago Defender*, August 29, 1953, 12, ProQuest.
13. "Tan Delegates Hold Balance," *Afro-American*, July 5, 1952, 1, ProQuest.
14. "Seek Way to Bolster Gop's Weak FECP Plank," *Chicago Defender*, July 11, 1952, 2, ProQuest.
15. "Funeral Services for Dr. T. L. Zuber," *Pittsburgh Courier*, August 25, 1958, 29, newspapers.com.
16. "Seek Way to Bolster Gop's Weak FECP Plank," (photo), *Chicago Defender*, July 9, 1949, 28, ProQuest.
17. History of Clay County, Mississippi, Clay County History Book Committee, 1988, 811–812.
18. "Plaque to Honor Zuber Park Namesake," *Daily Times Leader, February* 20, 2015, 1.

Epilogue

They Were Extraordinary

Most of these men lived long and productive lives. A few died soon after returning from war, suffering from the lingering and damaging effects of exposure to phosgene and mustard gas and diseases such as tuberculosis. Their impact in their communities was felt for decades following their return from France in 1919. The last of them didn't die until the early 1980s. They proved to be a long-lived group. Only 22 of them died before the age of 50. Forty-one lived into their 70s or 80s with four in their 90s.

With few exceptions, they led their communities and the national move toward racial equality. They would become "firsts" in a host of roles: first black head of the NAACP, first black chairman of a veterans hospital, first to establish a hospital for all citizens in a number of U.S. cities, first black on the staff of many hospitals, and first black on the staff of several major medical schools. They became national and local leaders in the National Medical Association (NMA). They were among the first African American "Fellows" admitted to the American College of Surgeons and the International College of Surgeons.

They pioneered medical procedures that were adopted nationally, helped establish integrated public housing, served on school boards, and were appointed superintendent and principals of schools, and chairmen of many municipal and community organizations. They founded life insurance and other service companies for the African American community.

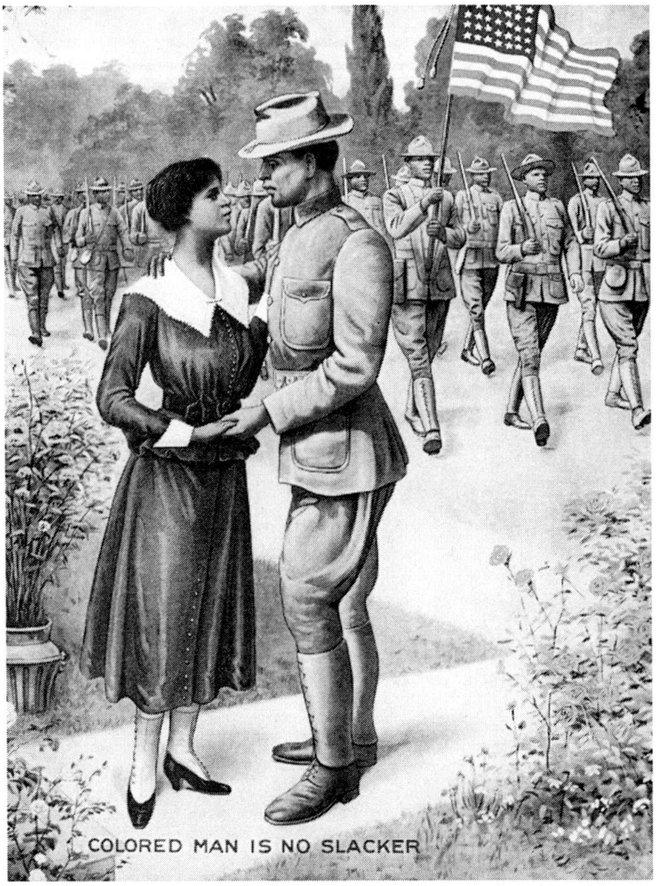

World War I "No Slacker" recruitment poster (courtesy Wolfsonian, Florida International University).

These veterans often maintained contact following the war. Some even entered medical practice together. Los Angeles, Memphis, New York, Chicago, Indianapolis, Cleveland, Kansas City, Boston, Nashville, Washington, D.C., and Philadelphia were the most popular destinations for their post-war careers. Those who settled in smaller cities like Natchez, Tuskegee, Shreveport, Tuscaloosa, Gary, and Tampa positively affected the lives of nearly everyone in their communities.

These men were Alain Locke's "New Negroes," educated and skilled. They were patriots and progressives who refused to submit quietly to the practices and laws of Jim Crow racial segregation. They pursued their rights as citizens and leaders in their communities in the charge for change in post-war America.

Once the decision was made to include African American citizens as combat troops in the First World War, those in positions of responsibility for the war effort realized they would need physicians, medics, nurses, dentists and clergy to tend to their sick and wounded in France. It is no secret that this was a terribly bloody war. It ultimately saw the deaths of tens of millions of civilians and combatants. More than 100,000 American soldiers died from battle and disease. Slightly more than 5,000 of the dead were African Americans.[1]

The research required to create 104 biographies of these men, who were born more than 125 years ago, was a real challenge. It also revealed there are thousands more untold stories buried in these words. It is our hope that this work will start that process of further discovery, as it answers many questions and raises many more.

NOTE

1. Bispham, Col. William N., M.C., *The Medical Department of the United States Army in the World War*, Vol. VII, Training (Washington, DC: US GPO, 1927), p. 263.

Appendix: Physicians Not Able to Serve on Active Duty and Dentists Who Did

Of the 130 medical officers who reported to the Medical Officers Training Camp (MOTC), 14 did not serve on active duty because of physical disability or other factors.

Blackburn, Morris A., Louisville, KY
Bugg, George W., Nashville, TN
Burnett, Foster F., Wilmington, NC
Cornish, Louis A., Cincinnati, OH
Davis, Van J., Paducah, KY
Johnson, Robert L., Jackson, MS
Jones, Daniel W., Columbus, OH
Martin, Edgar H., Atlanta, GA
Oliver, Robert L., Louisville, KY
Raby, William G., Memphis, TN
Stokes, Hugo B., Montgomery, AL
Stroud, James R., Jersey City, NJ
Thompson, James S., Dunn, NC
Williamson, B.T., Greenwood, MS

These 12 dentists entered the MOTC programs and qualified successfully.

Butler, Lucius A., Cumberland, MD
Booth, George C., Chicago, IL
Bouden, Harry E., Philadelphia, PA
Carter, Frank C., Logansport, IA
Cobb, Edward J., Iowa City, IA
Crawford, James L., St. Joseph, MO
Davis Thomas B., Sumter, SC
Dowdell, Crawford B., New Haven, CT
DeHaven, Burrell B., Columbus, OH
Jones, Edward C., Nashville, TN
Peebles, William W., Omaha, NE
Rosenburgh, Samuel H., Indianapolis, IA

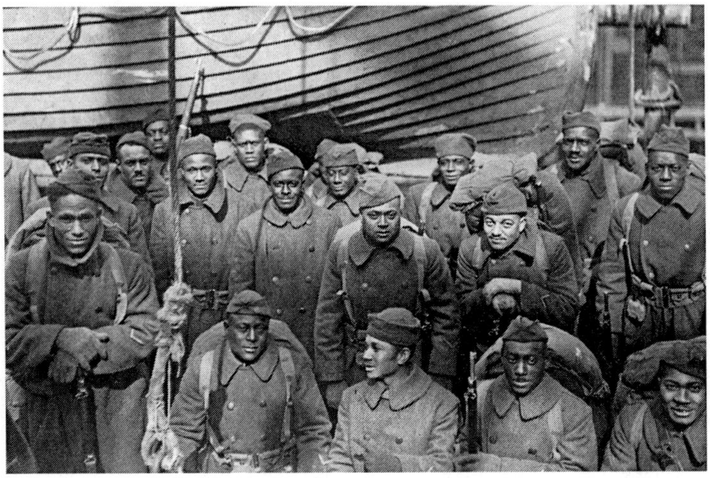

The 92nd Division aboard the SS *Ulua* returning home, 1919 (National Archives).

Bibliography

Medical Sources

A.C. Long Health Sciences Library, Columbia University Medical Center, New York, New York
AMA Deceased Physicians Masterfile Cards, 1906–1969, National Library of Medicine, Bethesda, Maryland
Charlotte (North Carolina) *Medical Journal*
Genesee County (Michigan) *Medical Society Bulletin*
Journal of the National Medical Association (JNMA)
Meharry Medical College Annual Reports
Palmetto Medical, Dental and Pharmaceutical Association, Waring Medical History Library, Medical College of South Carolina, Charleston, South Carolina
Public Health Reports, U.S. National Library of Medicine, National Institutes of Health, Washington, D.C.
Wayne County Medical Society of Southeast Michigan
West Virginia Biennial Report, State Board of Health, June 1913–1914

Manuscript and Oral History Collections

A.C. Long Health Sciences Library, Columbia University Medical Center, New York, New York
The Cape May (New Jersey) *County Magazine of History and Genealogy*
Detroit African American History Project, Wayne State University
Dunn-Landry Family Papers Collection, 1872–2003, Amistad Research Center, Tulane University, New Orleans, Louisiana
Evansville African American Museum, Evansville, Indiana
Fort Des Moines Museum and Education Center
Harold D. West Collection, Meharry Medical College Archives, Nashville
Hinton, West Virginia, Veteran's Museum
Howard University, Moorland-Spingarn Research Center, Washington, D.C., Louis T. Wright Papers
Iowa Collection, Public Library of Des Moines
Isaac E. Moore, Jr., Papers, Blair-Caldwell African American Research Library, Denver Public Library, Colorado
Jersey Room, Jersey City Free Public Library, New Jersey
Kansas Collection, Kansas City, Kansas Public Library
Missouri Valley Special Collections, Kansas City, Missouri, Public Library
Notable Kentucky African Americans Database, University of Kentucky Libraries, Lexington
Pennsylvania State Archives, Harrisburg
Phillips Exeter Academy, Alumni Records, Exeter, New Hampshire
Pikes Peak Library District, Special Collections, Colorado Springs, Colorado
Rosenwald Papers, Minutes, National Archives, College Park, Maryland
St. Croix Landmarks Society Research Library & Archives
Shaw University Library, Shaw University Archives and Charles Meserve Papers, Raleigh, North Carolina
South Carolina Department of Archives & History, Reference Library, Columbia, South Carolina
Southern Historical Collection, University of North Carolina, Chapel Hill, WPA Federal Writers Project: North Carolina
University of South Florida Oral History Program
William Henry Smith Memorial Library, Indiana Historical Society, Indianapolis
Williston Northampton School Archives, Easthampton, Massachusetts

Military Records

Center for Military History (CMH), U.S. Army in the World War, 1917–1919, U.S. Army Center for Military History, Fort McNair, Washington, D.C.
National Personnel Records Center, National Archives, St. Louis, Missouri
92d Division, Summary of Operations in the World War, Prepared by the American Battle Monuments Commission, United States Government Printing Office, Washington, D.C., 1944
The Official Roster of South Carolina Soldiers, Sailors and Marines in the World War, 1917–18, South Carolina Department of Archives & History
Record Group 120, Records of the American Expe-

ditionary Forces (World War I), Records of Combat Divisions, 1918–1919, 92d Division, 317th Sanitary Train, National Archives, College Park, Maryland

Record Group 120—93rd Division Regiments & Medical Detachments Manifests, National Archives, College Park, Maryland

U.S. Army Medical Department, Office of Medical History, Vol VIII, Field Operations, Chapter IV, Medical Service of the Division in Combat, GPO 1925, Washington, D.C.

World War I Draft Registration Cards, 1917–1918, Ancestry.com

Magazines

Du Bois, W.E.B., ed. *The Crisis*. New York: Official Publication of the National Association for the Advancement of Colored People (NAACP), 1910–1934

Jet Magazine. Chicago: Johnson Publishing Company, 1951–

The Oracle. Semi-annual publication of the Grand Chapter of the Omega Psi Phi Fraternity. Washington, D.C.: Murray Bros. Publishers, 1919–

Newspapers

The Advocate, Kansas City, Kansas
Alton Evening Telegraph
Asheville Gazette-News
Atlanta Constitution
Atlanta Daily World
Baltimore Afro-American
Beckley (WV) *Post-Herald*
The Bystander (Des Moines, IA)
California Eagle
Charleston News & Courier
Charlotte News (NC)
Chicago Daily Tribune
Chicago Defender
Cleveland Call & Post
Coffeyville (KS) *Weekly Journal*
Colorado Springs Gazette
Colored American Newspaper (D.C.)
Daily Times Leader (West Point, MS)
Dallas (TX) *Express*
The Daily Intelligencer (Atlanta)
Evansville Courier and Journal
The Flint (MI) *Journal*
Florence Morning News (SC)
Gary (IN) *Post-Tribune*
Goldsboro (NC) *Daily Argus*
Hamilton Daily News (OH)
Harrisburg (PA) *Telegraph*
The Herald-Press (St. Joseph, MI)
Hinton (WV) *News*
Index-Journal (Greenwood, SC)
Indianapolis Freeman
Jefferson City (MO) *Post Tribune*
The Jersey Journal (Jersey City, NJ)
The Journal News (OH)
Kansas City Star
The Kansas City Sun
Laurel (MS) *Leader-Call*
The Lima News
Los Angeles Sentinel
Memphis World
Nashville Banner
The Negro Star (Wichita, KS)
New Journal and Guide (Norfolk, VA)
The New York Age
New York Amsterdam News
New York Times
Newark Evening News
The News-Palladium (Benton Harbor, MI)
Miami (OK) *News Record*
Oxford Public Ledger (NC)
Philadelphia Daily Tribune
Pittsburgh Courier
Plaindealer (Kansas City, KS)
The Public Ledger (Maysville, KY)
The Quincy (IL) *Daily Journal*
The Quincy (IL) *Whig*
St. Thomas Daily News
The Salisbury Times (MD)
Savannah Evening Press
Savannah Morning News
Savannah Tribune
Scranton Republican
The Times-Picayune
The Topeka Daily Capital
Tuscaloosa (AL) *News*
The Tuskegee Student, Tuskegee Institute
The Vindicator (Coffeyville, KS)
The Warren Record (Warrenton, NC)
Washington Bee
Washington Evening Star
The Washington Herald
The Washington Post
The Watchman and Southron Newspaper (Sumter, SC)
Xenia Daily Gazette

Published Works

Ballard, Claudius. "After Its Victories." *California Eagle*, November 29, 1919.

Banner, Melvin E. *Short Negro History of Flint*. M. E. Banner, publisher, 1964.

Barbeau, Arthur E., and Florette Henri. *The Unknown Soldiers*. Philadelphia: Temple University Press, 1974.

Beasley, Delilah L. *The Negro Trail Blazers of California*. Los Angeles, 1919.

Bingham, Darrel E. *We Ask Only a Fair Trial*. Bloomington: Indiana University Press, 1987.

Bodenhamer, David, and Robert G. Borrows. *Encyclopedia of Indianapolis*. Bloomington: Indiana University Press, 1994.

Boris, Joseph J., ed. *Who's Who in Colored America*. New York: Who's Who in Colored America Corp., 1929.

Brawley, James S. *The Rowan Story 1753–1953*. Salisbury, MD: Rowan Print Co., 1953.

Brinkley, Velma Howell, and Mary Huddleston Malone. *African-American Life in Sumner County (TN)*. Images of America. Mount Pleasant, SC: Arcadia, 1998.
Brown, Albert J. *History of Clinton County, Ohio*. Indianapolis: B. F. Bowen & Company, 1915.
Bundles, A'Lelia. *On Her Own Ground: The Life and Times of Madam C. J. Walker*. New York: Simon & Schuster, 2001.
Burton, Willie. *On the Black Side of Shreveport*. 1983.
Caldwell, Arthur Bunyan, ed. *History of the American Negro and His Institutions*. Atlanta: A. B. Caldwell Publishing, 1917 and 1921.
Clay County History Book Committee. *History of Clay County, Mississippi*. Dallas: Curtis Media, 1988.
Cleaveland, Clif, M.D. *That Democracy Might Reign: The Story of Billie Dyer, Healers & Heroes*. American College of Physicians, 2004.
Fenner, F., D.A. Henderson, I. Arita, Z. Jezek, and I.D. Ladnyi. "Smallpox and Its Eradication." Geneva, World Health Organization, 1988.
Ferrell, Robert H. *Unjustly Dishonored*. Columbia: University of Missouri Press, 2011.
Fitzbutler, Henry. *The Encyclopedia of Louisville*. Lexington: University Press of Kentucky, 2001.
Fitzgerald, Ruth Coder. *A Different Story: A Black History of Fredericksburg and Spotsylvania, Virginia*. Unicorn Press, 1979.
Flavin, Jeanne. *Our Bodies, Our Crimes: The Policing of Women's Reproduction in America*. New York: New York University Press, 2009.
Ford, James E. *A History of Jefferson City*. Jefferson City: New Day Press, 1938.
Gamble, Vanessa Northington. *Making a Place for Ourselves: The Black Hospital Movement, 1920–1945*. New York: Oxford University Press, 1995.
Gloster, Hugh Morris. *Who's Who in Colored America*, 7th ed. 1950.
Glynn, Robert L. *How Firm a Foundation, A History of the First Black Church in Tuscaloosa County, Alabama*. Friends of the Hunter's Chapel African Methodist Episcopal Zion Church and the City of Tuscaloosa, Alabama Bicentennial Committee, 1976.
Harris, Stephen L. *Harlem's Hell Fighters*. Washington, D.C.: Brassey's, 2003.
Hayden, Robert C. *Mr. Harlem Hospital*. Littleton, MA: Tapestry Press, Ltd., 2003.
Holley, John Stokes. *The Invisible People of The Pikes Peak Region: An Afro-American Chronicle*. Colorado Springs: The Friends of the Colorado Springs Pioneers Museum, 1990.
Holt, Annye S. *The Black Physician's Presence in Asheville, North Carolina*. Self-published, Annye S. Holt, Asheville, NC 28801.
Hughes, Ruth Anita Hawkins. *Contributions of Vance County People of Color*. Sparks Press, 1988.
Hunton, Addie W., and Kathryn M. Johnson. *Two Colored Women with the American Expeditionary Forces*. Brooklyn Eagle Press, 1920. Reprinted by G. K. Hall & Co., New York, 1997.
Keene, Jennifer D. *Doughboys, the Great War, and the Remaking of America*. Baltimore: Johns Hopkins University Press, 2001.
Lapp, Rudolph M. *Afro-Americans in California*. New York: Boyd & Fraser, 1987.
Lentz-Smith, Adriane. *Freedom Struggles, African Americans and World War I*. Cambridge: Harvard University Press, 2009.
Lightfoot, G. M., A.L. Locke, and M. Maclear. *Howard University in the War*. Washington, D.C.: Howard University Press, 1919.
Logan, Rayford W., and Michael R. Winston. *Dictionary of American Negro Biography*. New York: W.W. Norton, 1927.
Mjagkij, Nina. *Loyalty in Time of Trial*. Lanham, MD: Rowman & Littlefield, 2011.
Manning, Kenneth R. *Black Apollo of Science: The Life of Ernest Everett Just*. New York: Oxford University Press, 1983.
Maxwell, William. *Billie Dyer and Other Stories*. New York: Knopf, 1993.
McCarthy, Kevin M. *African American Sites in Florida*. Sarasota: Pineapple Press, 2007.
McFarland, Patricia LaPointe, and Mary Ellen Pitts. *Memphis Medicine: A History of Science and Service*. Westbrook, ME: Legacy Publishing, 2011.
Mead, Fredrick S., A.B., ed. *Harvard's Military Record in the World War*. Boston: Harvard Alumni Association, 1921.
Millender, Dharathula (Dolly). *Gary's Central Business Community*. Images of America. Charleston, SC: Arcadia, 2003.
Morris, Robert V. *Tradition and Valor: A Family Journey*. Manhattan, KS: Sunflower University Press, 1999.
Patton, Gerald W. *War and Race*. Westport, CT: Greenwood Press, 1981.
Reagan, Leslie J. *When Abortion Was a Crime*. Berkeley: University of California Press, 1996.
Remnick, David. *The Bridge: The Life and Rise of Barack Obama*. New York: Vintage, 2010.
Roberts, Frank E. *The American Foreign Legion*. Annapolis, MD: Naval Institute Press, 2004.
Ross, Sgt. William O., and Cpl. Duke L. Slaughter. *With the 351st in France, A Diary*. Afro-American Company, Baltimore, Maryland, Pennsylvania State Archives, Harrisburg.
Sammons, Vivian Ovelton. *Blacks in Science and Medicine*. New York: Hemisphere Publishing Corporation, 1990.
Savitt, Todd L. *Race and Medicine in Nineteenth- and Early-Twentieth-Century America*, Kent, OH: Kent State University Press, 2007.
Scipio, L. Albert, II. *With the Red Hand Division*. Silver Spring, MD: Roman Publications, 1985.
Scotland, Thomas, and Steven Heys. *War Surgery 1914–18*. West Midlands, England: Helion & Company, 2012.
Scott, Emmett J. *Scott's Official History of the American Negro in World War I*. Chicago: Homewood Press, 1919.
Shust, Alex P. *West Virginia's McDowell County and the Industrialization of America*. Harwood, MD: Two Mule Publishing, 2010.

Silag, Bridgford, and Hal Chase. *Outside In: African-American History in Iowa*. Des Moines: State Historical Society of Iowa, 2001.

Simms, James N., comp. and pub. *Simms Blue Book*. Chicago, 1923.

Solberg, Winton U. *Reforming Medical Education: The University of Illinois College of Medicine*. Urbana: University of Illinois Press, 2009.

Summerville, James. *Educating Black Doctors: A History of Meharry Medical College*. Tuscaloosa: University of Alabama Press, 1983.

Sweeney, W. Allison. *The American Negro in the Great World War*. New York: Negro Universities Press, 1969.

Thompson, John L. *History and Views of Colored Officers Training Camp*. Des Moines: The Bystander, 1917.

Udogu, E. Ike. *African American Politics in Rural America*. Lanham, MD: University Press of America, 2006.

Vihlen, Sally P. *The Black Physician in Florida*. Gainesville: University Press of Florida, 1994.

Ward, Thomas J., Jr. *Black Physicians in the Jim Crow South*. Fayetteville: University of Arkansas Press, 2003.

Williams, Chad L. *Tourchbearers of Democracy*. Chapel Hill: University of North Carolina Press, 2010.

Wilson, Adam P. *African American Army Officers of World War I*. Jefferson, NC: McFarland, 2015.

Wright, Amos. *Hidden Legacies: I. African-American Physicians in Alabama*. www.uab.edu.

Wynn, Commodore. *Negro Who's Who in California*. San Francisco: California Publishing Co., 1948.

Yenser, Thomas, editor and publisher. *Who's Who in Colored America*. New York, 1938–1939–1940–1944.

Index